'I am a totally changed person. I feel incredible. Before, I didn't have a cut-off switch. I could just eat and eat and would still be hungry throughout the day. After two months on your diet I now feel full and can leave food on the plate because I'm full.'

Adrian

'It's as if someone has given me a magic pill and said, "You'll have more energy, you'll feel calm and you'll feel less stressed." It's worked better than I would have believed. I am full of energy, my skin has improved dramatically, my cholesterol level has dropped by a third in seven weeks and I've lost 14lb [6.3kg], mostly from around my middle.'

Marianne

'Well, I have now been on it for ten weeks and have lost 10.4kg [1st. 9lb]. It has been the easiest way to lose weight and stay healthy that I have ever tried.'

Glynda G

'When we first started I thought it would be difficult. The thought of cooking three meals a day with all these new foods was daunting. But it's been so easy. We used to be total chocaholics, eating sweets and chocolate every day. None of us have eaten any chocolate or sweets since the diet. It's a miracle. We've had no cravings. I would never have believed this is possible. It's quite unbelievable. My daughter, who loses weight very slowly, has lost between 5kg [11lb] and 6kg [13¼lb], I've lost 7.5kg [16½lb]; my husband has lost 8kg [1¼st.] and my son, who is not so overweight, has lost 5kg [11lb] all in the last six weeks. The other thing is the energy. I was permanently tired. I could have spent the whole day in bed. Now my energy level is incredible. My blood sugar is well under control (I'm diabetic) and I've been able to halve my medication. It's been so easy.'

Linda B

'I lost 13lb [5.9kg] in a month and, amazingly, I lost my craving for sweets! My energy also increased so much.'

John G

'It feels as though a shroud has been lifted from me. Not only have I lost the weight, but I also have 100 per cent more energy. It used to be an effort to go up the stairs. I used to get headaches most days, and they have gone. I used to get sinus twinges almost every day, and that has cleared up. I used to sweat a lot, and thought I was just a sweaty person. But now I can walk and run and just don't sweat. My skin used to be cold all the time but now it's nice and warm. I feel more relaxed as well. It had got to the stage where I couldn't even think clearly, but now I can do so again.'

Fenton R

'I am becoming more and more adept at making the yummy recipes in the book! Seriously, I cannot understand why everyone hasn't adopted this way of eating! Healthy, interesting and, most importantly, utterly delicious!'

Ciara S

patrick
HOLFORD

THE
LOW-GL
DIET
BIBLE

THE PERFECT WAY TO
LOSE WEIGHT, GAIN ENERGY AND
IMPROVE YOUR HEALTH

piatkus

PIATKUS

First published in Great Britain in 2005 as *The Holford Low-GL Diet* by Piatkus Books
This updated and expanded version first published in 2009 by Piatkus
Reprinted 2009 (four times), 2010 (twice), 2011

A CIP catalogue record for this book
is available from the British Library.

ISBN 978-0-7499-4167-3

Typeset in Plantin Light by Phoenix Photosetting, Chatham, Kent
Printed and bound in Great Britain by CPI Mackays, Chatham, ME5 8TD

Piatkus
An imprint of
Little, Brown Book Group
100 Victoria Embankment
London EC4Y 0DY

An Hachette UK Company
www.hachette.co.uk

www.piatkus.co.uk

About the author

Patrick Holford BSc, DipION, FBANT, NTCRP is a leading spokesman on nutrition in the media, specialising in the field of mental health. He is the author of over 30 books, translated into over 20 languages and selling over a million copies worldwide, including the *Optimum Nutrition Bible* and *Optimum Nutrition for the Mind*.

Patrick Holford started his academic career in the field of psychology. In 1984 he founded the Institute for Optimum Nutrition (ION), an independent educational charity, and was involved in groundbreaking research showing that multivitamins can increase children's IQ scores – research that was published in the *Lancet* and the subject of a *Horizon* TV documentary in the 1980s. He was one of the first promoters of the importance of zinc, antioxidants, essential fats, low-GI and -GL diets and homocysteine-lowering B vitamins such as folic acid.

He is Chief Executive of the Food for the Brain Foundation and director of the Brain Bio Centre, the Foundation's treatment centre. He is an honorary fellow of the British Association for Applied Nutrition and Nutritional Therapy, as well as a member of the Nutrition Therapy Council.

BY THE SAME AUTHOR

100% Health
500 Top Health and Nutrition Questions Answered
Balancing Hormones Naturally (with Kate Neil)
Beat Stress and Fatigue
Boost Your Immune System (with Jennifer Meek)
Food GLorious Food (with Fiona McDonald Joyce)
Hidden Food Allergies (with Dr James Braly)
How to Quit Without Feeling S**t (with David Miller and Dr James Braly)
Improve Your Digestion
Natural Chill Highs
Natural Energy Highs
Natural Highs (with Dr Hyla Cass)
Optimum Nutrition Before, During and After Pregnancy (with Susannah Lawson)
Optimum Nutrition for the Mind
Optimum Nutrition for Your Child (with Deborah Colson)
Optimum Nutrition for Your Child's Mind (with Deborah Colson)
Optimum Nutrition Made Easy
Say No to Arthritis
Say No to Cancer
Say No to Heart Disease
Six Weeks to Superhealth
Smart Foods for Smart Kids (with Fiona McDonald Joyce)
Solve Your Skin Problems (with Natalie Savona)
The Alzheimer's Prevention Plan (with Shane Heaton and Deborah Colson)
The Fatburner Diet
The H Factor (with Dr James Braly)
The Holford 9-day Liver Detox (with Fiona McDonald Joyce)
The Holford Diet GL Counter
The Holford Low-GL Diet Cookbook (with Fiona McDonald Joyce)
The Little Book of Optimum Nutrition
The Optimum Nutrition Bible
The Optimum Nutrition Cookbook (with Judy Ridgway)

Contents

PART THREE Five Simple Principles

PART FOUR The Action Plan

PART FIVE Food, Menu Plans and Recipes

Appendices

Acknowledgements

This book has been a continual evolution over the past 15 years and I would like to thank the people who have been involved at every stage and the many scientists around the world who have contributed to our understanding of weight loss and blood sugar. Most of all, I would like to thank the thousands of people who have tried my diet approach and volunteered for the trials you'll read about in this book. No doubt this approach will continue to evolve, thanks to your invaluable feedback.

Specifically, I'd like to thank nutritionists Shane Heaton, Natalie Savona, Deborah Colson, Liz Efiong, Fiona McDonald-Joyce (thank you for your excellent recipes!), who have all trained at the Institute for Optimum Nutrition. Also Paul Bedford from the YMCA for his help with the exercise chapters. I would also like to thank Jan Cutler, and Gill Bailey and Jillian Stewart at Piatkus, for their skilful and patient editing. Also, thanks to Wendy Nagle and Carolyn St. John at Zest4Life.

Finally, I'd like to thank Gaby, my wife, for acting as guinea pig for the diet and supporting my crack-of-dawn lifestyle that gives birth to books!

Guide to Abbreviations and Measures

Vitamins

1 gram (g) = 1,000 milligrams (mg) = 1,000,000 micrograms (mcg, also written as µg)

Most vitamins are measured in milligrams or micrograms. Vitamins A, D and E used to be measured in International Units (iu), a measurement designed to standardise the various forms of these vitamins, which have different potencies.

Six mcg of betacarotene, the vegetable precursor of vitamin A is, on average, converted into 1mcg of retinol, the animal form of vitamin A. So, 6mcg of betacarotene is called 1mcgRE (RE stands for retinol equivalent). Throughout this book betacarotene is referred to in mcgRE.

1mcg of retinol (1mcgRE) = 3.3iu of vitamin A
1mcgRE of betacarotene = 6mcg of betacarotene
100iu of vitamin D = 2.5mcg
100iu of vitamin E = 67mg

Metric	**British (imperial)**
(Note: these figures are rounded up or down a little to make measuring easier: 28.3 grams equals 1oz)	
25g	1oz
55g	2oz
85g	3oz
115g	4oz
140g	5oz
175g	6oz
200g	7oz
225g	8oz

British (imperial)	Metric	USA
1 teaspoon (0.17oz)	5ml	1 teaspoon
1 dessertspoon	10ml	2 teaspoons
1 tablespoon (0.5oz)	15ml	1 tablespoon
2 tablespoons (1oz)	30ml	2 tablespoons
4fl oz	125ml	½ cup
⅘ Imperial pint (16oz)	450ml	2 cups
⅘ Imperial quart	900ml	1 quart
⅘ Imperial gallon	3.6 litres	1 gallon
1 pound	454g	1 pound

CONVERSION SUMS

Ounces to grams:
Multiply oz figure by 28.3 to get number of g

Grams to ounces:
Multiply g figure by 0.0353 to get number of oz

Ounces to millilitres:
Multiply oz figure by 30 to get number of ml

Calories
Carbohydrate has 3.75 calories per gram
Protein has 4 calories per gram
Fat has 9 calories per gram

In each part of the book, you'll find numbered references. These refer to research papers listed in the References section on page 415, and are there for readers who want to study this subject in depth.

Introduction

It is a wonderful thing to discover that a radical idea, based on absolute logic and supported by science, actually works far better than you could have dared to hope.

Since the first edition of this book, written in 2004, thousands of people from around the world have successfully lost more weight than they, or I, would have thought possible, and in the process have gained health and solved long-standing health problems such as diabetes, heart disease and high cholesterol. Gone is the constant battle to stem the tide of weight gain and the craving for food (especially sugar and carbs), the energy dips and the need to diet.

Lesley N from England, lost 38kg (6st.) in nine months:

> *This is the diet I'll be following for life. And the best thing is, it doesn't really feel like a diet – because I don't feel like I'm missing out. In fact, I can't think of a single reason to go back to my old way of eating.*

Lesley, like many, had tried every diet under the sun and over 20 years had been in a cycle of losing weight, then gaining it again. But now she has achieved her dream – great health and a stable, perfect weight.

Defying convention

For many years there has been a widely accepted belief that the correct way to lose weight is to follow a low-fat, low-calorie diet and do lots of exercise. The problem is, as you probably know from experience, this method doesn't work particularly well. My low-GL diet (the Holford Diet), in contrast, defies conventional wisdom on diet and brings amazing results! Many people can testify to its effectiveness for weight loss – not only that but it also sets you on the path for good health and vitality for the future, so that you look good, feel good and can avoid many of today's prevalent health problems.

How can this be possible you may ask. The simple reason is that many of the dietary conventions that you have probably accepted as fact are slowly but surely being overturned. Let's look at these conventions in turn.

Convention: on an ongoing basis, even if you starve yourself, you can't lose more than 1kg (2lb) a week. I'd always assumed this to be true – until time and time again I witnessed people on this diet losing more. Adrian, who is diabetic, is a case in point. His doctor put him on the Holford Diet and he lost 12kg (1st. 8lb) in the first four weeks – and completely normalised his blood sugar. Six months on he'd lost 38kg (6st.), an average of 1.5kg (3.2lb) a week – and 25cm (10in) off his belly. That's heresy according to conventional calorie theory. Yet it's what so many people are reporting on my low-GL diet. Adrian told me:

> ❝ I am a totally changed person. I feel incredible. Before, I didn't have a cut-off switch. I could just eat and eat and would still be hungry through-out the day. After two months on your diet I now feel full and can leave food on the plate because I'm full ... It's amazing. It's totally changed my life. ❞

Adrian is no exception. I see this all the time. A TV programme in Ireland recently presented me with six significantly overweight people who wanted to lose weight. Twelve weeks later all reported significant weight loss and four out of six had lost over 19kg (3st.) each. That's an average of over 900g (2lb) a week weight loss. None of them felt hungry.

Convention: the only way to lose weight is to eat a low-fat, low-calorie diet and exercise more. So how do you explain Julie, who was doing two body pump (weight-based group-fitness) classes a week, one spinning class, two body-attack classes and also walked for 4½ miles every Sunday, but still wasn't losing any weight? She took part in a televised British GMTV six-week diet trial that tested Britain's most popular diets, from the Atkins Diet to WeightWatchers. The runner up, who had followed a WeightWatchers diet (a low-fat, low-calorie diet with weekly support-group meetings), lost a perfectly respectable 4kg (9lb). That's 600g (1.3lb) a week. The winner, Julie, on the other hand, lost 8.6kg (1st. 5lb) in six weeks and dropped two dress sizes, losing 20cm (8in) off her waist! She had no weekly support-group meetings.

> 〈 *I started the Holford Diet and was amazed I was able to shed the weight so easily without feeling hungry.* 〉

All over the world we are facing a global epidemic of weight gain. In Britain 67 per cent of men and 57 per cent of women are overweight. In the US obesity has overtaken smoking as the number-one preventable cause of premature death. Once obese your risk of diabetes goes up 77 times. Up goes your cholesterol. And up goes your risk of heart disease and many other health problems as well, from breast and prostate cancer to arthritis and polycystic ovaries.

Convention: diet plays a small part in diseases such as cancer, diabetes, cardiovascular disease and high cholesterol, and medication is essential. The case of Kyra sheds some interesting light on this belief. She was diagnosed with diabetes in the January and told by her GP that she would need to be on medication for life. She saw me that April and, within six weeks, needed no medication. On re-running a battery of blood tests, her results showed not one single indicator of diabetes.

> 〈 *My doctor told me I'd be on medication for the rest of my life. I am really thrilled to have been able to come off medication and still have a stable blood sugar. My energy is much better. My skin is clearer, mood more stable and I've lost 12lbs [5.4kg] in a month. I feel in control of food instead of it being in control of me.* 〉

Kyra reversed her diabetes in six weeks simply by following my low-GL diet. One year on she's 20kg (3st.) lighter and has perfect blood sugar levels without drugs.

Andy was diagnosed with high cholesterol (8.8 mmol/l – it should be below 5 mmol/l). He was also gaining weight, feeling tired and stressed, and not sleeping well. He was prescribed statins, which are cholesterol-lowering drugs, but, six months later, his cholesterol was still 8.7. His lack of response to the medication, plus the unpleasant side effects he was experiencing, led Andy to stop taking the drugs. Instead, he attended one of my workshops and went on the Holford Diet as well as taking the recommended supplements. Three weeks later he had lost 4.5kg (10lb), his energy levels were great, he no longer felt stressed and he was sleeping much better – *and* his cholesterol level had dropped to a healthy 4.9 mmol/l!

Like me, you might be sceptical of case histories in books. Are they for real? Surely it can't be that easy? Aren't these people the exception, not the rule? Well, the case studies in this book are certainly real, and the Holford Diet *is* that easy, and it *does* work this well for the vast majority of people. If you want to prove it for yourself visit my website www.holforddiet.com. In the 'testimonials' section you'll see unedited personal testimonials and videos (some made by independent television stations) showing people whose lives have been transformed by this simple and doable approach. The Holford Diet, in every single televised trial to date, has been extraordinarily successful.

The perfect diet

If you're reading this book you are probably thinking, *can there really be a diet that works for weight loss, will make me feel great, and is easy to stick to.* I can tell you that the hunt for that perfect diet is over – this is it. This diet will stop you feeling tired, hungry and craving sweet foods or stimulants; it causes consistent short-term and long-term weight loss; it can prevent (and in some cases help reverse) diseases such as type-2 diabetes, cardiovascular disease, high cholesterol, breast cancer, prostate cancer and colon cancer; and it's so easy, delicious and sustainable that it rapidly stops being a diet and starts becoming a habit.

In this book you will not only learn how to lose weight and gain health but you will also discover why the five key principles in the Holford Diet, when applied together, have such extraordinary results. I'll show you the cutting-edge science behind these principles, the cornerstone of which is eating a low-glycemic load (or GL) diet, and why this approach is much better than the Atkins Diet and conventional low-calorie, low-fat diets. Once you truly understand the principles and the evidence to back them up, you'll understand why the Holford Diet is nothing short of a revolution.

But, you might say, if this low-GL approach is really so effective – and proven to be – why isn't every doctor and dietician recommending it over more conventional diets? It's a good question and one I'll explore in detail, providing you with the science that shows that low-GL diets are much more effective than the low-calorie, low-fat diets promoted by many well-meaning but ill-informed health professionals. I'm glad to say that those who lead the field are switching camps. For example, Dr David Haslam, a GP and Clinical Director of Britain's National Obesity Forum says: 'There is no question that low-GL is pushing back the boundaries in terms of safe, rapid and permanent weight-loss diets. Although the scientific evidence has been mounting for some time, what Patrick Holford has done for the first time, is to create a totally simple, easy-to-follow guide, which helps to naturally integrate GL into our diets so that it's easy to follow for both short-term weight loss and long-term maintenance.'

My diet is not a low-calorie diet (although you may end up eating less because you don't feel hungry). Nor is it a low-fat diet (as I'll be recommending good fats, from fish and seeds). In fact, I'm going to show you that it is sugar, and foods containing fast-releasing sugars, that make you fat. So, this is why the diet is a total revolution – and revolutions change the status quo.

Leading weight-loss researchers around the world are waking up to the GL revolution. In Norway, diabetes expert Dr Fedon Lindberg, author of the *Greek Doctor's Diet*, also recommends a low-GL diet along very similar lines. Not only do his patients lose significant amounts of weight but they also lose their diabetes. He recently published the case of a woman who had type-2 diabetes and had to inject insulin, but who lost 40kg (6st. 3lb) on a low-GL diet and now has stable blood sugar and no need for any medication.

These are the words of Dr Iris Shai of Ben Gurion University in Israel: 'I'm reading my daughter's high-school health textbook and it's like a religion: "Everyone should follow a low-fat diet", and "Saturated fats kill you", and that's just wrong, plain wrong. I think that what we're soon going to find is that no one's going to be defending the low-fat diet any more.'

Dr Shai is an expert in weight management, and director of a recent research trial published in the *New England Journal of Medicine*, one of many that clearly show a low-GL diet is more effective than a low-calorie, low-fat diet.

Where do you fit in?

The question is: are you ready to join the GL revolution? The chances are you are already an expert in what doesn't work. You've no doubt tried many diets, cut out entire food groups, followed the culinary habits of far-flung tribes and spent a fortune on 'miracle' foods. But, however wonderful these regimes seemed when you began them, the fact that you picked up this book probably means that none of them gave you what you need – a diet for life that you enjoy, that you can stick to and that works.

Chances are, you're still carrying extra pounds, but that's just for starters. You may also often feel gnawingly hungry, beset by cravings for foods you shouldn't have, and tired much of the time. And, above all, you're tired of those hollow promises and 'sure-fire' methods that are soon unmasked as just another gimmick.

Fifteen years ago I proposed a way out of this wilderness. *The Fatburner Diet* pinpointed the secret to successful weight loss and weight control: balancing blood sugar. It was based on eating low-GI (glycemic index) foods, together with protein foods. That was the prototype. Thousands of people have benefited from this diet, but now, there's something even more effective. The core principle, however, remains the same.

Put simply, when your blood sugar is too high you turn the excess into fat, and when your blood sugar is too low, you feel lethargic and hungry. This is when you're likely to grab a sugary, refined snack to boost your energy, only to find that you sink back into exhaustion soon afterwards. This pattern of eating can be seriously bad for your health, not only causing weight gain but increasing your risk of many diseases. That's the bad news.

But there is good news. You can break out of this vicious circle forever. One step beyond low-GI diets is low GL. I'll explain the difference in detail in Chapter 13. Combined with the other key principles of the Holford Diet, this is the Rolls-Royce of diets. The magic of it is that you don't have to avoid carbohydrates, just get the balance right in a meal, which means eating 10 ⓖⓛ. Again, I'll explain exactly how you do this. And, when you do, the weight will fall off easily and your energy will spring back to optimum levels.

Evolution of an idea

This discovery grew out of a growing conviction that I gradually developed at the Institute for Optimum Nutrition (ION), which is a not-for-profit educational charity in Richmond, Surrey. I founded ION in the mid-1980s with the support and encouragement of Dr Linus Pauling, recipient of two Nobel Prizes and forty-eight PhDs, who famously declared that 'optimum nutrition is the medicine of the future'. He was the maverick who, in the 1970s, discovered that high-dose vitamin C had remarkable anti-cancer effects. Although ridiculed at the time, according to a series of studies reported by the National Academy of Sciences[1] last year he was, as usual, on the right track. A friend of Einstein, Pauling was to chemistry what Einstein was to physics. He believed that many prevalent diseases of our time were the consequences of sub-optimum nutrition. The future of medicine would be about discovering what an individual's optimum nutrition is, both to maintain and restore health.

I established ION to explore the remarkable insights of this nutritional maverick further. With the ION team, I worked with hundreds of overweight people to find the key to losing weight.

Back then, of course, calorie counting was really the sacred cow of weight loss and, in some people's minds, it still is. The dominant belief was that the number of calories you ate, minus what you burned off through exercise, ended up as a wodge of fat around your middle. Diets aimed to cut calories – usually by cutting fat, since fat has the most calories per gram.

But I was seeing something very different – that eating different *kinds* of foods, such as what we call 'low-glycemic-load' foods, can lead to more weight loss than 'high-glycemic-load' foods, even if the calorie intake stayed the same. At the time, it was sheer heresy.

However, we were right. There are specific foods and food combinations that cause rapid weight loss, and I used this knowledge to devise my low-GL diet. I soon realised that people who balanced their blood sugar not only lost weight but they also kept it off, felt superb and had all the signs of improved health and vigour.

Followers of the diet happily slipped into a new way of eating, but, more importantly, they found that it works for life. The food on offer is so delicious and varied that boredom and hunger are not an issue. Now, many years on, hundreds of thousands of people have followed the system with great success, and numerous scientific trials since then have validated our original research findings.

Today's Holford Diet takes this tried-and-tested method into another dimension. With ongoing advances in nutrition, and feedback from users, *The Low-GL Diet Bible* is a cutting-edge guide to optimal health, containing new studies that have confirmed the health benefits of a low-GL diet combined with all-round healthy eating and a healthy lifestyle. These elements are the core of the Holford Diet. And what's more, it's a breeze to follow, with menus and wonderful recipes that are delicious as well as straightforward to prepare.

Beyond Atkins

Overall, we owe a lot to the late Dr Atkins, who boldly stated that you could lose more weight by eating a high-protein, high-fat, low-carbohydrate diet. He claimed, as I do, that obesity results from losing blood sugar control, and he knew that the body's 'cleanest' fuel is carbohydrate, which is simply digested down into glucose – the substance your cells need to run on.

Fat and protein, however, are much harder to metabolise and turn into useable fuel, so Atkins proposed that you would lose some of the energy or calories they contain as ketones – breakdown chemicals – in the urine. In this way, he said, you could eat more calories and still lose weight.

Atkins was almost on the right track, but for the wrong reasons. Despite all the hype about miracle diets, we now know that high-protein diets work for a very simple reason. It isn't because fat and protein are so hard to break down for energy that you lose calories by eating them. This theory has been proved wrong.

High-protein diets work because people actually eat less. You tend to feel much fuller when you eat meat and cheese than when you eat carbohydrates, because a high-protein diet does help keep your blood sugar even – and an even blood sugar means less hunger. However, there are some serious consequences for health with this approach (we'll look at these in Chapter 2, page 35). Meanwhile, there is an easier, safer, healthier and tastier way to lose weight – and you'll see amazing results in just 30 days, as well as sustainable long-term results.

On your marks, get reset ...

Although you will lose weight right from the start, I recommend you commit to this diet for 30 days. That's because, if your blood sugar is out of balance (and there's a 95 per cent chance if you are overweight that it is), it takes up to 30 days to 'reset' your system to work properly. Then, not only do the pounds continue to fall away but you start to feel fantastic as well.

How can you tell whether you've lost control of your blood sugar? Check out this page from the food diary of someone who has:

❛ Woke up tired. Staggered out of bed on remote control to the kettle. Made a strong cup of tea. Had a piece of toast and jam. Avoided eating anything substantial till lunch to cut down on calories. Got really hungry. Craved some bread, pasta, biscuits. Had a big bowl of tuna pasta for lunch. Wanted something sweet to end the meal. Felt depressed in the afternoon and really lethargic. Had another coffee and some chocolate. Felt better. Got home and had some toast. Meant to go to the gym but felt too tired … ❜

If this sounds like you, let me ask you a few simple questions:

- Do you find it hard to get going in the morning without a cup of tea or coffee, a cigarette or something sweet, perhaps cereal or toast with jam?

- Do you crave something sweet after meals?

- Does your energy dip during the day, and do you find yourself craving a stimulant (such as tea, coffee, a cigarette or chocolate) or something sweet?

- Do you feel too tired to exercise?

- Does your mood go up and down?

- Are you gradually gaining weight, and finding it hard to lose, even though you're not noticeably eating more or exercising less?

If you answered 'yes' to any of these questions, the Holford Diet is perfect for you. The diet is also radical enough to change the way you eat and live forever.

At this point, you might be prompted to ask who I am, and why you should trust what I have to say. The fact is, the kernel of the Holford Diet began as a personal experience that transformed my life long before I even set up ION.

Life study

When I was 19 and studying psychology at York University, I met two extraordinary nutritionists, Brian and Celia Wright. Like Linus Pauling, they had realised that most disease was the result of suboptimum nutrition. At the time, I found this hard to swallow, but, being an adventurous spirit, asked them to devise a diet for me, which they duly did.

So there I was, a university student, eating a virtually wheat-free diet, masses of fruit and vegetables, and taking a daily handful of supplements shipped in from the US (they weren't yet available in Britain). It was a far cry from the usual fish and chips, cigarettes and pints of bitter usually enjoyed at university! My colleagues, friends and family thought I was crazy but I persisted.

Within two months I had lost 6kg (1st.) in weight, which has never returned; my skin, which had resembled a lunar landscape, became clear; and my regular migraines virtually vanished. But, most noticeable of all, was the extra energy. I no longer needed so much sleep, my mind was much sharper and my body full of vitality. I started to investigate this 'optimum nutrition', and I haven't stopped since.

I set up ION, now an educational charity, with no funding from food, supplement or drug companies, and it has grown into Europe's largest and most respected training school for nutritional therapists. Here are some of the breakthroughs:

- In 1986 I researched and helped put zinc on the map as the most deficient mineral in the British diet. Deficiencies can cause bad skin, poor appetite control, depression and even schizophrenia. In those days virtually no one had heard of zinc, there was no RDA for it, and few supplements contained it.

- In 1988 we ran an experiment, filmed by the BBC's *Horizon* programme and published in the *Lancet*, which proved vitamin supplements could boost children's IQs by a massive 9 per cent. This was a world first. Since then 14 out of 16 trials have shown that multivitamins really do improve children's IQs.

- In the 1990s we showed that a high antioxidant intake reduces the risk of cancer, heart disease and Alzheimer's and slows down the ageing process. No one had heard of antioxidants then, but now they're the big buzzword.

- In 1993 I went public as saying that HRT causes breast cancer and advised women to use safer and equally effective natural alternatives. (An estimated 20,000 women in Britain have got breast cancer because of HRT between 1994 and 2004 alone.) Ten years later doctors were advised to stop prescribing it.

- In 1998 I wrote *The Optimum Nutrition Bible*, now translated into 17 languages and sold in 30 countries, with sales of over a million copies worldwide.

- In 2003 I put the spotlight on homocysteine – an amino acid more important than cholesterol, your blood pressure and even your weight as a gauge of health risk. It is your single most important health statistic, measuring where you are on the scale of health, from superhealth to heading for an early grave. In recent years high homocysteine has proven to be a reliable indicator of risk for heart attacks, strokes, memory decline and Alzheimer's. High homocysteine levels are easily reversible by upping certain B vitamins but, like so many important discoveries that don't have a patentable, profitable drug as the treatment, the value of giving inexpensive B vitamins to counteract disease will no doubt be resisted for many years to come. In Germany ten times more people have their homocysteine levels checked each year than in the UK.

- In 2004 I published the first edition of the *Holford Low-GL Diet*, saying that eating a low-GL diet, and specifically eating no more than 40 🌀 a day, was the healthiest and most effective way to lose weight. As you'll see this prediction is coming true.

In short, I've been walking my talk for 30 years – during which time my weight, size, blood pressure, pulse, homocysteine and cholesterol levels have barely changed. (I'm 7lbs heavier at the age of 50, compared to when I was 21.)

So, after a quarter of a century at the cutting edge of diet and health – having studied thousands of research trials, tested my theories on myself and on more than 200,000 people, and gained more than a million readers worldwide – I can say with confidence that there is a simple way to lose weight, feel and look great, and stay young. And that is the Holford Diet.

How to use this book

Part One gives you the background, and tells you why the diet is scientifically proven, safe and better for you. It also reveals why it will give you the easiest and most sustainable weight loss and is truly a revolution.

Part Two shows you why the Holford Diet is also the best way to improve your health and energy, prevent and reverse diabetes and heart disease, and naturally lower your cholesterol without drugs. It will also help you to improve your mood and memory, slow down the ageing process and look younger.

Part Three explains the five key principles of the Holford Diet – which are just as applicable to kids as well as adults – and how to discover your 'good' foods and 'bad' foods. Once you've read this you'll understand why the Holford Diet is the state-of-the-art weight-loss and maintenance strategy.

Part Four tells you exactly what you need to do on the Holford Diet, and will answer all your practical questions.

Part Five provides lots of easy, delicious fatburning recipes and menus for you to enjoy.

Wishing you the best of health, and looking forward to seeing less of you!

Patrick Holford

PART ONE

Dieting – The Bottom Line

1

Why the Holford Diet Works

Imagine this...

You've just woken up. You feel full of energy. Your mind is clear. You get up, have a healthy breakfast and, throughout the day, your energy is good, your mood is stable, you're mentally sharp and your concentration is good. You haven't once experienced a single craving. You haven't had energy dips or got cranky and irritable.

But that's just the *inside* story. You also look great. Your weight is more or less where you want it to be. You're well toned. Your skin has a healthy glow. People often comment on how slim and well you look and how young you look for your age. You feel young, both physically and mentally. And this is how you feel every day!

Welcome to the new you. Not only is this how you *could* be but it is also how you *should* be. More importantly, it's how you *will* be when you follow the Holford Diet. And all it takes to see a dramatic difference is 30 days.

I realise that you may have spent the last decade trudging through a succession of diets with nothing to show for it but a slimmed-down bank balance and more fat than you started with. Every bookshop bristles with 'miracle' weight-loss techniques, and 'guaranteed' recipes for everything from longevity to cellulite control. So I know you may be feeling cheated by claims and promises that have never panned out. Why, then, should you believe what I'm saying?

You can be thin *and* healthy

This is why. The Holford Diet works because it is much more than just a way to lose weight. It is a holistic system for attaining optimum health – and a healthy, self-regulating body is naturally slim. Unlike most diets it works with your body's natural design, not against it.

The fact is that many of the people who discovered my diet, followed it and wrote to me reporting substantial weight loss, didn't actually set out to lose weight in the first place. They wanted to be healthy and thought the optimum-nutrition approach made sense. And, as their health improved, the weight dropped off. Optimum health, they found, also means optimum weight.

The body will naturally reach its ideal weight when given the chance. You'll eat less if your blood sugar is stable, and your metabolism will be better able to burn off excess weight.

I have yet to see any diet work better in the long run than this approach. I teach doctors, healthcare practitioners and nutritionists all over the world, but none are as slim, energetic and healthy as the thousand nutritionists we have trained at ION – the Institute for Optimum Nutrition.

At ION, decades of work with more than 100,000 volunteers first revealed how overall health determines weight by showing that overweight is a symptom of a much wider condition. We sometimes call it 'twenty-first-centuryitis'.

Exhaustion, moodiness, depression, bloating – twenty-first-centuryitis is a response to our polluted, urbanised, speeded-up world, and overweight is a common symptom of it. Could you be suffering from twenty-first-centuryitis? Check yourself out by answering the questions below, scoring 1 point for each 'yes' answer.

How do you feel now?

Are you:

☐ Tired most of the time? (76%)*

☐ More than 3.2kg (7lb) over your ideal weight, and rising? (74%)

☐ Prone to mood swings or PMS? (58%)

☐ Suffering from poor memory and concentration? (43%)

☐ Quite often low or depressed? (42%)

☐ Plagued by dry skin, in need of daily moisturisers? (58%)

☐ Having difficulty sleeping? (47%)

☐ Often feeling anxious or stressed? (50%)

☐ Prone to indigestion or bloating after food? (54%)

☐ Often constipated – that is, you rarely go twice a day?   (90%)

☐ Worried about your dry, dull or oily hair?   (34%)

*In Britain, the average person will tick seven of these boxes. The percentages on the right represent people who answered 'frequently or always' in our ONUK health-and-diet survey of over 30,000 people – Britain's largest ever – which we carried out in 2004.[1]

You may have ticked a few boxes yourself. And the reality of being, say, tired all day, uncomfortably overweight and not feeling well is no joke. Remember, though, that all this can change in just 30 days. Your load could be significantly lightened. And three months on the Holford Diet will leave you completely free of these symptoms, as well as much lighter.

A diet for life

The point is that we already know how to cure twenty-first-centuryitis, and that is my goal for you. I want you to lose weight fast, keep losing weight until you reach your goal, and maintain your weight once you get there – but always within the context of optimum energy and well-being. This is what you can look forward to:

- Within 7 days you will start to lose weight as quickly as you'll gain energy.

- Within 20 days you'll notice your skin has dramatically improved.

- Within 30 days you'll be starting to feel like a new you.

- And within three months? You'll have seriously undamaged your health.

We put the Holford Diet to the test with 16 volunteers over eight weeks.[2] Body-fat percentage dropped by an average of 2 per cent. In addition, 94 per cent reported greater energy; 67 per cent had greater concentration, memory or alertness; 67 per cent had less indigestion or bloating, with clearer and less dry skin; 50 per cent reported fewer feelings of depression and more stable moods. There was also a significant drop in blood pressure.

Marianne, one of the participants in this trial, is a case in point.

❛ *It's as if someone has given me a magic pill and said, "You'll have more energy, you'll feel calm and you'll feel less stressed." It's worked better than I would have believed. I am full of energy, my skin has improved dramatically, my cholesterol level has dropped by a third in seven weeks and I've lost 14lb [6.3kg], mostly from around my middle.* ❜

Of course, if you just want to lose weight there are plenty of ways to do it. I've studied them all. I was there with the rise and fall of the F Plan Diet, the Hip & Thigh Diet, the Atkins Diet, the South Beach Diet and many others. I advised Rosemary Conley back in the 1980s, as her original diet was dangerously low in essential fats. I challenged Dr Atkins when the science just didn't seem to stack up.

I know the pros and cons of them all. I know why high-protein diets work better for some people but not for others, and why they don't work so well for anyone in the long run. I've tested Atkins dieters and I believe that his original regime can actually seriously damage health. I know why you can lose weight on low-fat diets, only to end up with dry and wrinkly skin. I know why most diets leave you exhausted. Most of all, I know why the weight you lose keeps coming back and, why, year on year you get fatter around the middle!

For me to get excited about a diet that claims to be successful, it must fulfil the following criteria:

It works in both the short and the long term

Instant results may be thrilling, but they're usually not sustained. What you want is steady weight loss, week after week. Many diet trials show no more weight loss at one year than at three months. In contrast, Holford dieters report steady, ongoing weight loss ranging from 680g (1½lb) to 1.3kg (3lb) a week. In one survey, we found that those following the Holford Diet with high compliance, and taking the supplements I recommend, lost an average of 900g (2lb) a week. As I pointed out in the Introduction, the convention is that the body can't burn more than 900g (2lb) of actual fat in a week, unless you go into total starvation mode. But many people on the Holford Diet do lose more weight than this on a long-term basis, without starving and without any evidence of harm. In fact, their health invariably improves. I wish I had a good explanation for this, but I don't. That said, you can lose up to 2.7kg (6lb) of excess water if you have given up eating foods you've developed an intolerance to. That's probably why some people lose 3.2kg (7lb) in the first week of the Holford Diet.

You never feel hungry

If a diet leaves you feeling famished, you won't stick to it. So from day one it has to satisfy your appetite. The Holford Diet specifically recommends the foods that are scientifically proven not only to satisfy your appetite the best but also to end your cravings, and I'm going to tell you exactly which those foods are.

It's enjoyable

If you can't eat a wide variety of foods or if you have to actively avoid eating certain food groups, a diet will start to feel boring very fast, and it will be neither enjoyable nor sustainable. My low-GL diet allows a cornucopia of delectable foods containing good fats, protein and carbohydrates. You'll be able to eat bread and pasta, mayonnaise, meat – the lot. You'll just pay more attention to quality and type. Although there are loads of recipes in this book, you can also use *The Holford Low-GL Diet Cookbook* and *Food GLorious Food* (see Recommended Reading) to back them up.

It's safe

I'm not interested in helping people lose weight by cheating the body. Sure, you can lose weight with slimming pills or by cutting out all carbohydrates, but it just isn't good for you and, in the end, crime doesn't pay. The only side effect I want you to experience is added health. This diet is safe for children (although, depending on their age the quantities needed will be less), in pregnancy (although you might want to up the portion sizes a little) and for you, forever.

It makes you feel great

If a diet is working with the body's design, not against it, you should start to feel better, with more energy, improved mood and concentration and better skin within days. I hear this all the time. For example, one Holford dieter, Diana A, said:

Within four days of starting the Holford Diet I felt much clearer and more alert, without the fuzziness that I'd lived with for years. Then I started feeling more flexible. By the second week I was sleeping much better. I'm more optimistic, my mood is better and my energy is loads better.

She lost 5.4kg (12lb) in four weeks. This is a typical weight loss on the Holford Diet.

There's no rebound weight gain

If you massively restrict food intake, you can lose weight – but the body thinks starvation is imminent and slows down your metabolism. So, as soon as you start eating enough for your needs, the weight boomerangs back. The same is true with stimulants such as caffeine. They can suppress your appetite so that you lose weight in the short term, but in the end they slow down your metabolism. As you'll see, these give short-term weight loss, but rebound weight gain.

The reason that this doesn't happen with my low-GL diet is that it doesn't cause the same drop in metabolic rate that low-fat, low-calorie diets do. That's what the science shows. For example, in a study published in the *Journal of the American Medical Association*, 39 overweight or obese adults were assigned to one of two diets.[3] One group was on a low-GL diet, the other group followed a conventional low-fat, low-calorie diet. Each person had their metabolic rate measured once they had lost 10 per cent of their body weight. The group on the conventional low-fat, low-calorie diet had almost twice the reduction in metabolic rate compared with the low-GL group.

It's easy to follow

At the end of the day, if a diet becomes as easy and natural as breathing, you'll stick to it for life. So, if the food is delicious, is easy to find and prepare, and leaves you satisfied and feeling wonderful, you're far more likely to make it part of your life. Here's what one Holford dieter said:

> ❝ I can't think of a single reason to go back to my old way of eating. This is the diet I'll be following for life. And the best thing is, it doesn't really feel like a diet – because I don't feel like I'm missing out. ❞

This is how you will feel.

The word from the weight-loss coalface

The Holford Diet scores ten out of ten for each of the criteria given above. But you don't have to take just my word for it. Here are the stories of a handful of the many thousands who have followed my diet and achieved, or exceeded, their goals:

Keano K is a radio presenter in South Africa. He contacted me because he needed to lose weight and wanted my advice. He was overweight at 91kg (14st. 5lb) and lacked energy:

❝ I wanted to slim down. I also felt unhealthy and fat, and had a complex about the way I looked, and I decided that it was time to make a change. I religiously stuck to Holford's basic principles. For example, replacing sugar with xylitol, no fizzy drinks, no coffee, and replacing this with water and rooibos tea. I snack on almonds and fresh fruit. The Holford Low-GL Diet Cookbook *has become my cooking bible. ❞*

After one month Keano lost 11kg (1st. 7lb) and has since lost a further 7kg (15½lb), achieving his goal weight of 74kg (11st. 9lb) and is delighted:

❝ I feel great, I have more energy and have even learnt to cook through using your cookbooks. ❞

David F, a business consultant, had almost resigned himself to being overweight:

❝ For the last 30 years I have always been heavier than I should be by as much as a couple of stone. Other diets I've tried were either really hard to follow or didn't work, and I'd resigned myself to just being overweight and blaming my genes. Since last November I have followed the Holford Diet, removing wheat, which I discovered I am intolerant to, out of my diet. I've lost 9.5kg [2st.], look 15 years younger and have the energy levels I had when I was in my thirties. To say it's been transformational for me is an understatement! ❞

Tracy P attended our Zest4Life club, which is based on the Holford Diet principles:

❝ Thanks for all your support at the Holford Diet Club and for educating me in healthier ways of eating. I am now 9st. 7lb [60.3kg] and have lost 22in [55cm], and my body fat has gone down by 16½lb [7.5kg] – all in 12 weeks! I can fit into size 10 again – this all from a starting point of 11st. 8lb [73.5kg] and size 16! I almost can't believe it, but the proof is the mirror and scales, and also my health. Another benefit is that I don't seem to suffer from airborne allergies any more, such as hay fever. ❞

Nikki P and Fiona D gained weight with each of their children – a depressing experience many women can relate to. Here's what happened:

Nikki P:

❝ *I went from a comfortable size 10 before the first child to being a tight size 12 with my third. My self-esteem fell dramatically and I just didn't feel I had my body back from becoming a mum. I started going to the gym several times a week to try to shift the weight, but lost nothing over three years. I began the Holford Diet around the middle of August. By the middle of December (four months later) I had lost the 'baby tummy'. My body-fat percentage went from 21.5 per cent to 16.2 per cent. I lost 4in [10cm] from both my chest and hips, 5in [13cm] from my waist and 1¼in [3cm] from each of my thighs. I went from weighing 11st. [69.8kg] to weighing 8½st. [54kg] – a loss of 2½st. [15.8kg]. I now feel great and am still getting compliments from people about how good I look, which has obviously increased my self-esteem no end. I have kept the weight off by basing my diet on your low-GL recipes and then having the odd treat and days where I don't worry so much about it. The important thing for me is that the food is full of flavour and there are no calories to count – life is too short for that.*

Your recipes are there simply to be made, most of them incredibly easily. If I do put on the odd pound I simply go back to eating the diet recipes consistently and the weight comes off again. Fantastic! I have had to replace my entire wardrobe and am now a size 8 for trousers, etc, and a size 10 in tops. I even tried on my wedding dress a little while ago – we got married in 1992, three years before I had my first child – and I managed to do the zip up really easily! ❞

Fiona D:

❝ *I have two children aged two and three and a half. I had put on a lot of weight from the pregnancies and I was continuing to gain weight. So at the beginning of 2006 I made a promise to myself that I would lose all the weight I had gained during my pregnancies and my target was 57kg [9st.], which is what I weighed when I got married in August 2000. Well, my starting point was 72kg [11st. 5lb] and I wasn't sure if I would ever reach my target, but I was going to try! The low-GL diet is easily understood; best of all it has great recipes that are really easy to make, which is so important when you have two young kids. I learnt to cook using delicious foods I had not tried before, and so had more choice in what I was eating, not less. I also found it was easy to adapt the diet to suit your lifestyle. I took up Pilates and squash, as I now had energy that I didn't have before. It is surprising how the diet made me feel – I now feel alive with much more energy than I had before, and my skin glows. In a period of one month my weight dropped to 68kg [10st. 10lb] and I lost several inches from all over. In five months I was down to 62kg [9st. 10lb] and in ten months I reached my goal weight of 57kg [9st.], so from beginning to end I lost in total 15kg [2st. 5lb], 4cm [1½in] off my waist and 15cm [6in] off my hips, which to me was awesome! I feel as alive as I did when I was first married, and at Christmas I was able to wear my going-away dress that I wore at my wedding – a dress that I thought I would need surgery to get into again! I continue to eat the low-GL way, as I now know it is the right way to eat, and I have introduced it to my family who, surprisingly, are happy to be eating in a healthier way. My two children actually prefer the food, especially the snacks! What more can I say? If in doubt try it, you certainly won't be disappointed!* ⟩

Lesley N also achieved her goal, and lost her menopausal symptoms in the process:

⟨ *I started this way of eating when I was a year away from my fiftieth birthday and my goal was not to be fat at 50. My goal was to lose 2st. [12.7kg]. In under a year I actually lost about 3½st. [22.2kg]. I never looked on it as a diet. It was easy. It was very straightforward. The recipes were fantastic, and I just kept going, and in the end I lost about 5st. [31.7kg]. But that's not all. As part of that I have better nails, better skin, better hair, much more energy, and it's just a way of life for me now. I followed all the recipes and I took all the supplements, and I got rid of any menopausal symptoms that were lurking in the background – in fact, I can't even remember what they were, now!* ⟩

Linda H was just 1.57m (5ft 2in) tall, but had gradually expanded sideways in her twenties, weighing 59kg (9st. 4lb). She had tried every diet under the sun and finally settled on WeightWatchers, with some success. She had been a member of WeightWatchers for five years and had managed, with much sacrifice, to get down to and maintain a weight of 55.3kg (8st. 10lb). But she found she couldn't get below this. She wasn't quite at the right weight for her and it was a frustrating impasse. Then she discovered my diet.

⟨ *On your diet I began to lose weight at once. Within 30 days I came down to 8st. 4lb [52.6kg] – a thing I thought impossible! However, I was totally unprepared for the new energy levels. I cannot believe how marvellous I feel – I am no longer tired – no matter what I do or how active I am. I have stopped falling asleep at odd moments when I relax. I no longer feel bloated and tired after eating. Your diet has changed my life!* ⟩

I now get letters from all over the world from people wanting to share their health transformations. Glynda G, from South Africa, said this:

⟨ *Well, I have now been on it for ten weeks and have lost 10.4kg [1st. 9lb]. It has been the easiest way to lose weight and stay healthy that I have ever tried.* ⟩

But the long-term results are the most important. Kay B, from Australia, reports on her success one year on:

⟨ *It is exactly one year since I read your book* The Holford Low-GL Diet *and started eating my way to optimum nutrition. Over the past year I have lost 18kg [2st. 11lb]: 15cm [6in] from my bust, 16cm [6¼in] from my waist, 18cm [7in] from my hips and 9cm [3½in] from each thigh – two dress sizes. (I am 1.65m [5ft 5in] tall and 51 years old.) I am delighted to be able to look at myself in the mirror and to shop for size 12 clothes once again. My skin is much clearer too and my sleeping has improved. My family and friends tell me that I look "fantastic". I have also stopped drinking all fizzy drinks – diet colas were a large part of my old life. Thankfully, I have lost the taste for those. I am very proud of my achievement, as I didn't believe I would ever manage to lose so much weight.* ⟩

But can this way of eating really solve the obesity epidemic? Wayne P had been gaining almost 6.3kg (1st.) a year, and was now dangerously obese. ITV's *Tonight with Trevor McDonald* asked me to help him. Here's what happened:

⟨ *As a teenager I was very fit. By the age of 17 I was playing ice hockey for England. When I hit my twenties and went to work I stopped exercising, but kept eating and drinking – curries, lager and takeaways. I reckon I put on close to 1st. [6.3kg] for every year I was alive. By the age of 33 I was 27st. 9lb [175.5kg] and basically addicted to junk food. I met Patrick when I became a volunteer for ITV's* Tonight with Trevor McDonald, *testing whether junk food was addictive. I started following Patrick's Fatburner System [the earliest Holford Diet].*

In the first four months I lost 32lb [14.5kg], a little more than 2lb [900g] a week, and I'm still losing weight, week by week. I'm still following your principles, and I'm not even that strict. I eat more fresh food and less packaged food, and I snack more on fruit. My downfall is drinking – I still knock back a few lagers and a bottle of wine at the weekends. But I feel better. I have more energy. I feel happier and more comfortable and have gone down two sizes. I'm also becoming more active and my weight is still reducing. ❩

The one consistent finding is the big health improvements beyond weight loss. I receive letters like the following on a regular basis:

❨ *Since following your diet I have totally cured my migraines. For eight years I suffered incredibly badly from rheumatoid arthritis. I could barely walk without suffering from pain and exhaustion.* ❩

❨ *Following your advice has enabled me to control arthritis and to lead a full and active life: I am eternally grateful.* ❩

❨ *I was both surprised and pleased to see a rapid reduction in the wrinkly skin under my eyes.* ❩

❨ *Following your diet and supplements my cholesterol has dropped from 6.5 to 5.1. My GP couldn't believe it!* ❩

❨ *I used to have constant pain in my knees and joints, could not play golf or walk more than 10 minutes without resting my legs. Since following your advice my discomfort has decreased 95 to 100 per cent. I never would have believed my pain could be reduced by such a large degree, with no return, no matter how much activity in a day or week.* ❩

❨ *Within two weeks, I had much more energy. My mood is very positive – no panic or depression. I feel buoyant, energetic and enthusiastic. I haven't had any colds or infections. I'm sleeping much better, my PMS is much better, I experienced no breast tenderness in my last period, and no mood swings or tearfulness.* ❩

And this is how you should feel all the time. I call it 100 per cent health, and there's no reason why you can't claim it for yourself. You can lose weight and feel great.

You know the definition of insanity? To keep doing the same things but expect different results. And that's what millions are doing: eating the same foods and expecting to feel better and magically shed the excess weight. But the real magic lies in a very different means to this end.

The science of slimming

Your body has evolved over millions of years to work perfectly with a certain kind of diet. Our ancestors weren't fat because they kept active and ate this optimum diet, as do the lucky ones such as the Hunzas in the Himalayas, whose average lifespan is over 100 and who never get fat or suffer from diabetes, heart disease, cancer, Alzheimer's or any other of the diseases plaguing the twenty-first century. This is, in all its essentials, my diet.

If you follow my low-GL diet, you will lose weight, gain energy, improve your skin, sharpen your mind and balance your mood – *and* add years to your life, and life to your years. Let's look at why.

The role of glucose

The science behind the Holford Diet is very simple. Your body is designed to burn glucose for energy, which is carried by blood to the cells. Carbohydrates such as grains and fruits are broken down into glucose in the body. However, carbohydrates figure hugely in today's typical Western diet, and if you eat too much of them – particularly the refined type – you'll end up with more blood glucose than you need. Too much glucose in your blood is dangerous, because it damages arteries. So the minute there's too much it's removed, sent to the liver and turned into fat. That's what fat is: stored energy in reserve for a rainy day when there's no food to eat. The trouble is, that day never comes and you end up with a large reservoir of stored fat.

Foods such as sugar and refined foods have a high 'glycemic load' which means that they raise your blood glucose level big time. As you'll come to see, this is a more important criterion to understand than calories, because high-GL foods turn rapidly into fat.

In a study published in the *Lancet*, two groups of mice were fed either low-GL or high-GL diets.[4] The researchers controlled their feeding to ensure that the mice from both groups maintained the same average body weight throughout. At the end of 18 weeks the group on the high-

GL diet had almost twice the body fat compared to the low-GL group. Sugar really does make you fat.

If you keep your blood glucose levels even, you'll have a steady supply of energy and a healthy but stable appetite. This is the reason why you'll have no problem maintaining the correct weight. But, if your blood glucose levels are sometimes high and sometimes low, you'll see the beginnings of twenty-first-centuryitis. When levels are too high, you'll lay down fat; when they're too low, you'll feel lethargic, and, in time, it will become harder and harder to burn fat. A quarter of all people, and nine out of ten people with weight problems, have difficulty keeping their blood sugar level even. The result is exhaustion and overweight.

And this is just the beginning. Obese people are 77 times more at risk of developing diabetes than non-obese people – a statistic that alone tells you how strongly linked weight gain is to blood sugar control.

So the best way to lose weight is to regain blood glucose control, which heralds the return of your body's ability to burn fat. You'll lose weight effortlessly without having to starve, and gain health and vitality at the same time.

The five key principles

My low-GL diet – the Holford Diet – is based on five key principles, which, taken together, form the fastest, safest and most effective way to lose weight and gain health. Each is explained in detail in Part Three, but let's take a look at them now.

1: Balance your blood sugar
This is the crux: once you achieve it, weight loss is inevitable. Keeping your blood sugar even depends not only on what you eat but also on how and when you eat it. In Chapter 13 I'll explain exactly which foods and food combinations stabilise your blood sugar best and help to burn fat. I'll be introducing you to the glycemic load, or GL, of a food. This is a much superior method of measuring a food's suitability than the 'glycemic index' (GI) or 'carbohydrate points'.

I give an in-depth explanation of GI and GL in Chapter 4, page 67, but here's a summary. Put simply, the GI of a food is a *qualitative* measure that tells you whether the kind of carbohydrate in the food converts rapidly or slowly into glucose, thus being 'fast' or 'slow' releasing. It doesn't tell you, however, how much of the food is carbohydrate. Carbohydrate points or grams of carbohydrate are *quantitative* measures that tell you how much of the food is carbohydrate, but they don't tell you what that particular kind of carbohydrate does to your blood sugar – whether it's fast or slow releasing.

The GL of a food takes both the *quality* and *quantity* into account – it is literally the quantity of carbs in the serving of food multiplied by the quality of its carbohydrate (it's GI score). Foods with a higher GL can lead to weight gain if you eat too much of them.

Take the example of watermelon. It contains very fast-releasing sugar. It has a GI (glycemic index) of 72. That's high. Most low-GI diet books recommend avoiding foods with a GI above 70. But this would be bad advice, because a nice big slice of watermelon – weighing about 120g (4¼oz) – contains only 6g (⅕oz) of this fast-releasing sugar. The GL is therefore 6 × 0.72 = 4.32 ⓖⓛ. You'll see that, on my diet, I recommend two snacks a day of no more than 5 ⓖⓛ. So watermelon is in, not out.

You may be amazed by some of the foods that have a high-GL score. But it's important to know the truth: if you understand why you gain weight, you hold the key to losing it. Cornflakes and corn chips, for instance, have a very high GL, whereas ice cream and peanuts do not. One single date has the same effect on your blood sugar and weight as a whole large punnet of strawberries. So be ready for some surprises.

Your goal will be to eat no more than 40 ⓖⓛ a day – that's 10 per meal and 5 each for two snacks (though you can, if necessary, have an extra 5 for drinks – or desserts). So knowing your GL points is essential. Just look at this comparison of two typical breakfasts.

Breakfast	**ⓖⓛ**		**ⓖⓛ**
A bowl of porridge oats (30g)	2	A bowl of cornflakes	21
Half a grated apple	3	A banana	12
Half a small tub of yoghurt	1	Milk	2
Tablespoon of pumpkin seeds	0		35
And some milk	2		
	8		

The two may seem broadly similar, but in GL terms they are worlds apart. The breakfast on the left will keep your blood sugar level even and stop you feeling hungry for hours. It will push your body's metabolism one giant step towards fatburning and away from fat-storing – and you will feel fuller and more energetic for longer.

And there will be masses to choose from. Part Five is packed with zesty, delicious recipes and menus, including Crunchy Thai Salad, Cod Roasted with Lemon and Garlic, Chicken Tandoori and even Beefburgers. In case you're wondering, I've done all the adding up of the GLs for you. You'll find that 'GL awareness' swiftly becomes second nature; before you know it you'll be doing your own mixing and matching of low-GL foods at every meal. In fact, we even have a website that helps you mix and match, creating your own low-GL recipes (see www.holforddiet.com).

You'll note that the fatburning breakfast combines porridge oats with seeds and yogurt. These contain protein. Mixing carbohydrates with proteins is another important way of regulating blood sugar. This is because eating protein with carbohydrate slows down the release of the carbohydrate into your bloodstream, because protein takes longer to digest. Effectively, it lowers the GL of the meal. Don't worry, it's very easy to master: there's a full discussion in Part Two, but, basically, it means you'll eat low-GL carbohydrates with good-quality protein – for example, brown basmati rice with organic, free-range chicken; wholewheat pasta with wild salmon; or rye toast with scrambled egg; or fruit with some seeds or nuts.

Consider this. If you eat an apple when you're hungry, does it satisfy you? Most people say 'kind of' but still you feel hungry for something. Now try eating an apple with a few almonds or pumpkin seeds. You'll notice a different level of satisfaction – in fact, you won't notice it because you won't feel any craving or hunger.

Fibre plays a starring role, too, because a food's fibre content lowers its GL. So you'll find plenty of high-fibre choices, from beans to brown rice. Lastly, *when* you eat is very important. Unlike most diets, which are snackless deserts, mine encourages you to eat two snacks a day along with your three meals. (You can also have a 5 **GL** drink every day.)

These are the three golden rules on my low-GL diet:

- Eat no more than 40 **GL** a day (10 for main meals; 5 each for two snacks).

- Combine protein with carbohydrate in every meal and snack.

- Graze rather than gorge. Have five food intakes a day – three main meals, two snacks.

2: Eat good fats and avoid bad fats

If you have become conditioned to be fat phobic already you'll be reacting to any mention of nuts or seeds. A voice in your head will say,

'Fat is bad. Fat is calories.' I'm here to tell you that, not only will you lose weight eating fat (within limits), but that you *need* to eat fat. Essential fats may be a bit of a buzzword these days, but they thoroughly deserve their celebrity status. These are the 'good fats' I've talked about for years, and, although it may seem counterintuitive, there's evidence that eating them can actually help you to lose weight.

The reason is very simple. Your body and brain depend on omega-3 and omega-6 essential fats. In fact, excluding water, one-quarter of your brain is made up of omega-3s. So almost nothing works well without them. Your brain can't function, leading to lower IQ, poor memory and a tendency to depression. Your hormones go up the creek, possibly leading to mood swings, PMS, sugar cravings and weight gain. Your skin dries up, and your heart and arteries suffer.

This is why these fats are called 'essential'. And, since we can't manufacture them ourselves, it's as if our body and brain are designed to seek them out. We literally have an instinct to eat fat. We are instinctively drawn towards the creamy texture of fats, sauces, cheese and cream – and that's not all, the body's 'fat sensors' are in your mouth, there to tell you when you've hit nutritional gold. Think about it. If the body needs anything (water, air, essential fats, vitamins) there's always an instinct that makes you crave it. That's why fat-free diets are such a titanic struggle for most of us.

But our need for fats has also spawned a legion of 'bad' fats: fried fat, processed fat in junk food, saturated fats, even 'fake' fats (processed fats called hydrogenated fats – these look like the real thing but no longer work as essential fats). And the body response these fats set up is bad news. When you eat essential fats, your body's fat sensors tell the brain that your essential fat needs are satisfied. But, when you eat bad fats, your fat sensors remain unconvinced, even though your eyes and taste buds may have been fooled. The sensors respond much more strongly to essential fats than to processed or saturated fats. So, if you've packed away a burger and chips or several doughnuts, you'll find yourself craving fats the next day because your body hasn't received what it needed. And you'll keep on craving them until it has.

The Holford Diet gives you exactly the right kind and amount of essential fats, not only to help you stay healthy and glowing (and cellulite-free!), but also to reduce your desire to eat unhealthy fatty foods. But that's not all. The essential fats also tune up your metabolism and help you burn unwanted fat. So it's not true to say that a calorie of *any* fat has the same effect on weight gain. You'll hear the whole story and the latest research in Chapter 14.

3: Eliminate your hidden allergies

Each one of us is unique. Think about your friends. They probably look very different from each other. Some will be night owls, others skylarks. They'll have different blood types. A number of them may be natural carnivores, others natural vegetarians. And most of us have different intolerances or allergies to certain foods, but very few even know it. Weight gain, however, is a common reaction to foods we're intolerant to.

It follows, then, that eliminating the food that you are unknowingly allergic to can lead to dramatic weight loss. Lisa M, for instance, lost 13cm (5in) off her waist in three days and 19kg (3st.) in three months by discovering and avoiding what she was allergic to.

Rebecca S also lost 19kg (3st.) simply by avoiding the foods she was allergic to. In her twenties Rebecca had a stable weight, and exercised three or four times a week. But in her thirties she started to pile on the pounds. Over three years her weight drifted from 63.5kg (10st.) up to 82.5kg (13st.) and her dress size went up to 16.

> ❛ *I started feeling tired and lethargic and generally unwell. I didn't have the energy to go to the gym any more. But it seemed the foods I ate were blowing me up, which is why I thought I could have a food allergy.* ❜

She decided to test herself for a food allergy, which you can do using a home test kit, involving a pinprick of blood. The results showed that she was reacting to milk, egg white and gluten (the protein found in wheat). Within a week of excluding these foods her skin and mood improved and the weight started to fall away.

Don't think that all allergies are for life. After three months strictly avoiding the foods Rebecca had become allergic to, she reintroduced egg whites and then milk to see if there was a reaction. Now she's fine on both foods, but still reacts to wheat.

> ❛ *I can't tell you how much better I feel. I'm 100 per cent. Eliminating my food allergies has transformed my health. I just wish I'd done it sooner.* ❜

Why did she lose so much weight? Because water retention, bloating and puffiness are all common allergic symptoms, and they make you feel and look fatter.

This is great news because, once you've singled out and eliminated the 'bad' foods, you can see dramatic changes very fast. It's not unusual to lose up to 3.2kg (7lb) within three or four days.

Aside from weight gain and bloating, food allergies also cause many other niggling problems: aches and pains, headaches, sinus problems, fatigue, mood dips, itchy skin and digestive conditions such as bloating and IBS (irritable bowel syndrome). These also go when you identify and avoid what you are allergic to. You'll find out how to pinpoint the 'baddies' lurking in your larder in Chapter 15.

It's reassuring to know that, as in Rebecca's case, most food allergies aren't for life. You can often 'unlearn' your intolerances in as little as three months, which means that you can reintroduce previously 'bad' foods back into your diet.

4: Take the right supplements

By now you're probably realising that calorie intake and weight loss are not all that firmly linked. In fact, one of the biggest lies in nutrition today is, 'You can lose weight only by eating fewer calories.'

The other is, 'You can get all the vitamins and minerals you need from a well-balanced diet.' This is untrue. You simply can't guarantee that the nutrients you need are in your food.

Take vitamin C, which not only protects against degenerative diseases such as cancer and heart disease but also helps stabilise your blood sugar and speeds your fatburning. For example, you have half the risk of being diabetic if your blood level of vitamin C is high.[5] At ION, we've examined hundreds of studies – including the 'gold standard' type, which are known as 'randomised, double-blind, placebo-controlled' – that have led us to conclude that the optimal intake of vitamin C is around 1,000mg a day. This is what our jungle-dwelling, fruit-eating ancestors could have got from leaves, berries and fruits.

But how much vitamin C is there in a supermarket orange? The 'average' orange contains 60mg of the precious vitamin, but some contain much less. And, even if your supermarket orange contains 60mg, you'd need to eat 22 of them to achieve 1,000mg.

So I recommend that you supplement 1,000mg of vitamin C a day, along with eating vitamin-C-rich foods such as strawberries. You can eat strawberries until the cows come home and never gain weight. (Not all fruits are this useful for fatburning or general health, however, as we'll see.)

There are some 30 vitamins and minerals that are essential for health, and along with vitamin C a number will help you burn fat, too. Essentially, they boost your metabolism, reprogramming your body to turn food into energy rather than fat. For example, the mineral chromium helps to even out appetite and energy dips by stabilising your blood sugar. It's so effective that it's given to diabetics, with amazing results. There are also amino acids and herbs that really can give you the edge when it comes to losing weight. Hydroxycitric acid, or HCA, is a herbal extract from the tamarind plant, which makes it harder for your body to turn glucose into fat. There's another herbal extract from a bean called griffonia, which is naturally high in an amino acid called 5-hydroxytryptophan. Known as 5-HTP, this amino acid has an extraordinary capability to ease excessive appetite and sugar cravings. I'll show you the evidence, and also our own results from people following the Holford Diet, with or without supplements, in Chapter 16.

There's no question, the right supplements make a difference, tuning up your metabolism and reducing cravings. They are not drugs and they don't have side effects – except for better health, mood, sleep and energy.

5: Do 15 minutes of exercise a day
If you exercise just to burn calories, quite frankly you might as well just not eat that piece of toast. The real value of exercise is that it helps stabilise your blood sugar levels and reduce your appetite. And the great news is that you don't have to do much to achieve this result – just 15 minutes a day, in fact.

The single greatest reason people give for not doing even 15 minutes a day is that they feel 'too tired to exercise'. On my diet that will become a thing of the past. In fact, you'll have so much energy you'll positively want to exercise.

It has been found that people who don't exercise eat more than people who do a little exercise or just have active jobs. The human body is programmed to need physical activity to work properly, in the same way that it needs water or vitamins. Certain kinds of exercise boost the rate at which you burn fat for up to 15 hours afterwards.

That's the immediate effect, but there's a long-term effect too. With the right kind of exercise, you'll put on more muscle and lose fat – and a pound of muscle burns many more calories a day than a pound of fat. So every pound of fat you lose and every pound of muscle you gain increases your body's long-term ability to burn fat.

To kick-start this process, you'll do 15 minutes a day, or 21 minutes five times a week, or 35 minutes three times a week, of the right kind of muscle-building and fatburning exercise. I explain all this in Chapter 17. And, fortunately, the fatter and less fit you are right now, the easier it will be to get the same benefits! For example, if you are overweight and underfit, jogging 0.8km (½ mile) slowly can burn 300 calories, whereas if you are fitter and lighter you'd need to jog 1.6km (1 mile).

★ ★ ★

Following these five principles is easy, and enjoyable – yet they'll revolutionise the way you live, simply because of the way you'll feel and look, day by day. And, if you feel and look great, that's the best motivation for making it a diet for life.

Meanwhile, the dieting industry continues to make money from you by selling quick fixes that are destined to fail. That's what keeps you coming back for more. How many diets have you been on and how many have worked? I want to make sure that the Holford Diet is the last diet you'll ever go on.

2

Why So Many Diets Fail

Dieting can be like negotiating a minefield of misconceptions. Many methods for losing weight have no basis in science whatsoever. So, if your dieting life has been one long string of depressing failed attempts, it's hardly surprising.

Here, I'd like to debunk some of these 'methods' and expose them as myths (the biggest of all being that the best way to lose weight is a conventional low-fat, low-calorie diet). That way, you'll have the knowledge to prevent a life of yo-yo dieting and long-term health problems.

Myth number 1: the only way to lose weight is to eat less fat and less calories

Hard-wired into our culture is the false idea that the best way to lose weight is to eat a low-calorie diet. We all know the simple equation: calories in, minus calories out, equals your weight. Since fat has more calories per gram/ounce than protein or carbohydrate, the easiest way to cut the total number of calories you eat is to eat less fat. That's what you are told.

Low-fat, low-calorie diets have become the orthodox approach to weight loss, jealously guarded by doctors and dieticians the world over. But orthodoxy doesn't necessarily mean it's right, just that it won the battle of the diets. In fact, it's wrong. As you will see, whichever way you look at it, low-GL diets work better. Let's examine the evidence, both by looking at the big picture, then at what the latest science shows us about burning fat.

Let's start with the big picture. America leads the world's obesity epidemic. In fact, obesity has recently overtaken smoking as the number-one preventable cause of premature death. Flying the low-fat, low-cal flag back in the 1970s they set out to reduce the total percentage of calories eaten from fat. In 1977 fat averaged 42 per cent of calories. Their campaigns were extremely successful, and by 1997 fat averaged 32 per cent of calories. Did the decrease in fat intake stop the obesity epidemic? No. It's accelerated.

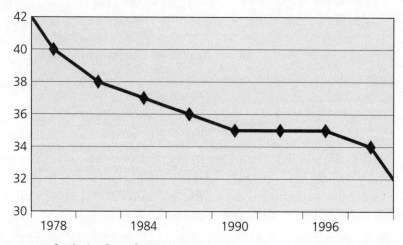

Percentage of calories from fat In the US, there has been a drop in fat intake as a percentage of calorie intake yet rates of obesity continue to rise.

So, what about the UK? Government diet surveys conducted between 1985 and 2000 show that, like the Americans, we have been successful, both in cutting the percentage of fat and the total intake of calories.[6] People are eating less. Calorie consumption has gone down, and fat intake has gone down even more. Just like the Americans, these changes haven't halted our escalating epidemic of weight gain one iota. Just watch a movie from the 1980s and notice people's size. Something is going seriously wrong in the twenty-first century, and clearly the blame cannot be laid at the level of fat intake.

Not only have we been told that eating fewer calories is the best way to lose weight but we've also been told that a calorie is a calorie and that's all that counts.

Myth number 2: a calorie is a calorie is a calorie

It's not easy to control rigidly how many calories a person eats, but you can do it with animals. So let's look at what happens to animals given identical diets in terms of calories and all other nutrients – with only one

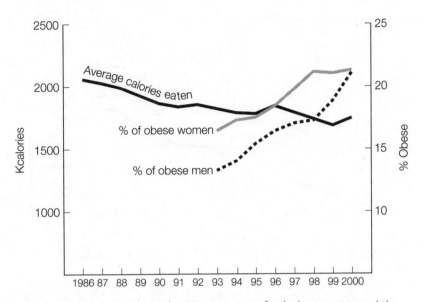

UK Government statistics show that the amount of calories we eat, and the percentage of calories we eat from fat, has steadily decreased, whereas the percentage of obese people has steadily increased.

difference: GL. In the chart on page 38 you'll see what happened to one group of rats. Half were given a high-GL diet, the other a low-GL diet. They couldn't cheat. They had exactly the same number of calories – and there weren't any sweetshops round the corner.

In this strictly controlled study by one of the world's leading experts on weight loss, Professor Jennie Brand-Miller from the University of Sydney, the low-GL rats gained no weight.[7] But the high-GL rats gained weight week on week, and pound on pound. By the end of 32 weeks, the high-GL group were not only 16 per cent heavier but they had gained 40 per cent more body fat on the same number of calories!

Another study, published in the *Lancet* medical journal, found that mice with a low-GL diet lost almost *twice* the body fat in nine weeks as mice given identical calorie-controlled diets, the only difference being that one group was on a high-GL diet, the other a low-GL diet. The low-GL dieters were substantially leaner and slimmer.[8]

Same calories, very different results. Yet, of course, this is nothing short of heresy for conventional calorie theorists.

But, you may be asking, does the same thing happen to us? After all, rats and humans don't always respond in a similar way. The answer is yes. Here's a couple of examples, although there are more in Chapter 4.

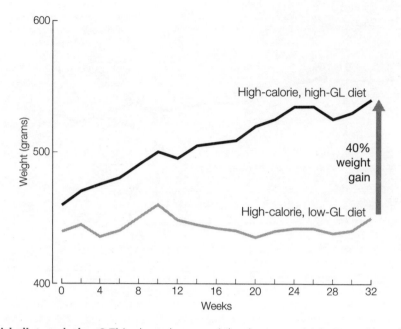

Which diet works best? This chart shows weight change on high-GL and low-GL diets of equal calories and fat/protein/carbohydrate percentage.

Researchers in the human nutrition department at South Africa's University of the Orange Free State assigned 15 volunteers to a low-GL diet and 15 others to a normal calorie-controlled diet for 12 weeks.[9] Both diets contained identical numbers of calories. The two groups then switched diets for 12 more weeks. As you can see from the chart opposite, during the first 12 weeks both groups lost weight, but those on the low-GL diet lost more weight. During the second 12-week period, the group that switched to the low-GL diet lost 40 per cent more weight than the group that switched to the normal diet. Yet the caloric content of both diets remained the same.

Another recent study published in the *New England Journal of Medicine* put volunteers on to one of three diets: a conventional low-calorie, low-fat diet; a Mediterranean diet, restricted for calories and high in fibre and monounsaturated fats; and a high-protein, high-fat, low-carb diet, similar to the Atkins Diet, but emphasising vegetarian sources of protein rather than meat and dairy products.[10] Both the Mediterranean diet and the low-carb diet were effectively lower-GL diets.

Despite similar calorie intakes the participants lost 4.5kg (10lb) on the low-carb diet, 4.3kg (9½lb) on the Mediterranean-style diet and only

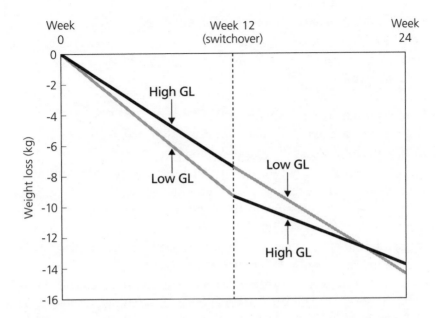

Weight loss on a high-GL vs. low-GL diet Two groups of overweight women were given a low-calorie diet, with equivalent amounts of protein, fat and carbohydrate. One group ate low-GL carbohydrates and the other group ate high-GL carbohydrates. Both groups lost weight, but those on the low-GL diet lost considerably more weight over 12 weeks. Those on the low-GL diet were then switched to the high-GL diet, and vice versa. During the second period of 12 weeks, again, those on the low-GL diet lost considerably more weight.

2.7kg (6lb) on the low-calorie, low-fat diet. The fact is that low-fat, low-calorie diets were not as effective for weight loss as the low-GL diets.

Despite all this evidence (and there's a lot more given in Chapter 4 and in Part Two), some so-called experts still say 'a calorie is a calorie', as far as weight loss is concerned. Whichever way you slice it, this is simply not true. You can lose weight by changing the quality of what you eat, even if you don't change the quantity. Of course, if you change both the quantity and the quality by eating fewer calories of lower-GL foods, that will trigger the most rapid weight loss.

But that's not all. We now know that people who eat low-GL food eat significantly less anyway, simply because they feel much more satisfied.[11] One study compared hunger between those on a conventional low-calorie, low-fat diet with a low-GL diet. Those on the low-GL diet reported much less hunger.[12]

Adrian, a chef, is a case in point. He was diagnosed with diabetes and his doctor recommended the Holford Diet:

❛ I am a totally changed person. I feel incredible. Before, I didn't have a cut-off switch. I could just eat and eat and would still be hungry throughout the day. After two months on your diet I now feel full and can leave food on the plate because I'm full. ❜

Adrian lost 84lb (6st.) in six months.

So, if you eat a low-GL diet, you not only lose weight but you also tend to want to eat less. It's a double whammy in your favour.

But calories can't just vanish. If two people eat the same number of calories and one, eating the high-GL diet, stores some of the calories as fat, what happens to the calories in the low-GL dieter? Think about those animals that lost more weight on the same calories. A calorie is a unit of energy and, if it's not going into fat, it must be burnt off as energy. This either means that the body's metabolism speeds up, 'burning' up the calories, or the person becomes more active and burns them off through exercise, or possibly both. We'll never know in those animal studies because they didn't fit the animals with pedometers! But, either way, it's good news.

I believe that that is why people on the Holford Diet always talk about how marvellous they feel.

Linda B says:

❛ Now my energy level is incredible. ❜

She lost 7.7kg (1st. 3lb) in six weeks. I hear this kind of feedback all the time from people who have followed my diet. You really can, and you will, lose weight and feel great. This is precisely why the Holford Diet works so amazingly well.

Myth number 3: you can't change your metabolism

Your metabolism is the way in which you turn your food into energy or into storage as fat. We are each programmed to respond differently to the food we eat. This programming is partly inherited: some people's metabolism rapidly turns food into fat, for example. But your metabolism is primarily down to what you eat and how active you are.

Because of this, you can change both the efficiency of your metabolism and your metabolic rate – the speed at which you burn calories. Crash diets usually lower your metabolic rate dramatically, for instance, whereas intensive aerobic exercise can increase it tenfold, and leave it raised for up to 15 hours.

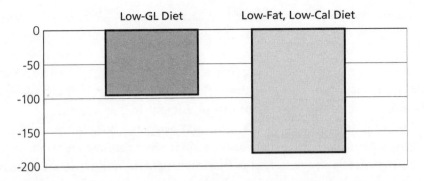

The effects of a low-GL vs. low-fat, low-calorie diet on metabolic rate A low-GL diet causes half the reduction in metabolic rate of a low-fat, low-calorie diet.

By changing the kinds and combinations of food you eat, and exercising, you can reprogramme yourself to burn fat more rapidly. And the less fat and the more lean tissue you have, the more calories you burn off just keeping your body alive. In other words, your metabolic rate has increased, and you've changed from fat-storer to fatburner. This is what a low-GL diet, together with exercise, will do for you over the long term.

The dramatic drop in metabolic rate is one of the main problems with low-calorie diets, not only because you burn fewer calories but also because you feel tired and sluggish. This means that dieters find it increasingly difficult to lose weight the lower their calorie intake, because they don't have the energy to exercise and raise their metabolic rate. Low-GL diets cause half the reduction in metabolic rate compared to a typical low-fat diet and consistently increase energy levels.

This was shown in a study published in the *Journal of the American Medical Association*.[13] The researchers assigned 39 overweight or obese adults to one of two diets. One group was on a low-GL diet, the other group followed a conventional low-fat, low-calorie diet. They were then followed for two years while on these diets. Each person had their metabolic rate measured once they had lost 10 per cent of their body weight. The group on the conventional low-fat, low-calorie diet had almost twice the reduction in metabolic rate compared with the low-GL group.

Myth number 4: if you eat a high-protein diet you lose calories in urine, so you will shed more weight

When you're on a high-protein, low-carbohydrate diet, your body switches from using carbohydrates as its primary fuel to using fat and protein instead – including the body's fat reserves. As the body burns fat, ketones – a by-product of the process – are excreted in the urine. This process is called *ketosis*.

Supposedly, since fat and protein constitute a less efficient fuel than carbohydrate, you can eat more. The thinking is that the body will excrete some of the calories of this inefficient fuel as ketones.

Nice theory, but wrong. It is true that people do lose more weight on high-protein diets. But the reason is that they eat less on those diets. And the reason they eat less is that high-protein diets help to stabilise blood sugar.

The high-protein-diet camp, led by the late Dr Atkins, was one of the first to say that sugar makes you fat. But its solution was to say that carbohydrates are bad and protein is good, so you should eat a high-protein, high-fat diet that's very low in carbohydrates. Now, a high-protein meal has a low-GL, which, as we've seen, is the key to stabilising blood sugar, which in turn balances our appetite and helps us lose weight. But a meal with some protein and some low-GL carbohydrate works in the same way. There is absolutely no need to avoid or massively restrict carbohydrates to lose weight, provided you are eating the right low-GL kind, plus protein.

Let's take a look at three weight-loss trials published on the Atkins-type high-fat, high-protein diet versus a conventional low-fat diet. The first showed that, after six months, those on the high-fat, high-protein diet lost 5.8kg (12lb 11oz), compared with 1.8kg (4lb) on the low-fat diet. That's a rather unexciting 225g (8oz) a week. However, after 12 months, there was no significant difference.[14]

The other trial showed no real difference in weight loss between the high-protein approach and conventional dieting, with an average weight loss of 4.5kg (10lb) after six months.[15] That's less than 225g (8oz) a week.

The third compared the Atkins Diet with the Slim-Fast plan, WeightWatchers and Rosemary Conley's Eat Yourself Slim diet and fitness plan in a community-based sample of otherwise healthy overweight and obese adults. Weight and body fat changes were measured over six months.

Results showed that all diets resulted in weight loss, averaging 5.9kg (13lb) over six months, or a rather unimpressive 225g (8oz) a week. The Atkins Diet resulted in significantly higher weight loss during the first four weeks, but by the end was no more or less effective than the other low-fat, low-calorie diets.[16]

A review of all the high-protein/low-carbohydrate diet studies done to date concluded, 'Weight loss was principally associated with decreased calorie intake.'[17]

In other words, an Atkins-type diet works, but the results aren't spectacular and are principally due to eating less in general. Moreover, there are problems, and even serious dangers, associated with eating high-protein, low-carbohydrate diets, which I go into in detail in Appendix 3 (page 402), but here's an overview.

The problem with high-protein, low-carbohydrate diets

High-protein diets are usually high in meat and dairy. High meat intake is strongly linked to increased risk for cancer of the colon, breast, prostate, pancreas and kidney, according to the World Cancer Research Fund. They also recommend, 'If eaten at all, limit intake of red meat to no more than 80 grams a day.' High-dairy diets also dramatically increase the risk of breast cancer and prostate cancer. High-protein diets are also proven to tax the kidneys and can tip older people with less than perfect kidney function into kidney failure. Since high-protein diets first became popular, kidney problems have increased. Another problem with high-protein diets is bone mass loss. What's more, high-protein diets are often designed to produce ketones, which are toxic by-products of running your body on protein.

In excess, ketones can be very toxic and in extreme cases ketosis can be fatal. Reports suggest that 58 deaths have been associated with very low-calorie, very high-protein diets. Moreover, recent research has proved that the amount of calories lost through ketosis is negligible. One study put people on a ketone-producing very low-carb diet (5 per cent of calories as carbs) versus a non-ketone producing low-carb diet (40 per cent of calories as carbs) for six weeks.[18] This second diet is closer to the Holford Diet. Both lost weight – 6.3kg (1st.) vs. 7.2kg (16lb) respectively – but those on the ketone-producing diet had an increase in markers for inflammation and felt worse. So, if you don't lose more weight, and it makes you feel worse, *and* the risks are high, why do it?

These high-protein diets promise more than they deliver in other ways too. As I've said, I think the switch to ketosis triggers weight loss by stabilising blood sugar, and it's known that ketosis also suppresses appetite. A low-carbohydrate diet also kick-starts weight loss because you use up your short-term stores of glucose, which are stored in the muscles and liver as glycogen, bound up with water. In fact, for every pound of glycogen, you store 1.3–1.8kg (3–4lb) of water. The net result is an immediate weight loss of up to 2.25kg (5lb) – just one reason why people claim spectacular short-term weight loss. But it's not sustainable. The glycogen and water will come back, as will your appetite. Many people on high-protein diets lose weight, get bored, then gain it all back.

A diet lacking in carbohydrates such as fruit and green leafy veg will leave you deficient in antioxidants and vitamins, unless you are very careful about what you eat and take supplements. You won't get enough fibre, and could get constipated as a result, which can lead to digestive problems. Additionally, many people feel ill as they go through sugar withdrawal and switch to ketosis. Nausea and tiredness continue for some people, making it hard to stick to the diet.

Nowadays, there are many variations on the original low-carb Atkins Diet, from America's South Beach Diet to Australia's Total Wellbeing Diet, supposedly based on good science.

The South Beach Diet is really the Atkins Diet with an emphasis on polyunsaturated fats and low-glycemic index (GI) carbohydrates. In a sense, this might be a step in the right direction if the advice on those fats and carbohydrates were up to date. Like Atkins, South Beach emphasises a 'ketogenic' diet of minimum carbohydrates for the first two weeks. Ultimately, this doesn't seem to result in more fat loss, but it may cause greater initial weight loss as the body sheds water. (If you avoid carbohydrates, the body has to break down glucose for energy, which is stored as glycogen. Glycogen is stored with water.) This benefit is immediately attractive and may add to the diet's short-term popularity; however, the weight will come back because it's not a loss of fat. The only published trial I could find on the South Beach Diet appeared in a 2004 issue of the *Archives of Internal Medicine,* and it reported an average weight loss of 6.1kg (13lb 9oz) over 12 weeks, or 500g (1lb 2oz) per week.[19]

The Australian Total Wellbeing Diet, researched and developed by Australia's Commonwealth Scientific and Industrial Research Organisation (CSIRO), and funded by Meat and Livestock Australia and Dairy Australia, is another high-protein diet that has hit the headlines. It recommends scoffing no less than ten portions of meat and two portions of fish, plus six eggs and a few servings of cheese in a week. This makes a total of 300g (10½oz) protein a day, just like the Atkins Diet.

The Australian Total Wellbeing Diet is said to be based on solid research. The research in question involved 120 people put either on the

Total Wellbeing high-protein diet or a high-carbohydrate diet for 12 weeks. The trial, published in the *American Journal of Clinical Nutrition*, found no difference in weight loss at all![20] What it did find, although this isn't mentioned in the conclusion, was signs of kidney stress (decreased creatinine clearance) and potential bone mass loss (increased bone mass turnover) in only 12 weeks! I guess that's not something the high-protein diet brigade want to shout about.

The bottom line is that high-protein diets, especially those based on meat and milk, can be dangerous. They potentially increase the risk of bone and kidney problems, and breast and prostate cancer. And as we've seen, the weight-loss results are little different to conventional dieting in the long run. In my opinion the high-protein approach to stabilising your blood sugar, and hence your weight, is certainly not worth the risk.

Myth number 5: don't eat protein with carbohydrates; these foods fight

Food-combining diets separate protein foods from carbohydrate foods. Nature doesn't. Beans, lentils, nuts and seeds all contain both. And the healthiest nations of the world are the nut, bean and seed eaters.

Despite this, a number of food-combining diets abound, based on the principles of Dr Hay, a physician writing back in the 1930s. He emphasised eating wholefoods and lots of fruit and vegetables; he also advocated eating fruit separately from other foods, since, if trapped in the stomach after a steak for example, fruit can ferment. So far, so good.

Dr Hay also recommended never eating carbohydrate-rich foods with protein-rich foods. So, for example, fish with rice or chicken with potatoes is out. The only study I've seen recommending that overweight or obese people follow this kind of diet showed a 3.5 per cent average body-weight change over 12 weeks. Although subjects in this trial were not advised to eat less or change the kind of food they ate, there was no measure to indicate whether this weight loss was solely due to food-combining or changes in the quantity or quality of food.[21]

It is now known, however, that combining protein with carbohydrate slows down the release of sugars from a meal to the bloodstream, helps stabilise blood sugar levels and hence helps to control weight (see Chapter 12). Since the majority of overweight people have blood sugar problems, it would seem that combining protein with carbohydrate would be better, not worse for you. So, in my book, fish with rice is in, not out. This is the staple diet, along with fruits and vegetables, of many island and coastal people around the world, many of whom are exceedingly healthy and slim.

Dr Hay's approach, if followed strictly, is probably best for those with digestive problems and worst for those with blood sugar problems. I remain to be convinced that the benefits reported by those on food-combining diets aren't largely due to changes in the kind of foods eaten, rather than their non-combination.

Myth number 6: it's eating fat that makes you fat

We've already seen many examples of low-fat diets causing less weight loss than low-GL diets, and how cutting fat intake hasn't worked. Yet most people still believe that the fat you eat turns into fat in your body. It isn't just fat that makes you fat. All sugar or carbohydrates and all alcohol, as well as all fats, are turned by the body into glucose. (Protein, too, can be turned into glucose, but not so easily.) Glucose, remember, is the fuel our bodies run on, and any excess is turned into fat. So, too much fat, protein, carbohydrate or alcohol can all lead to fat gain and weight gain. As you'll see in the next chapter the main culprit is sugar and refined carbohydrates, not fat.

What is more, looking at fat alone, as far as your body is concerned there's a world of difference between, say, 100 calories of saturated fat from meat and 100 calories of essential fat from seeds or fish. Saturated fat can only be burned for energy or stored as body fat. But essential fats are used by the brain, the nerves, the arteries and the skin, and they balance your hormones and boost immunity into the bargain. Only if there's any left over does it make sense for the body to burn it or store it. Although the research is in its infancy, it appears that omega-3 fats EPA and DHA (which is what's found in oily fish), and monounsaturated fats (as in olive oil), as well as possibly medium-chain triglycerides (MCTs – as found in coconut), are easier for the body to burn and less likely to be converted to body fat than animal-based saturated fats.[22] So you are more likely to gain weight eating a diet full of animal-based saturated fat or damaged fat in fried or processed foods than you are eating essential fats in fish and seeds.

One big reason for this is that the body craves essential fats, precisely because it needs them to function. This craving means we are drawn to fats in general, and, as we're surrounded by saturated and processed fats the minute we enter the average supermarket, we may well end up eating them. Yet, afterwards the body still keeps craving fat – so we eat more fatty foods. But, if you eat essential fat-rich foods such as fish and seeds, you'll fully satisfy the craving and will end up eating less.

Does eating fat make you fat? Of course it does, in excess, but fat isn't the main culprit. As we saw earlier, the number of calories we eat from fat has dropped, but it hasn't curbed the obesity epidemic.

Low-fat diets arose out of the belief that fat is the prime culprit in weight gain. But, as with high-protein diets, there are two potential problems with this approach. First, most low-fat diets are high in carbohydrates, so sugar and refined foods replace fatty foods. This encourages a blood sugar problem that, in turn, makes it harder to maintain weight control. For this reason, very low-fat, high-carbohydrate diets can often cause fatigue, mood swings and sugar cravings.

But the worst aspect of a low-fat diet is that it cuts out essential fats. Ann Louise Gittlemann is the former director of nutrition at the Pritikin Longevity Center in Florida, which emphasised low-fat eating. In her book, *Beyond Pritikin,*[23] she notes certain conditions in people placed on low-fat diets, such as allergies, yeast problems, mood swings, a lack of energy, and dry skin, hair and nails, that she believed were caused by the lack of essential fats.

Although most of us could do with cutting back on fat, the real emphasis should be on reducing foods rich in saturated fats and devoid of essential fats (meat and dairy produce), and instead eating foods rich in essential fats (seeds, their oils and fish).

Myth number 7: the best way to lose a lot of weight fast is to eat a very low-calorie diet

I'm dead against very low-calorie diets and calorie counting. Not only does it encourage obsessive eating but also the maths are patently wrong.

Consider this simple example. A banana is approximately 100 calories. So, if you eat a banana fewer every day for a year, you'd lose 36,500 calories. A pound of body fat is equivalent to around 4,000 calories. That means you'd lose nearly 4.5kg (10lb) in the first year, 22.7kg (3½st.) by the fifth year, and 45.3kg (7st.) after ten years – and vanish completely after 15 years!

The calorie equation for exercise is equally ridiculous. Cycle vigorously for 15 minutes each day and you will lose 4.5kg (10lb) in the first year. Quite possibly. But 45.3kg (7st.) after 10 years? No chance. However, according to calorie theory, merely a banana every day undoes all that hard work anyway.

According to Dr Michael Colgan, nutritionist to many Olympic athletes, some athletes burn off more than 7,000 calories a day, but eat only 3,500 calories. Going by calorie theory alone, these athletes should have completely disappeared by now.

An investigation by Dr M. Appelbaum of people living in famine in the Warsaw ghetto during World War One came up with the same contradiction.[24] With an average calorie intake of 800 calories a day, and a requirement of around 2,500 calories, a deficiency of 1,241,000 calories would have built up over two years. The average body has 13.6kg (2st. 2lb) of fat, representing 120,000 calories, to dispose of. Even if all the fat were lost, what happened to the other million calories?

If you still believe it's all down to calories, listen to this. The *Sunday Times* put two similarly overweight people on diets, one on an earlier version of the Holford Diet (called the Fatburner Diet, which had approximately 1,500 calories), and one on the Cambridge Diet (330 calories in those days). The volunteer on my diet lost more weight after six weeks.

The missing link in the low-calorie approach is metabolism – the process of turning the fuel in food into energy that the body can use, and burning off unwanted fat. As we've seen, people's metabolism can vary considerably. Having a slow metabolism means you'll turn more food into fat.

If you start out this way, a low-calorie diet can simply exacerbate the problem. With crash diets below 1,000 calories a day, the body sees this reduction in food as a threat, and slows down the metabolic rate dramatically.[25] According to Dr John Marks from Cambridge University, 'As weight falls, the metabolic rate always falls too.' In the short term you can lose around 3.2kg (7lb) of body fluid and, if you're lucky, an absolute maximum of 900g (2lb) of body fat a week, which together could account for as much as 4.5kg (10lb) in two or three weeks. But the minute you go back to what you were eating before, the fluid returns. And so will the fat, because your metabolic rate has slowed down, meaning that you now need to eat less food to maintain a stable weight.

This 'rebound effect' is good business for mortuaries. A report by the National Institutes of Health, using the findings of a 22-centre study called the Multiple Risk Factor Intervention Trial, illustrated that people whose weight showed a wide variability over six to seven years had a higher death rate.[26] It's also good for food-replacement programmes (using special drinks or bars in place of food), whose customers try crash-dieting on average three times a year.

To see how dramatically unpleasant the rebound effect can be, hark back to the *Sunday Times* trial I mentioned above. Michelle, who was on the Cambridge Diet, said:

> ❝ *The first three days were torturous, but from then on it got worse. Walking down the road required serious will: I was constantly exhausted and couldn't concentrate, so my work suffered badly. Weight loss came slowly – I'd expected miracles after reading the publicity boasts – but in the final week it finally plummeted … I blew up like a balloon when I resumed eating, and seemed to retain gallons of water; conversely, 'loose' skin has appeared, creating an under-arm bat-wing effect. When I first stopped the diet, irresistible bingeing took over, but after six weeks, with the exercise of limbs and discipline, I've managed to limit the damage to a gain of 5lb [2.25kg].* ❞

Michelle lost 4.5kg (10lb) over the month and gained 2.25kg (5lb) in the weeks that followed – making her net weight loss 2.25kg (5lb).

However, Caroline, on my diet, also lost 4.5kg (10lb) in a month. She then put 900g (2lb) back on while on holiday. She commented:

> ❝ *One of the hardest – but best – things about it was the insistence on giving up coffee and stimulants. I had caffeine-withdrawal headaches for the first few days, but began to feel wonderful after that – alert and fit, and thoroughly detoxified, with no more puffy eyes staring back from the bathroom mirror. I regained 2lb [900g] while on holiday, but will whittle it off by eating sensibly.* ❞

The bottom line is that the body is intelligent. If you try to starve it, it will turn down your metabolic fire. If you work with its natural design you'll burn unwanted fat easily. (By the way, you don't have to give up all stimulants and caffeine-containing drinks on the Holford Diet, but there's no question that it helps to speed up weight loss if you do. More on this in Chapter 13.)

Very low-calorie diets do more, however, than make you feel bad and gain weight afterwards. They can be dangerous, and are now required to provide at least 400 calories and 40g (1½oz) of protein per day for women and 500 calories and 50g (1¾oz) of protein per day for men, to ensure the dieter's body will not be breaking down muscle tissue or vital organs to meet calorie requirements. These diets do not encourage the re-education of eating habits. And they leave you very hungry.

The solution in the eyes of the people designing these diets is wheat bran, which fills you up while at the same time supposedly triggering weight loss. But does that make dieters want to stick to the regime? To find out, I put ten people on a diet of 1,000 calories per day, plus high fibre, for three months. Only four lasted the course, with an average weight loss of a measly 1.4kg (3¼lb). The high dropout rate is a reflection of how difficult it is to stick to a low-calorie diet for a long period of time.

In another study we put ten slimmers on high-fibre tablets – claimed to induce weight loss – for a period of three months. Five completed the three months with an average weight loss of 680g (1½lb). Not very impressive.

However, some special kinds of fibre do assist weight loss, and having a high-fibre diet by eating wholefoods – not by adding wheat bran – is definitely good for you. This is explained in Chapter 13.

Myth number 8: stimulants help you lose weight by reducing your appetite

It's true that stimulants such as caffeine, nicotine and the body's own adrenalin all help to reduce your appetite. They do this by releasing stores of sugar held in your body. So, sure, you can lose weight by just drinking coffee – in the short term.

However, long-term use of stimulants messes up your blood sugar control. When your blood sugar dips, this leads to fatigue, mood swings, anxiety, sugar craving, weight gain and, of course, dependence on stimulants. The best way to control your appetite, and your cravings, is to eat a low-GL diet.

Myth number 9: slimming pills work

Every year there is a new pill or potion that claims to do it all for you – starch blockers, fat blockers, appetite suppressants, slimming pills. Avoid them at all costs. You can't cheat the body without paying a price.

Starch blockers inhibit the digestion of carbohydrate. The theory is that if you can't digest it you can't gain weight. But having a whole lot of undigested carbohydrate in the digestive tract is bad news. It feeds the wrong kind of bugs, causing bacterial and yeast infections as well as terrible gas.

Much touted as an answer to weight loss is a supplement called chitosan, sometimes called the 'fat attractor' or 'fat magnet', which inhibits the digestion of fat. It apparently works because it has a positive charge and attracts fats, which have a negative charge. Once bound together with chitosan, the fat is less likely to be absorbed and passes through the body, so it is claimed, and cholesterol levels decrease.

However, three studies have found no significant differences in either weight or cholesterol levels in people taking chitosan or a placebo. One study involved 30 overweight people who took chitosan or a placebo for 28 days while eating their normal diet. There was no difference in weight or cholesterol.[27] The second study, involving 51 obese women, found that the chitosan group had slightly greater cholesterol reduction than the placebo group, but no difference in weight loss after eight weeks.[28] Another study, with 68 obese men and women, found no improvement in weight or cholesterol.[29]

The latest fat blocker to hit the market is a patented fibre extract from the prickly pear (*Opuntia ficus indica*) called NeOpuntia®. Although some studies do show that it binds to fat, and also lowers cholesterol, I've not been able to find any evidence to date that it causes weight loss.

Drug companies are also cashing in on the weight-loss market with drugs that stop you from digesting fat. An example is Xenical, the drug name for a chemical called orlistat. This drug does actually work, in the sense that it does reduce fat absorption. The immediate potential side effects are gas with discharge, oily or fatty stools, oily discharge and an inability to control bowel movements. If that doesn't put you off, more worrying are the effects on essential fats, so vital for heart, brain and skin, but whose absorption is also reduced when taking Xenical. Since essential fats are probably the most commonly deficient nutrient in the West, the last thing you want to swallow is something that stops you from using the little essential fat there is in your diet. Also, it probably isn't a good idea to have undigested fat in your digestive tract.

Some slimming drugs are basically stimulants that suppress appetite and wire you up, inducing anxiety and hyperactivity. Similarly, if you drink 15 cups of coffee a day, it would also work in the short term. In the not-so-long term, stimulants mess up your body's metabolism as well as your physical, mental and emotional health (see also Myth Number 8). Even if it sounds 'natural', avoid any herb or supplement whose active ingredient is caffeine – and that includes guarana.

Myth number 10: there's nothing wrong with being overweight

The health risks associated with weighing more than you should accumulate as soon as you are as little as 3.2kg (7lb) overweight. With over half of people in Britain overweight and 20 per cent obese, that's a lot of extra health risks.

And these are serious risks: heart disease, high blood pressure, diabetes, kidney problems, osteoporosis, cancer, polycystic ovaries and arthritis. One study showed that about 40 per cent of heart disease in women is linked to overweight, whereas others connect it to higher risks of breast cancer, arthritis, osteoporosis and other complications.[30] Diabetes is strongly linked to obesity – your risk of developing diabetes goes up 77 times if you're obese. With over 200 million obese people in Europe alone, that's a lot of sick people.

In fact, every year obesity causes the premature deaths of 30,000 people, costs Britain's National Health Service £1 billion and is responsible for the loss of more than 20 million working days. According to Dr Susan Jebb of the Dunn Clinical Nutrition Centre in Cambridge in the UK, 'Obesity is a serious medical condition that reduces life expectancy by increasing the risk of many chronic and potentially fatal diseases.'

And with a thousand people becoming obese every day, we need to wake up to the fact that there's a disaster in the making here – but only potentially. It only *looks* like a slippery slope: there is a way out.

Why the Holford Diet works where others fail

You can lose weight on a low-calorie diet, a high-protein diet, a low-carb diet or a no-fat diet. But you are stacking the odds against you. Why? Because...

- You get short-term weight loss as your body burns its essential store of glycogen – that's 2.25kg (5lb) gone, but it all comes back!

- None of these diets satisfy your appetite better than the Holford Diet, so you have to fight hard to stay on them.

- All of these diets are highly restrictive in some way – who wants to live without carbohydrates or fats?

- None of these diets have been shown to trigger as much weight loss in the short term or long term as the Holford Diet.

In a trial comparing my original diet to Unislim (a low-calorie, high-exercise regime, with weekly support meetings), on average, the volunteers on my diet lost four times more weight than the other dieters: 6.3kg (1st.) in three months. Every single trial by third parties has proven highly successful, with many reports of additional benefits besides consistent weight loss, such as 'increased alertness', 'concentration improved', 'no wobbly feeling', 'never felt hungry', 'easy to stick to', 'extra energy', 'thoroughly detoxified'. In these trials, not one person failed to lose weight. When GMTV compared the effects over six weeks of WeightWatchers (based on a low-fat, low-calorie diet) with the Holford Diet, the WeightWatchers' dieter lost 4kg (9lb) and the Holford dieter lost 4kg (9lb). The Holford dieter, however, had none of the benefit of weekly support group meetings as had the WeightWatchers' dieter. The benefits of the Holford Diet, with its increased feeling of good health and well-being, are enough to encourage dieters to continue.

Although the Holford Diet might mean slightly fewer calories than you are eating now, slightly less fat and slightly more protein, the major emphasis is on quality, and there will be plenty of it – all delicious.

Now you know what *doesn't* work, in the next chapter you'll find out what does.

Summary

- The major cause of the obesity epidemic is an increase in sugar and refined carbohydrate, not an increase in fat.

- Different sources of calories have different effects on weight loss.

- Eating a low-GL diet triggers the most rapid weight loss.

- If you eat too few calories your metabolic rate slows down to conserve your fat, so you have to suffer to lose weight and will inevitably develop rebound weight gain.

- High-protein diets stabilise your blood sugar levels and reduce your appetite, but they don't work better than conventional diets and they're not good for you in the long run.

- Low-fat diets are bad for you because the body needs essential fats and keeps craving fats until it gets them.

- The best diet for long-term weight loss is a low-GL diet, in which low-GL carbohydrates are combined with protein and essential fats – in short, the Holford Diet.

3

Why Sugar and Carbs Make You Fat

Losing extra inches is very simple. It's all about keeping your blood sugar even, a balancing act your body is designed to do. The trouble is we don't eat what our species is designed to eat. Our genes haven't changed. What's changed is our environment – both what we eat and how we eat it.

Take a look at the chart below. As you'll see, today's average diet is slightly higher in fat, much higher in carbohydrate, and slightly lower in protein than our caveman ancestors. But, of course, it's not just quantity but quality that counts. We eat more saturated fat and less essential fats, more refined and simple sugars, less complex low-GL carbs and fibre, and less lean meat or vegetable protein.

	The Stone Age	Today
Proteins	34%	13%
Fat	21%	35%
Carbs	45%	52%*
Fibre	46g	21g/day
Sugar	0%	14%
Salt	1.7g	about 10g/day

If, like many dieters, you've been following low-fat diets in the past you will almost inevitably have been eating more carbohydrate. That's because when you get hungry you choose low-fat foods, but they are most likely to be high in carbs instead.

Most people, probably including you, have unwittingly created a set

*Includes 14% sugar, as indicated below.

of circumstances that have led your body to lose its natural balance. The result is roller-coastering blood sugar, energy and weight.

It's the massive increase in the consumption of both sugar and refined carbohydrates that's fuelling the obesity epidemic – and your bulging midriff. In Britain, for example, carbohydrate intake has gone up, while fat intake has gone down. But, most noticeably, sugar and refined carbohydrate intake has gone up massively. Much of this is hidden in food and you won't even know about it.

Officially, the average person in Britain eats 22kg (48lb) of sugar a year. But this is likely to be a gross underestimation. According to government sources, 2.3 billion tons of sugar go into the British food supply every year.[31] That amount translates as an average of 38kg (84lb) per person per year, almost double what the government diet survey above shows. This makes a lot more sense because more comprehensive surveys in the US, which tops the world in obesity, show that the intake of sugar there went from 56kg (124lb) in 1975 to 71kg (157lb) in 1999.

So where is all this sugar lurking? You'd be amazed at the amount not just in cakes and sweets but in soft drinks, convenience foods, flavoured crisps and other savoury snacks, condiments, many breakfast cereals and most of the food you eat in restaurants or cafés, hidden in sauces and dips. Whichever way you slice it, there's obviously an awful lot of hidden sugar being consumed, and our bodies simply can't cope with it.

Exercise is obviously a factor too. Our ancestors had to work hard to get their food. Most people think the Mediterranean diet will solve all ills. But, today, there's a greater percentage of overweight men in Greece than in America. Part of the Mediterranean lifestyle of old was walking everywhere. The average Cretan walked 11.25km (7 miles) a day! The same was true in Britain. The Victorians in the early 1800s ate a diet very similar to the Mediterranean diet – high in vegetables with much more fish than today – and they were also much more active.[32]

Today, we just dial up for a takeaway. But this alone doesn't explain the explosion in weight gain in the last 20 years. Some surveys estimate that women increased their level of physical activity between 1994 and 1998, from 22 to 25 per cent. For men it seems there has been little change.[33]

The fact is, every time your blood sugar level goes too high, the hormone insulin floods into the bloodstream and escorts the excess glucose off to your liver, which turns it into fat and puts it into storage. There are two reasons for this. Firstly, having too much sugar in your bloodstream is dangerous because sugar damages your arteries, so your body protects itself. Secondly, we are programmed to store food as fat for a rainy day. It's called survival of the fattest. Those genetically best programmed to do this have survived. Unfortunately, these days, rainy days never come, so we just keep storing the excess as fat, and especially abdominal fat. What's even worse is that recent research shows that a high-carb diet switches off brain signals that tell you when you're full[34] – so you keep eating.

The roll of stimulants

It isn't just sugar that messes up your blood sugar balance. So does caffeine, alcohol and stress. For example, do you need to kick-start the day with coffee, cigarettes or something sweet? Do you gravitate towards bread, biscuits, pasta and sweet foods? Do you drink caffeinated drinks or alcohol every day? Are you often stressed? If so, the chances are you have significant peaks and troughs in your blood sugar. When your blood sugar level dips, you feel hungry or crave a stimulant. Then, when you've satisfied the craving with a big plate of pasta, a cola, a large glass of wine or a couple of pastries, your blood sugar levels shoot up – and you dump the excess as fat. Then it dips down and you're tired and hungry again.

If you lose blood sugar control, you gain weight, yet feel hungry and tired. If you can keep your blood sugar level on an even keel, you'll gravitate towards your natural weight, stay there and have a consistently high energy level.

If you have poor blood sugar control you are three times more likely to have difficulty losing weight. That's what we found in our health-and-diet survey in 2004, when we surveyed 37,000 people using the web-based 100% Health Questionnaire (see page 433 for details on how you can assess your own health on-line using my 100% Health Check).[35] We also found that when you gain blood sugar control you lose weight.

The question is, how do you regain blood sugar control? To tell you, I need to introduce you to the key players in this drama. First we'll meet the villain: insulin.

Insulin stores sugar as fat

Carbohydrates are turned into glucose by the body, which is conveyed through the bloodstream for delivery to cells, where it's used as fuel. The trouble is that glucose is the equivalent of high-octane fuel, and is dangerous stuff.

If glucose levels in the blood are too high, it can be very harmful – that's why people with diabetes can get nerve, eye, kidney and artery damage. So, as soon as your blood sugar level shoots beyond a certain level, the body moves quickly to get it out of your blood and, if you don't need it for energy, stores it as fat.

Insulin, a hormone produced by the pancreas, moves the glucose out of your blood. So, why is it the villain of the piece? The more frequently your blood sugar is raised, the more insulin you produce. The more insulin you produce, the more sugar you dump as fat. As a result, insulin can be thought of as the fat-storing hormone.

But there's more bad news. Having a high insulin level doesn't only encourage your body to turn food into fat, it also inhibits the body's breakdown of stored fat. So, once you're fat, you stay fat. If you're

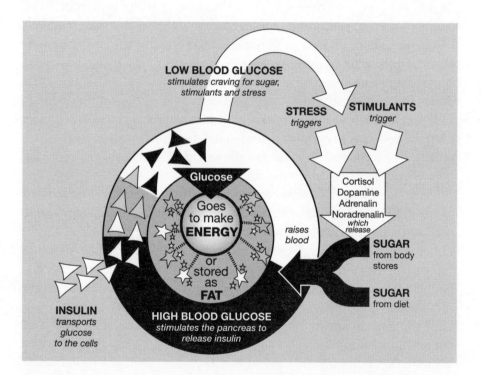

The sugar cycle Eating sugar increases blood glucose levels. The body releases insulin into the blood to help escort glucose out and into body cells, to make energy or convert into fat. The result is low blood glucose. Either stress, causing more adrenalin, or induced stress by consuming a stimulant such as caffeine, which raises adrenal hormones, causes breakdown of stores of sugar in the liver and muscles, called glycogen, which raises blood sugar levels. Low blood glucose causes stress or cravings for either something sweet or a stimulant.

overweight, you've probably got elevated insulin levels. Also, we are now learning that too much insulin itself is dangerous and may contribute to damaging your arteries. This discovery is important, because a new anti-diabetes drug called rosiglitazone, aimed at increasing the amount of insulin in the blood to curb blood sugar highs, actually led to increased cardiovascular disease and deaths.[36] A sure case of 'out of the frying pan, into the fire'. Rather than trying to cheat the body, by eating my low-GL diet your blood sugar level is much more even, so you naturally don't need to produce so much insulin.

Insulin is implicated in another factor that messes up your blood sugar level – 'insulin resistance'.

In the grip of resistance

Let's say that, during the day, you're snacking or bingeing on sugary foods, drinking several cups of coffee, or smoking a few cigarettes. Every time you get a 'hit' of sugar or a jolt from caffeine or nicotine, your blood sugar peaks. And, if this is happening a lot, more and more insulin will be rushing out to escort the glucose out of your blood as quickly as possible and into your cells. In effect, insulin will be subjecting your cells to a constant cry of, 'Open the door!'

Eventually the cells become so bored with hearing the same old message that it's as if they have become deaf to it. So your body has to produce more and more insulin, just as if it were shouting louder and louder to be heard. The end result is that you become insensitive to your own insulin – a condition called *insulin resistance*.

According to Professor Gerald Reaven from Stanford University in California, one of the world's leading experts in blood sugar problems, the majority of obese people and 25 per cent of non-obese people are insulin-resistant.[37]

This means that they, and quite likely you, need to produce even more insulin to lower blood sugar peaks. So you will eat even more carbohydrate before your body says 'Stop!' and then, by the time the insulin does kick in, you have so much in your bloodstream that your blood sugar levels will plummet too low, leaving you once again craving something to give you a lift.

When you're in the grip of this vicious cycle that lift is likely to be something high-GL, such as refined pasta, and, for up to four hours afterwards, insulin resistance will mess up your body's response to it. So you could either suffer from brain fog, sleepiness and low mood after a meal, or cave in to the cravings for something to raise your blood sugar levels once more. Most people choose the latter, either eating more carbohydrate such as pudding or homing in on a stimulant such as a cup of tea or coffee. Meanwhile, with all these inefficient peaks and troughs in blood sugar levels, you're turning the excess glucose to fat and feeling exhausted.

And there's an even more insidious downside. Remember, glucose is very damaging, so, as your insulin becomes more ineffectual at getting it out of your bloodstream fast to keep your blood sugar on an even keel, you spend more time with too much glucose in your blood. This literally damages your arteries, and paves the way for heart disease.

Diabetes is another direct result. This condition arises when you've become so insulin-resistant that the insulin doesn't work well enough, or when, eventually, the cells in the pancreas that make insulin become exhausted, and you can't produce enough. So you can't lower your blood sugar level very well, and some actually spills over into the urine (normally, the kidneys filter all glucose out, leaving it in the bloodstream, but even your kidneys have limits). Thus too little or defective insulin is also bad news. As always in the body, it's a balancing act.

The plain truth is that most of us are digging our own graves with a knife and fork by eating too many carbohydrates. And if you follow government guidelines, that's not about to change. Despite all this evidence in favour of low-GL eating, the UK's Food Standards Agency is running a campaign to get people eating *more* starchy foods – bread, rice, potatoes and pasta. Standard dietetic advice, quoting from the Manual of Dietetic Practice,[38] is to encourage 'a 50 per cent increase in the consumption of potatoes and bread', and the UK government's £372 million strategy for tackling obesity emphasises cutting calories and fat, and doesn't even mention the words 'glycemic load' once![39] There's a fat chance that this outdated way of thinking is going to do anything to reverse the obesity epidemic. But it doesn't have to be this way for you. The Holford Diet can literally save your life.

You can get a good idea of where you stand on the road to insulin resistance, loss of blood sugar stability, and ultimately diabetes – which is what happens to an estimated one in seven people over 40 – by completing the questionnaire below.

Are you insulin-resistant?

1   Are you rarely wide awake within 20 minutes of getting up?

2   Do you need tea, coffee, a cigarette or something to get you going in the morning?

3   Do you really like sweet foods?

4   Do you crave bread, cereal, popcorn or pasta most days?

5   Do you feel as if you 'need' an alcoholic drink on most days?

6   Are you overweight and unable to shift the extra pounds?

7   Do you often have energy slumps during the day or after meals?

8   Do you often have mood swings or difficulty concentrating?

9   Do you fall asleep in the early evening or need naps during the day?

10   Do you avoid exercise because you haven't got the energy?

11   Do you get dizzy or irritable if you go six hours without food?

12   Do you often find you overreact to stress?

13   Do you often get irritable, angry or aggressive unexpectedly?

14   Is your energy now less than it used to be?

15   Do you get night sweats or frequent headaches?

16   Do you ever lie about how much sweet food you have eaten?

17   Do you ever keep a supply of sweet food close to hand?

18   Do you ever go out of your way to make sure you have something sweet?

19   Do you feel you could never give up bread?

20   Do you think of yourself as addicted to sugar, chocolate or biscuits?

If you answered 'yes' to 10 or more questions, there's a very good chance that you are insulin-resistant, and struggling to keep your blood sugar level even. You are also three times more likely to have trouble losing weight. If you'd like to find out more about insulin resistance, read *The Insulin Factor*, by Antony Haynes, published by Thorsons (2004).

The single best way to know where you stand is a blood test of what's called glycosylated haemoglobin (technically called HbA1c). This is a measure of how often your blood sugar level peaks too high. When it does, red blood cells effectively become sugar-coated. That's what glycosylated haemoglobin stands for: sugar-coated red blood cells. And it's the 'glycoslaytion' of cells that causes damage in the long run. This test is much better than a single blood glucose test because it provides a long-term measure of your blood sugar control rather than just a single point in time. You can measure your glycosylated haemoglobin using a home-test kit (see Resources). You want to have a level below 5 for optimal blood sugar control and certainly below 6.5 per cent. Once your level is 7–8 per cent your risk of developing diabetes is substantial (read Chapter 10 for more details), and therefore I would advise seeing your doctor and checking for this. Most diabetics have a level above 6.5 per cent. It's a good measure to know so you can chart your progress as you follow my low-GL diet.

You'll notice, in the questionnaire above, that I've asked whether you need tea, coffee or cigarettes to kick-start your day. Obviously, these have nothing to do with carbohydrates, so let's take a closer look at the role stimulants play in blood sugar chaos.

How caffeine ties you to the vicious cycle

Let's say you find yourself in an energy trough triggered by low blood sugar. You may not have eaten for a while, or you're experiencing the rebound low blood sugar that happens after a high-GL meal. One of the effects is that your body releases hormones from your adrenal glands, which sit on top of your kidneys in the small of your back. These are adrenalin and cortisol, and, if your blood sugar levels are out of control, they're bad news.

You may have learnt about the 'fight-or-flight' mechanism at school. Adrenalin is the driving force behind this response, as it immediately makes stores of glucose available to give you fuel to fight back or run away. While adrenalin doesn't last long in the body, cortisol, another adrenal hormone, sticks around for much longer.

You can trigger adrenalin release by a stressful thought or situation, or by having too low a blood sugar level. This can happen either because you are starving, or as a rebound blood sugar dip after having something very sweet. In one study, researchers at Yale University gave 25 healthy children a drink containing the equivalent amount of glucose found in a can of fizzy drink. The rebound blood sugar drop boosted their adrenalin to over five times its normal level for up to five hours after ingesting the sugar. Most of these children had difficulty concentrating and were irritable and anxious, which are normal reactions to too much adrenalin in the bloodstream.[40] Adrenalin turns you into a hunter, which is good for fighting but lousy for solving problems.

When this kind of thing happened in our prehistoric past, of course, we'd have burnt off the extra glucose by either bashing that sabre-toothed tiger on the head, or legging it to the nearest cave. Our hormone levels would then return to normal and all would be well. But the twenty-first-century reality is that we may simply be sitting at our office desk hungry for lunch when adrenalin and cortisol start circulating. And, if we do nothing, they'll keep doing just that, leaving us anxious and stressed.

So what's caffeine got to do with all this? This stimulant also prompts the release of adrenalin and makes you more resistant to insulin.[41] If you combine a sugary, high-GL food with coffee the effects are disastrous on your blood sugar levels. Recent research at Canada's University of Guelph shows that Britain's most popular pick-me-up, a coffee and a croissant, is a dangerous combination and may be fuelling an epidemic of weight gain and diabetes. Participants were given a carbohydrate snack, such as a croissant, muffin or toast, together with either a decaf or caffeinated coffee. Those having the caffeinated coffee/carb combination had triple the increase in blood sugar levels, and insulin sensitivity was almost halved.[42]

Whereas coffee on its own has not been shown to increase weight or diabetes risk, today's most popular stimulant drinks often combine sugar with stimulants: Red Bull to a tea or coffee with sugar, mocha drinks, chocolate or colas, or a coffee with a muffin or doughnut. Some people become more addicted to carbohydrates, others more addicted to caffeine, but most are addicted to both. Either way, they further disrupt your blood sugar control, and make you less sensitive to insulin, keeping you in the prison of seesawing blood sugar, weight and energy levels.

The bottom line is that the body's and brain's sensitive mechanisms for keeping your blood sugar in balance simply can't cope with a daily onslaught of sugar and other high-GL foods and snacks, topped up with stimulants such as caffeine and nicotine. Although there's no evidence that a moderate daily consumption of coffee in and of itself increases your weight, I strongly recommend that, if you do drink coffee, to have it on its own, away from food.

In our ONUK survey we found that the two food groups most associated with low energy were caffeinated drinks and sugary food intake. Of course, this doesn't prove cause (it may be that tired people consume more caffeine, rather than caffeine causing tiredness – I suspect it's a bit of both) but countless Holford dieters, on quitting caffeinated drinks and following a low-GL diet, have reported big increases in energy. Coffee and caffeine also raise homocysteine, a risk factor for many diseases (see page 106) so, in any event, it is best to limit your intake. My advice is to keep your caffeine intake to a maximum of one or two caffeinated drinks a day and, if you are tired a lot of the time, have a month without any caffeine while following my low-GL diet. When your blood sugar level is stable you don't 'need' caffeine to feel full of energy.

Enter glucagon – a fatburner's best friend

There's good news. It doesn't take long to turn insulin resistance round and recover your fatburning ability. And glucagon is central to the process.

Although it's another hormone produced by the pancreas, glucagon is the hero to insulin's villain. It is, in fact, a fatburner's best friend, and will get you out of the vicious cycle of seesawing blood glucose levels.

Glucagon enters the picture when your blood glucose levels are very low. It evens up levels by telling the body to break down fat and burn it for energy. In the process, glucagon reduces any cravings for something sweet.

If insulin makes you store fat, glucagon makes you burn it. So glucagon is a fatburning hormone. The more glucagon you produce in relation to insulin, the more you are programming yourself to burn fat.

As we've seen, if you eat the kinds of foods that send your blood sugar rocketing, out pours the insulin and on creeps the fat. But, if you eat the kinds of foods that keep your blood glucose level in check, you'll produce only small amounts of insulin and, whenever your energy is low, release glucagon to burn some fat.

The Holford Diet is calculated to maximise glucagon release and minimise insulin release, thus literally reprogramming your metabolism to burn fat.

We've seen the inside story on hormones, sugar and fat. In the next chapter I'll frame it differently, and look at the dynamics of losing weight.

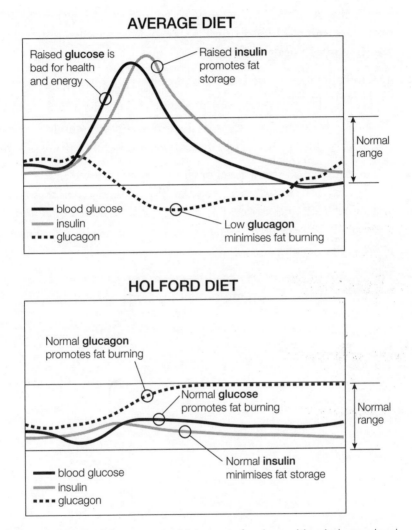

AVERAGE DIET

Raised **glucose** is bad for health and energy

Raised **insulin** promotes fat storage

Normal range

— blood glucose
~ insulin
••• glucagon

Low **glucagon** minimises fat burning

HOLFORD DIET

Normal **glucagon** promotes fat burning

Normal **glucose** promotes fat burning

Normal range

Normal **insulin** minimises fat storage

— blood glucose
~ insulin
••• glucagon

Blood sugar balance When you eat a high-sugar food your blood glucose level shoots up, followed by insulin. Insulin helps turn glucose into fat. When you eat a low-GL food your blood glucose level stays more stable, with less insulin release and relatively more glucagon.

Summary

- Sugar and refined carbohydrates can turn easily into fat and cause the release of an insulin overload.

- Eventually the body can become more and more resistant to insulin, leading to blood sugar peaks, followed by troughs, which lead to carbohydrate-and-sugar cravings.

- Insulin resistance is the hallmark of obesity and is present in most overweight people.

- Glucagon counters the effect of insulin and helps stabilise blood sugar levels and reduce appetite, sugar and carbohydrate cravings.

- When your blood sugar level crashes you release adrenal hormones. These further raise your blood sugar balance, making you more tired and stressed as a result. As a consequence you are more likely to become hooked on sweet foods, caffeinated drinks, or both as a result.

- The Holford Diet promotes glucagon and reduces insulin resistance, literally reprogramming the body to burn fat.

4

Why Low GL is Better than Low Fat, Low Calorie

There's a saying about new ideas: 'First they say it's not true and not important. Then they say it's true, but not important. Then they say it's true, it's important, but it's not new.' When I first went public with the Holford Diet I received a lot of criticism, especially from conventional dieticians who had been taught, and were defenders of the orthodox view, that conventional low-fat, low-calorie diets are the best way to lose weight.

They espoused that the best way to lose weight is to eat fewer calories. Since a gram of fat has the most calories, the best way to achieve this, we are told, is to eat less fat.

As logical as this may sound, this is bad advice, because if you cut back on your calories from fat, especially if you eat the many commercially available low-fat foods, you are inevitably going to eat more carbohydrates. So, a low-fat diet is usually a high-carbohydrate diet. And as we saw in the last chapter, eating more carbohydrates, especially sugar and refined carbohydrates, creates exactly the kind of seesawing blood sugar levels that spells disaster for your weight and your health.

Since the major driver of your appetite is your blood sugar level, instead of focusing on 'calories', which is an invented measure of the latent energy in food, focusing on GL is more likely to help you lose weight. It's not that calories don't count. Of course they do, but the easiest way to eat less is to feel full and that's how a low-GL diet makes you feel, because appetite and blood glucose levels are inextricably linked. Since low-GL diets cause more fat loss than low-fat diets of identical calories, as we saw earlier in undisputable animal studies, and since low-GL diets are easier to stick to because you feel fuller for longer, by focusing on the GL of your meal, rather than the calories, you are more likely to achieve your goal of long-term weight loss.

Since the first edition of *The Holford Low-GL Diet* there have been a number of well-designed studies that have directly compared conventional low-fat, low-calorie diets with low-glycemic-load diets. I'd like to tell you about these so that you can be confident that my low-GL diet is based on the latest science that proves it is a highly effective way to lose weight.

To cut to the chase, one 'Cochrane systematic review' of six such trials, published in 2007, considered by many to be the 'gold standard' of evidence-based medicine, concludes: 'Overweight or obese people lost more weight on a low Glycemic Load diet and had more improvements in lipid profiles than those receiving conventional diets.'[43]

This review compared the results of six well-designed trials comparing low-GL diets with conventional diets based on reducing calories. Other benefits were greater loss in body fat, reductions in bad LDL cholesterol, and an increase in good HDL cholesterol compared to those in the calorie-controlled diets. I'll go close up on the heart-protective effects of my diet in Chapter 11.

For now, let's take a look at some of these human studies, which have directly compared low-fat, low-calorie diets with low-GL diets for weight loss.

Low GL versus low fat, low calorie – the evidence

The first study to rock the boat was conducted back in 1994 at South Africa's University of the Orange Free State. I've already provided a diagram illustrating the results (see page 39) but their relevance to this debate makes it worth re-visiting them briefly here. Fifteen volunteers were put on either a low-GL diet or a conventional low-calorie diet for 12 weeks. Both diets contained identical calories. During the first 12 weeks those on the low-GL diet lost 9.3kg (1st. 6lb) whereas those on the conventional low-calorie diet lost 7.5kg (1st. 2lb). After the initial 12 weeks, the participants switched diets for 12 weeks. During the second 12-week period those placed on the low-GL diet had an average further weight loss of 7.4kg (16lb 5oz), compared to those on the low-calorie diet who lost a further 4.5kg (10lb). This is equivalent to 40 per cent more weight loss on the low-GL diet.[44]

A five-week study in France put overweight men on to a diet with high GI foods, or low GI foods. It wasn't strictly controlled for their glycemic load, but it was a step in the right direction. Those on the low-GI diet had a significant decrease in body fat and an increase in lean body mass, as well as lower blood sugar and insulin levels.[45]

In a longer study, published in the *Archives of Pediatrics and Adolescent Medicine,* involving obese teenagers, seven were put on to a conventional low-fat, low-calorie diet and seven were put on to a low-GL diet that recommended low-GL foods but wasn't calorie restricted as such.[46] They were put on these diets for six months, then followed up after 12 months to see whether they kept going with their dietary changes, and what difference that made to their weight. The low-fat, low-calorie group did eat less fat. The low-GL group did eat low-GL and, if anything, slightly increased their fat intake. At 12 months the low-GL group had lost weight and decreased their body-fat percentage, while the low-fat, low-calorie group had gained weight and body fat. During the second six months the low-GL dieters gained no more weight – so they maintained their weight loss, whereas those on the low-fat, low-calorie diet gained weight. So the low-GL diet, as well as being more effective, was more sustainable.

Another longer-term study, this time in Canada, put one group of people on a low-GL diet and another group on a conventional low-fat, low-calorie diet based on Canada's Food Guide to Healthy Eating.[47] Those following the low-GL diet lost significantly more weight compared to those following the conventional low-fat, low-calorie diet – 2.8kg (6lb 2oz) loss versus 200g (7oz). Once again, weight loss was sustained over 12 months.

According to the National Cholesterol Education Program (NCEP) in the US, we should cut back on saturated fat. In this study 60 volunteers were put on the NCEP's diet, effectively replacing saturated fat with carbohydrate, or alternatively, a diet with more protein and monounsaturated fat, and less carbs, in a modified low-carbohydrate (MLC) diet. This is lower in total carbohydrates and higher in protein, monounsaturated fat and complex carbohydrates, making it low GL. After 12 weeks those on the low-GL 'MLC' diet had lost significantly more weight than those on the conventional low-fat diet. There were also favourable changes in all fat levels within the MLC but not the NCEP group.[48]

There are other studies comparing even lower carb, high-protein diets with conventional low-fat, low-calorie diets that show greater weight loss, despite similar calorie intakes. For example, one such study, conducted by the University of Cincinnati, reported 8.5kg (18lb 12oz) weight loss at six months on the low-carb diet, versus 3.9kg (8½lb) on the low-fat diet, and double the fat loss.[49] Whereas low-carb diets are technically low-GL, longer-term studies tend to show that they are less sustainable than low-GL diets that include more of the right kind of low-GL carbs, probably because they are too restrictive on carbohydrates and hence harder to stick to.

Defining the perfect Low-GL diet

Now you know that low-GL diets in general do cause more weight and fat loss than low-fat, low-calorie diets, the question is what's the best *kind* of low-GL diet? One based on high protein and low carbs or one with more healthy low-GI/GL carbs? Two recent studies have explored this very question.

The first, published in the *Archives of Internal Medicine*, set out to answer this by placing volunteers on either a high-protein, low-carb diet or a higher carbohydrate, lower fat diet. Within each group half the volunteers ate only low-GI carbs, while the other half ate only high-GI carbs. Each of these four diets had the same number of calories. That made four diets in total:

Diet 1: higher carb, high GI	GL of 129 (effectively a conventional low-fat, low-calorie diet)
Diet 2: higher carb, low GI	GL of 89 (closer to the Holford Diet in balance, but still a lot higher in GL)
Diet 3: higher protein, high GI	GL of 75 (close to the original Atkins-type diet)
Diet 4: higher protein, low GI	GL of 59 (an Atkins-style diet, but with only low-GI carbs, so closer to the South Beach Diet)

As you can see from the chart opposite, the most effective for fat loss was Diet 2, which is the closest to the Holford Diet, although not as low GL, followed by Diets 3 and 4 – the high-protein diets. The least effective was Diet 1 (the conventional low-fat, low-calorie diet). By the end of the trial, more people on the low-GL diets achieved their target weight loss than those on the high-GL equivalents. Those on the low-GL diets lost fat faster, especially among the female participants. Women in this group lost 80 per cent more fat than those on the conventional low fat, low-calorie diet.

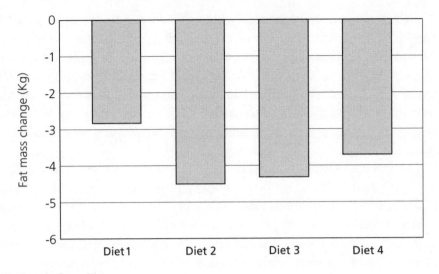

Fat loss in four diets

The researchers concluded: 'Our findings suggest that dietary glycemic load, and not just overall energy intake [calories], influences weight loss and postprandial glycemia [blood sugar levels after eating]. Moderate reductions in glycemic load appear to increase the rate of body fat loss, particularly in women ... Reassuringly, this advice can optimise clinical outcomes within current nutrition guidelines, without the concerns that apply to low-carbohydrate diets.'

This study strongly suggests that the best way to burn fat is to eat a diet that contains less carbs than a conventional low-fat diet, more carbs than a high-protein diet, and the right kind of low-GI carbs, with an overall low-GL score. That's a perfect description of my Holford Diet.

The next diet trial that gives us insight into the perfect diet was conducted by Dr Iris Shai of Ben Gurion University in Israel and published in the *New England Journal of Medicine*.[50] She put volunteers on one of three diets: a conventional low-calorie, low-fat diet; a Mediterranean diet, restricted in calories, high in fibre and monounsaturated fats, for example from olive oil; and a high-protein, high-fat, low-carb diet, but emphasising vegetarian sources of protein rather than meat and dairy products. Both the Mediterranean and high-protein diets were low GL.

Despite similar calorie intakes, the participants lost 4.7kg (10¼lb) on the low-carb diet, 4.3kg (9½lb) on the Mediterranean-style diet and only 2.9kg (6lb 6oz) on the low-calorie, low-fat diet. Again, the conventional low-fat, low-calorie diet came out worst.

Asked what she thought was behind the success of the low-carb and Mediterranean diets, Shai said that reducing calories may be slightly easier when moderate fat consumption is permitted, and the advantage of this strategy is that the 'enemy' (that is, carbohydrates) is well defined, and having learnt this, the dieter knows what to stay away from, without counting calories. 'I think that what we're soon going to find is that no-one's going to be defending the low-fat diet any more,' said Dr Shai.

My low-GL diet is a hybrid of the Mediterranean-type diet and a low-carb diet, with an emphasis on more vegetarian sources of protein, and slightly lower protein and higher carbohydrates. These help to mitigate the increased cancer risks associated with a high-meat, high-dairy diet, as well as the potential stress on the kidneys and loss of bone mass. It works and is easier to stick to by being more lenient on carbohydrate foods such as bread and pasta. It's very straightforward, as you will see, once you know what it means to eat 10 Ⓖ for main meals and 5 Ⓖ for snacks.

In summary, it took years for people to understand the concept of calories, which later became a mandatory statement on the label of foods. It took over a decade for people to wake up to the importance of the glycemic index (GI). I wrote my first book on low-GI eating in 1987. Scientists, doctors and nutritionists, and food companies, are gradually waking up to the discovery that the GL score of foods is probably the most important criteria for a healthy diet and the best way to control weight. No doubt it will take many more years before it becomes mandatory to put the GL score of a food on the packaging. But you don't have to wait. Be ahead of the curve. Become part of the solution, not part of the problem.

Of course, you could achieve a low-GL diet by eating only fat and protein but, as we've seen, that has considerable downsides and appears less effective for long-term fat loss. My Holford Diet provides the perfect balance of fat, protein and carbohydrate. It includes low-GL foods that aren't laden with calories, and which, compared with the average diet, are a little higher in protein and a little lower in fats, which come from healthy foods rich in essential fats. It is literally the last diet you'll ever need because it's perfectly balanced for both your weight and your health.

Understanding glycemic load

Glycemic load is a precise measure of the amount of available carbohydrate (excluding inabsorbable fibre) in the food in question multiplied by the glycemic index (GI) of that food. The problem with GI is that it only defines to what extent that type of carbohydrate in a food raises your blood sugar level, but it tells you nothing about how much of the food is carbohydrate. GL factors in both the quantity of carbs and their quality, or GI, so a food's GL value is the best way of predicting what that food serving, or meal or day's menu, will actually do to your blood sugar balance.

Since there are two components to GL (amount of carbs and type of carbs) there are two ways to lower the GL of your diet. One way is by eating less carbohydrates (an Atkins-style high-protein diet achieves this and is therefore low GL); the other is by eating low-GI carbohydrates instead of high-GI foods, as in a typical low-GI diet.

GL is not the same as GI

The problem with most low-GI diets is that they simply recommend you eat only low-GI carbs and not high-GI carbs, but they don't factor in how much of these foods are carbohydrate, or what quantity of these foods you can eat. You can get fat eating too many low-GI foods because the end result is that your diet becomes high GL.

Low-GI diets are also confusing, because high-GI foods with fast-releasing sugars but very little quantity of sugar or carbohydrate in them get unfairly maligned.

The only way you can see the truth, the whole truth and nothing but the truth is to multiply the GI (quality measure) by the amount of carbohydrate (quantity measure), which gives you GLs, or glycemic load. Take a look at the chart below:

Food	GI	Carbs per serving	GL
Watermelon	72	6 (120g/4¼oz)	4.3
Broad beans	79	5.2 (80g/2¾oz)	4.1
Pumpkin	75	5.7 (80g/2¾oz)	4.3
Carrots	92	4.2 (80g/2¾oz)	3.9
Sweet potato	48	26 (150g/5½oz)	12.5
White rice	56	42 (150g/5½oz)	23.5

continued

White spaghetti	57	44.3 (180g/6¾oz)	21
Pineapple juice	46	34 (250ml/9fl oz)	16
Ski yoghurt	33	31 (200g/7oz)	10
SlimFast	33	38.7 (325ml/11fl oz)	12.8

Let's say you wanted to eat a carrot (92 GI in some books) and pumpkin soup (75 GI), followed by some salmon, broad beans (79 GI) and sweet potato (48 GI), followed by a slice of watermelon (72 GI). Foods above 70 GIs are not allowed in a low-GI diet, as they are considered fast-releasing, so most of this meal would be disallowed except for the sweet potato.

This is entirely the wrong advice, because watermelon (4.3 **GL** per 120g/4¼oz serving), broad beans (4.1 **GL**), carrots (3.9 **GL**), and pumpkin (4.3 **GL**) all have a low GL, because there's very little carbohydrate in them, even though what's in them is fast-releasing.

Conversely, the one apparently 'good' low-GI food – sweet potato – is so packed full of sugars, albeit relatively low-GI sugars, that 150g (5½oz) sweet potato scores 12.5 **GL**!

If you had salmon and a decent serving of white pasta (57 GI, but 21 **GL**), with a sweet potato (48 GI, but 12.5 **GL**), followed by a Ski low-fat yoghurt (33 GI but 10 **GL**) and 250ml (9fl oz) of pineapple juice (46 GI, but 16 **GL**) you've just blown it big time as far as the net effect on your blood sugar is concerned, totalling 59.5 **GL** – that's almost two days' worth of carbohydrates! The net effect is a massive increase in your blood sugar and waistline. Yet, nothing you've eaten is above 50 GI, and is therefore classified as a low-GI diet.

Companies can manipulate the GI score of foods to be low by including slow-releasing sugars, but lots of it. Technically, it's 'low GI' which sounds good. Of course, you like it because it tastes sweet, but it doesn't do you good. A classic example is SlimFast. A 325ml (11fl oz) serving of this sugar-laden 'diet' drink has an impressive GI of 33, but a GL of 12.8 – above the 10 **GL** of an ideal meal that equates to optimum weight loss.

The fact is that no food is 'good' or 'bad' – it just depends on how much of it you can eat. It's unnecessarily restrictive to limit your intake based on the quantity of carbs only, as you would on the original high-protein, low-carb diets. To limit your intake based on GI only is inaccurate. GLs, on the other hand, don't lie.

continued

This is why some low-GI diet trials haven't worked so well. Some show weight loss, some show weight gain. The magic of GL as the yardstick is that it takes *both* the GI *and* the amount of carbs you consume into the equation.

Not all low-GL diets are equal

You are probably starting to realise that the term 'low GL' is itself a bit ambiguous, since it also is a matter of degrees. Some so-called low-GL diets provide up to 90 ⓖ a day, whereas mine delivers a maximum of 45 ⓖ (40 from food, plus 5 from drinks/desserts). It's the same with low-calorie diets – some provide 1,500 calories a day, others 1,000 calories and some only 500 calories. So, although studies tend to show that a low-GL diet, in principle, is the right way to go for weight loss, the lower the GL the greater the weight loss tends to be. The Holford Diet takes the winning principles that are being discovered in weight-loss research and gives you the exact way of eating that means you will have maximum weight loss without hunger and without any of the dangers of extreme diets that exclude healthy carbohydrates or fats, or that overload on protein. For most people that's no more than 45 ⓖ.

5

How to Lose Weight Forever

Losing weight isn't difficult as long as you work *with* your body's design, not *against* it. As you learned in Chapter 2, you can lose weight with 'extreme' diets, which are very low in fat, very low in carbohydrate or very low in calories. But your body and your mind fight back. Your body will crave all three – fat, protein and carbohydrate – and will signal its lack if you cut them down too far. This kind of diet fails because, in the end, your cravings win.

In fact, long-term studies have shown that 'dieters' gain more weight than non-dieters.[51] As we've seen, this is because just about any short-term extreme diet slows down your metabolism. It's because of this that many diets gradually move you from the unsustainable 'weight-loss' phase to a more sustainable 'weight-maintenance' phase.

The Holford Diet is sustainable from the start because it is scientifically calculated to satisfy your cravings and your appetite from day one. It's the Rolls-Royce of diets. Your body will love it, and will reward you with a myriad of super-healthy side effects – from extra energy to smooth, clear skin. On top of that it will cut your risk of the twenty-first century's most common diseases, including diabetes and heart disease, as you'll see in Part Two.

The trick with the Holford Diet is that *there is no trick*. It doesn't cheat or fool your body. Remember: given the right circumstances, your body will go to its ideal weight – and stay there forever.

Overweight or underlean?

We've looked at the crucial role hormones play vis-à-vis your blood sugar balance, and how an imbalance leads to weight gain. As you rev up to start the Holford Diet, I'd like you to understand how we actually lose weight, and to have realistic expectations about how fast you might lose it.

Although I will tell you about some rapid, miracle weight-loss results, the truth is that the body limits how quickly it can burn off fat without harming you. So there's no quick fix. Many popular diets cheat the body by kicking off with instant weight loss in the first week or two, but after this you pay the price. You don't feel full of health and energy, because these diets are not about optimum health, and, as time goes by, you actually begin to gain weight.

I don't want this to happen to you. I'm more interested in your reaching your ultimate goal and staying there, even if it takes months, not weeks. The Holford Diet will give your body what it needs to stay healthy and, as result, you will lose weight. You will be re-educating your eating habits to give your body what it needs, but this doesn't mean you will be restricting your food and eating bland and boring meals during the diet and beyond – quite the opposite. The diet provides exciting new foods and dishes that you will enjoy and that will positively make you glow with health.

At this point we need to look at how much you weigh, and how much you want to lose. But we won't look at poundage alone: we'll be sorting out the relative percentages of fat and lean tissue. This is because it's not so much being overweight that's the problem, but being underlean. Your body is made of both fat tissue and lean tissue (muscle and organs). A significantly higher proportion of fat increases health risk, so your body fat percentage is actually more important than overall weight.

Ideally, no more than 15 per cent of a man's body and 22 per cent of a woman's body should be made up of fat. Yet in the West the average man has a body fat percentage of a little over 20, and the average woman's is above 30.

Your body fat percentage is a little harder to measure than your weight. With a little patience and a tape measure, you can work it out roughly using the formula in Appendix 1 (see page 375). Some gyms work it out by making a few body measurements with callipers or with a piece of equipment that measures your electrical resistance. You can now buy body-fat scales that work it out for you. Since fat doesn't conduct electricity, the less 'electric' you are the more fat you've got.

But how can you measure the fat lost as your fatburning capacity really gets going? Fat is relatively light and bulky whereas protein is hard and heavy. So, as you convert fat into lean muscle, you may lose inches more quickly than you lose pounds. This is good news for several reasons. One is obviously that you'll look better. The other is that, when you follow the Holford Diet, you are giving your lean muscle a tune-up so it is ready to burn your excess fat. Exercise is an essential part of the plan (and remember, it's for only 15 minutes a day), and the more exercise you do the more efficient your muscles will become at fatburning.

So, as the diet progresses, you'll take a simple measurement with a tape measure once a week, as well as getting on the scales.

Measuring your body mass

The next best measurement to know is your body-mass index (BMI). To work this out, all you need to know is your weight and height; then look on the chart opposite. (There's another chart in Appendix 1, on page 378, that does this for you and shows you the ideal weight range for each height.) If your BMI is between 25 and 30 (Class 1) then you are technically overweight. If it's 30 (Class 2 or 3) or above, you are technically obese.

If you are technically obese, it may come as a shock. But you are not alone – the number of overweight and obese people doubled in the 1980s and continued to grow at the same alarming rate in the 1990s. In some parts of the US, as many as 50 per cent of women are now obese. By the end of this book you'll understand why. And you will have in your hand the best way out of the trap – forever.

If you are in Class 1, 2 or 3, then your risk of certain diseases, such as diabetes, is much higher. Weight-related diseases account for about as much of the total healthcare cost as the nation's cancer therapy or heart disease. By being close to your ideal weight, you will be healthier with less risk of life-threatening and debilitating diseases.

Top tip

Measure your waist. It's the best predictor of insulin resistance. Measure your girth 2.5cm (1in) above your belly button. For women, this should be less than 86cm (34in), for men less than 102cm (40in). Weight gain around the middle is much more harmful for your overall health than weight gain around the hips and thighs.

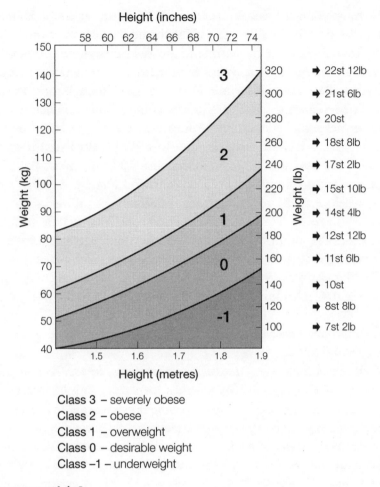

Class 3 – severely obese
Class 2 – obese
Class 1 – overweight
Class 0 – desirable weight
Class –1 – underweight

Are you overweight?

Statistics show that, if you're over 50, it may be better to be a little on the heavier side of the BMI range of 'desirable weight'.[52] Having a BMI below 23 has been associated with an increased death rate. This is partly because very sick people can lose a lot of weight. But if you are healthy, a BMI of around 20 to 24 is probably the best, whatever your age.

A pound of fat

Go to the supermarket and look at the size of 900g (2lb) of butter or lard. It's about four packets. Now imagine losing that amount of fat a week! Sound good? Read on.

The most you can easily lose in a week, without starvation, is between 450g (1lb) and 900g (2lb) of fat, according to conventional calorie theory. If you follow my recommendations strictly you'll probably lose, on average, 900g (2lb) a week. If you follow the general principles loosely, you'll probably lose 450g (1lb) a week. Although there are many cases of people losing 1.3kg (3lb) a week on the Holford Diet, it's better to have an achievable target. For example, in a survey of Holford dieters, those who said they stuck to the diet lost 775g (1lb 11oz) a week on average.[53] Those who followed it loosely lost 400g (14oz) a week. Those who also took the supplements I recommend lost an average of 900g (2lb) a week. A good goal to aim for is 680g (1½lb) a week.

So, if you're 12.7kg (2st.) overweight, and you decide to take on board what I've said in essence, you'll lose this weight in 19 weeks, a little over 4 months. With moderate exercise you can expect to lose at least 12.7kg (2st.) every three months. Here are three typical examples.

Della Y, from Maidstone, wanted to lose 19kg (3st.):

❝ *In February I weighed 13st. [82.5kg] and my dress size was 16. I have been trying to 'diet' for years. I may lose ½st. [3.2kg], only to put it back on. After following your fantastic GL diet, I now, in July (six months on) weigh 9st. 9lb [61kg], and can fit into a dress size 8 to 10. I am thrilled to bits, my sugar cravings have gone and my taste buds are definitely enhanced. I am exercising five days a week and everyone has commented on my weight loss. I am spreading the word and my family are also benefiting from optimum nutrition. I am positive my blood sugars were out of control, and I cannot believe that I am no longer bingeing. I feel so much happier on the inside as well as looking great on the outside. Thank you for giving me my life back.* ❞

Julia F, from Dubai, had tried every diet under the sun for the past 40 years but still the weight crept back:

❝ *My initial weight was 12½st. [80kg], and after following the Holford Diet strictly for 9 months, my weight has dropped to 9½st. [61kg]. I was very satisfied eating three meals and two snacks a day and it really helped that I had the constant reassurance of Patrick's book to read and re-read. I have yo-yo dieted for 40 years and out of all the diets, this is the first time I wasn't hungry during it. All together, this is an excellent approach to dieting. On top of that, my hiatus hernia has shrunk and I am now able to stop taking high-dose anti-acid drugs. I love my new life as a slim, fit 57-year-old woman. I have gone from a size 18 or 20 to size 12 and feel fit and happy. [You can see her 'before' and 'after' photos at www.holforddiet.com.]*

Linda R, from Leeds, desperately wanted to lose 4st. – and her sugar cravings:

My weight was spiralling out of control and, in January, I weighed 14st. [89kg]. By following Patrick's low-GL diet I have been able to shed about 900g (2lb) per week and by the end of August I was thrilled to have achieved my target weight of 10st. [63kg]. I have tried various diets in the past and have managed to lose weight on some of them. But, it has always been a struggle because of feeling hungry a lot of the time. There have been times on these other diets where I have gone to bed early, as I have been so hungry that I would have exceeded my allotted calories or points for the day had I not done so. And always, at the end of the diet, the weight seemed to return within a few months, once I started eating "normally" again. (I used to eat a lot of the foods I had felt deprived of during the diet – chocolate, crisps, etc.) I can honestly say that the Holford Diet has been the easiest diet I have ever followed. The diet is extremely healthy and has given me so much energy. The pain I used to suffer in my right knee has disappeared, as have my occasional back spasms. I have dropped four dress sizes and friends can't get over the "new me". Some of them are now successfully following the diet as well. But apart from all the health benefits, the beauty of this diet is that I have never been hungry at all, and this is what makes it easy to follow. In fact, I sometimes find it hard to remember to eat my two snacks as foods because my breakfast of porridge with blueberries is really filling. Also, all my cravings for sugar-loaded foods have completely disappeared. Now that I have reached a sensible weight that I am happy with, I have no intention of falling back into bad habits. I consider the diet as a permanent lifestyle change. I shall continue to eat healthily and take the supplements, although I can now add the occasional extra treat (there are some delicious desserts on this diet). You couldn't pay me to go back to my old eating habits! Many, many, many thanks.

Della, Julia and Linda all achieved their goals easily, lost their craving for sweet foods and are still slim today, and experiencing all the extra health benefits of my diet.

No 'miracle' weight loss

Between them they lost over 10st. (65kg), averaging 680g (1½lb) of weight loss a week. As the weight dropped off, they lost their craving for sweet foods, were never hungry, and their energy levels improved. They lost the excess pounds without taxing their bodies in any way. They also gained health benefits along the way, including better digestion and fewer aches and pains.

Don't be lured by diets that claim amazing weight loss in a couple of weeks. We all feel desperate sometimes – to fit into that outfit, look good on the beach, or just feel right striding to work. However, you don't want to add insult to injury. Being overweight isn't much fun, and it's bad for our health, but crash diets get rid of a lot of weight that isn't fat, and most of it comes right back afterwards. Let me remind you why.

We've seen how the body runs on glucose. It's the equivalent of four-star petrol, and it's why athletes rely on glucose drinks, not protein or fat, when they're practising endurance sports. Your body aims to use a lot of this immediately to power your cells, and you've seen how the excess is laid down as fat.

But, before that happens, excess glucose is first put into short-term storage in the liver and muscles in a form known as *glycogen*. It's only when stores of glycogen are full up that glucose is converted into fat and laid down for long-term storage. If you have insulin resistance, this will happen fast, and the excess fat will be dumped most readily around

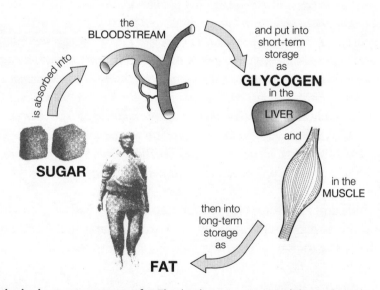

How the body stores energy as fat The body runs on sugar (glucose), and converts any extra into glycogen, which is stored in muscles and the liver. If glycogen stores are full the body can convert glucose into fat, our long-term energy storage.

the belly. So, carrying a lot of fat around the middle is a sure sign of insulin resistance.

Conversely, when you run out of glucose the body breaks glycogen back down into glucose. When glycogen stores are used up, the body burns fat for energy. If it has to, the body can also turn protein into fuel and burn this instead. That's why people on starvation diets lose muscle and possibly even damage body organs.

How losing fast is losing out

Each unit of glucose your body puts into storage as glycogen is bound together with three units of water. So, if you run out of glucose and start burning glycogen, you lose water. This is how you can get short-term rapid weight loss on a very low-calorie diet, say below 1,000 calories, or on a very low-carbohydrate diet. Since the maximum amount of glycogen in short-term storage in the body is about 1kg or 2lb, you could lose a maximum of 3.6kg (8lb) – but in reality you'd be more likely to lose 1.8kg (4lb). That's why, when you complete the first week of a diet with great gusto and enthusiasm, you may well be rewarded with a 1.8kg (4lb) weight loss. That's probably 450g (1lb) of fat and 1.3kg (3lb) of water.

However, the sad truth is that, when you start eating enough for your energy needs again, the glycogen and water stores are replenished, and the water weight comes back.

So the measure of a diet that's actually burning fat is not what happens when you starve yourself during the first week and temporarily run out of glycogen. Instead, it's a regular week-by-week loss of around 450–900g (1–2lb).

Look at the two charts on page 84. The top one shows the average weight loss, week by week, of a group of nine dieters on a regular low-calorie diet. In the first week there's 1.3kg (3lb) lost, in the second 900g (2lb). Things are looking good – 2.25kg (5lb) in two weeks. But most of this is water. By Week 4 there's no loss and, presumably as willpower wanes, the volunteers start eating what they need to eat for energy, restoring glycogen and, with that, back comes the water. The end result: an average of 900g (2lb) lost in 12 weeks.

The bottom graph shows the results of seven people on my original Fatburner Diet (the Holford Diet is even more effective). Once again, there's a sudden weight loss in the first week, but then it settles in at an average of 450g (1lb) a week. After 12 weeks, the average weight loss is

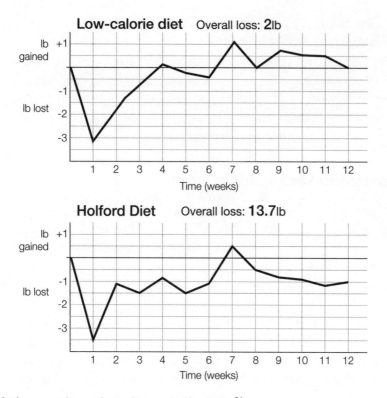

Weight loss on a low-calorie diet vs. Holford Diet[54]

6.2kg (13lb 7oz). This pattern of weight loss indicates fatburning – and, where there's fatburning, there's long-term, maintained weight loss.

And it is better not to lose weight a whole lot faster than this. Ultimately, the amount lost will be about 12.7kg (2st.) over three months. Weight loss of over 900g (2lb) a week is unlikely to be all fat loss. The body simply cannot burn off fat that fast. Of course, most of us want to lose 6.4kg (14lb) in a week, despite having taken a year to put it on!

A good target during the first 30 days is to lose 3.2kg (7lb) in weight. You'll probably lose more, but it's better to set yourself up for success. Even a weight loss of 450g (1lb) a week, maintained over a year, equals over 23kg (3½st.).

And this can be achieved, without any suffering, on my diet.

If you want to lose weight forever and turn yourself from a fatmaker into a fatburner, this is the essential framework for your new life:

How to lose weight instantly

There is, however, one way you can instantly lose weight and never put it back. It's by avoiding a food you are allergic to. One in three people has specific food intolerances, and some of these cause excessive weight gain – probably by triggering excessive fluid retention. Unlike the water that's stored with glycogen, which will come back once you stop starving yourself, this is *excess* water that the body lets go of when you avoid the foods you are intolerant to.

I remember my first overweight patient, Mary, who had struggled with her weight for years. I advised her to cut out wheat and within two days she had lost 3.2kg (7lb)! I'm going to tell you how to discover whether you are allergic to certain foods and what to replace them with in Chapter 15. This step is one of the five simple principles of my diet, which I introduce in Part Two.

1. Eat no more than 40 ⓖⓛ of carbohydrate foods (I'll show you how easy this is) with protein.

2. Eat essential omega-3 and -6 fats, and no saturated, processed or fried fats.

3. Find the foods you're allergic to and avoid them.

4. Take the right supplements.

5. Do the equivalent of 15 minutes' exercise a day.

Remember: you're unique

These principles work well for just about everybody – but it's important to remember that you're unique. For one thing, how much you need to eat will vary depending on how tall you are and how much exercise you do. If you are over 1.8m (6ft) tall or under 1.62m (5ft 4in), or exercise for an hour or more five or more days a week, you'll need to refer to Chapter 28, page 281 when the time comes, to adjust the Holford Diet according to your needs.

Summary

- You cannot lose more than 900g (2lb) of actual fat a week unless you are starving yourself or running for Britain.

- The body loses around 1.8kg (4lb) in water on a very low-calorie or very low-carbohydrate diet when you deplete your body's glycogen stores – but this inevitably comes back.

- You can lose 3.2kg (7lb) or more fast – and permanently – if you avoid foods you are allergic to.

- Losing inches is more important than losing pounds. Gaining lean body mass and losing fat, measured as your body-fat percentage, is the real goal.

- The body will naturally gravitate to its own ideal weight if you give it the right balance and kind of protein, fat and carbohydrate.

6

Why Fatburning is Easy

The Holford Diet is the state of the art of keeping you satisfied. For more than a decade, I've been researching exactly what keeps you replete – not only which foods but which foods in combination, and when to eat them.

And you'll be eating plenty of them. If all you've ever heard about weight loss is calorie cutting, this may make you wary. But eating little and often of low-GL foods will reduce, not increase, the number of calories you consume. And it will be easy and brilliantly satisfying, because you've got three meals and two substantial snacks a day, and no cravings brought on by low blood sugar.

Even better, the process will kick in fast. Most people's blood sugar balance begins to even out within three to seven days of starting the Holford Diet, which means less craving for sweet foods and less hunger, and within 30 days you should no longer be insulin-resistant – which means you are reprogramming your body's metabolism to burn fat.

Parts Three and Four of this book will get down to the nitty-gritty of the diet. This overview will show you how you can move from being a fatmaker to a fatburner with real ease.

Seven days to stop cravings

You may feel fantastic right from the start of the diet. But, the chances are, it'll take a few days for that feeling to kick in. This is because many people drink lots of coffee or regularly eat chocolate and sugary snacks – so if this is you, initially you are going to experience the effect of simultaneously launching out on a new diet and deciding to go cold turkey on caffeine.

Doing it like this is the quickest way to start the fatburning process, but it does mean that if you drink a lot of coffee or cola, or eat a fair amount of chocolate or sugary snacks, you will experience a withdrawal phase. You may feel a bit rough for the first three days, and a small minority of people might feel bad for the entire first week. The blood sugar dips that go with withdrawal can make you feel sleepy, mentally foggy, anxious, moody or tired, or spark cravings and headaches.

If you find yourself experiencing any of these sensations, be aware that it's all down to resistance. The more insulin, glucagon, adrenalin and cortisol you've been forcing your body to produce, the more resistant it becomes to their 'fine-tuning' effects. In Chapter 3 I explained about insulin resistance, but you also can become adrenalin resistant. Remember that stimulants such as coffee can kick-start the release of adrenalin. If you're downing four or five cups a day or more, you can become increasingly deaf to your own adrenalin. You might even find it tough to get out of bed in the morning. You can't hear your own inner adrenalin alarm because you've developed adrenalin resistance.

On the Holford Diet, it takes only a few days to overcome resistance – on three delicious meals and two snacks a day. I'm also going to be asking you to call in the cavalry: special supplements that work wonders for stabilising blood sugar and appetite.

If you feel you're very addicted to caffeine or chocolate, however, it is probably best to give yourself two weeks to give it all up before you actually start the diet. You'll see how to do that in Parts Three and Four.

You'll eat less without trying

After seven days you'll find that your desire to eat high-GL foods will rapidly fall away. You won't get the blood sugar dips after meals that lead you to crave the wrong foods. Even though I don't want you to try to eat less, you will naturally do so. Britain's first Holford dieter said this:

> ❝ I lost 3st. [19kg] and never felt hungry. I know I'll never go back to eating like I used to. ❞

Dr David Ludwig of the Department of Medicine at the Children's Hospital in Boston, Massachusetts, decided to put this to the test. He gave children one of two breakfast cereals. One was a low-GL cereal made from unadulterated oat flakes. The other was a processed 'instant oatmeal' that sounded good but actually had a high GL. Both groups of kids ate the identical calorie amount of each cereal and also had a calorie-identical lunch. In the afternoon and evening they were free to eat as they chose. The children on the low-GL diet ate 47 per cent fewer calories in the afternoon – they just weren't hungry.

The same thing will happen to you. That is why Holford dieters say that 'as far as hunger is concerned it's an easy diet to stick to' (*She* magazine).

The way it works

To get an idea of how the diet tackles hunger, first imagine a plate. Now divide it in half. In any main meal, one of those halves can be filled with vegetables chosen from a selection of almost a hundred.

Divide the other half in half again. One quarter is protein – fish, chicken, lamb or vegetarian proteins such as tofu or beans. Later I'll give you portion sizes of, say, a piece of chicken or a piece of fish.

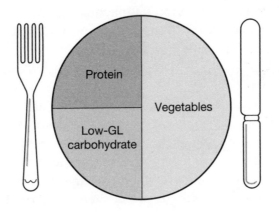

Dividing up your food

The remaining quarter is a low-GL carbohydrate food serving, equivalent to 10 ⒼⓁ. This could be bread, potatoes, pasta or any other of the foods that so many high-protein diets forbid. They're firmly part of the Holford Diet, but the serving size will vary depending on the GL of that carbohydrate. For instance, you can eat twice as much boiled potato as baked potato, and even more sweetcorn. You can eat twice as much whole rye bread as white wheat bread. You can eat twice as much wholemeal spaghetti as French fries. Very soon you'll learn which low-GL foods fill you up the best.

This is a sketch of a main meal. You'll roughly follow the same rules for your other two meals, allowing 10 ⓖ per meal – and don't forget there are two substantial snacks a day, at 5 ⓖ each (plus an optional 5 ⓖ extra for drinks or desserts/sweets). So the GL maximum for each day is 45, though 40 is the optimum amount for losing weight (and the minimum for not feeling hungry). (If you're very tall or very small, or doing loads of exercise this figure may not be right for you – see Chapter 28.)

Eating out is easy

I travel around the world, visiting an average of 30 cities in any given year. I've learned that I can follow this diet in every country anywhere in the world. Sure, some countries and types of food are easier than others. It's harder in the US, where more people are obese, and easier in Thailand, where most people are skinny. In general, pick restaurants from the countries where people are thinnest. The menus of Thai restaurants, Chinese restaurants, Indian restaurants and many others all around the world cater perfectly for people on my diet. You just need to make the right choices – I'll show you how in Chapter 25.

Effortless shopping

You may have encountered diets for which you had to buy foods by mail order, or hunt out exotic substances in specialist shops. Everything on my diet can be bought at the supermarket – including the organic foods I recommend – or, failing that, in your local health-food shop. (There is a website www.gloriusfood.com that tells you all about the best low-GL foods and where to get them.) Granted, you may be throwing a few things into your trolley that you've never cooked before, but I can guarantee it's all going to be delicious – and this may even become a culinary adventure. As it's a diet for life, it will never be dull.

Veggie heaven

The diet is a cinch for vegetarians. There's a vast and tasty array of vegetables and good, slow-releasing carbohydrates, as well as recipes for preparing them. On the protein front, vegetarians will just need to ensure they're eating the optimal amount for the diet to work.

Tofu, which is available in a number of delicious forms, features in a number of recipes, or can be substituted for fish or chicken in others. Beans and lentils figure large in the Holford Diet, as they are key to regulating blood sugar. Other vegetarian protein options – Quorn, soya mince, yoghurt, cottage cheese, eggs – are all well represented. So there's no shunting of vegetarian needs to the sidelines, which can happen with some high-protein diets.

Here's what one vegetarian, Barbara C from South Africa, said:

I have been a vegetarian for 15 years now and have always battled to keep the weight off. I read the Holford Diet book and it is really the first diet book that makes so much sense. I understand so much more about a balanced vegetarian diet now. I have managed to lose 1¼st.[8kg] in three months and I feel wonderful. I weigh myself once a week and I always feel apprehensive, because the one thing that does not happen on this diet is that you get hungry – ever. So I always imagine that I have eaten too much to have lost weight ... but the kilos are still going.

No forbidden foods

Never say never. So I'm not going to tell you never to eat chocolate, bread, pasta or potatoes. But I *am* going to tell you how much of these foods you can eat to keep within your 45 Ⓖ limit for the day. How you do that is up to you.

Let me give you an example. Below are four snacks. Each equal to 5 Ⓖ. The choice is yours.

Strawberries	1 large punnet
Apple	1 small apple
Peanuts	2 small packets
Chocolate	Less than a quarter of a bar (a bit more if you choose dark, low sugar chocolate)
Oatcakes	2 oatcakes with ⅓ tub of hummus

As you can see, high-GL foods such as chocolate aren't much fun because you can't eat much of them. Low-GL foods are the best value because they'll fill you up and stop food cravings.

So my advice is to eat mainly low-GL foods and food combinations, with occasional medium-GL foods. High-GL foods are probably more frustrating than they're worth. All in all, that's certainly the fastest way to lose weight and gain energy. You'll find the lists of foods, their GL scores and whether they're low, medium or high GL in Appendix 2.

This diet isn't just good for your weight and your waist, it's perfect for your health and well-being, as you'll discover in the next part. If you just want to get started, skip to Part Three to learn the five basic principles, then Part Four to put them into action.

Summary

- The Holford Diet reduces your appetite because it stabilises your blood sugar levels so you don't get hungry.

- Sugar cravings take no more than seven days to cure. After that, you'll find that your food cravings will virtually vanish.

- As long as you don't exceed 45 🅖🅛 a day you can eat or drink anything. However, you can eat much more of the best low-GL foods so you won't go hungry. Either way, you lose weight.

PART TWO

Undamage Your Health

7

Up Your Energy

With most diets, you will probably experience side effects when you've been following the regime for some time. On very high-protein diets, these may be constipation or bad breath, with increased risk of certain cancers associated with long-term use. On low-fat diets, they can include problems with skin or hair, and blood sugar problems that could lead to diabetes.

This diet, on the other hand, will seriously *undamage* your health. The only side effects you'll get on the Holford Diet are extra energy, better mood and memory, clearer skin and resistance to degenerative diseases such as diabetes, heart disease and cancer.[1] Your cholesterol level is also likely to normalise, as is your homocysteine level (this is explained below).

As I said at the start, weight loss, and the ability to maintain your optimal weight, is simply a side effect of giving your body optimum nutrition – which is exactly what the Holford Diet offers. Balancing your blood sugar and ensuring you're getting all the right nutrients will leave you in optimum health, slim, mentally fit and glowing with vitality.

Here's what you can expect:

- **An end to fatigue**. You'll never experience that weakened, lowered state that can creep up on you when you follow some low-calorie diets. Instead, you will wake up alert and clear-eyed – and, even better, get through the day without any energy slumps or exhaustion. This is the effect of cutting right back on stimulants and sugar, eating a low-GL diet, and supplementing nutrients known to boost energy.

- **Younger, smoother skin**. You'll discover the six secrets of having great skin, such as eating the right kinds of fruits (berries are tops), vegetables and omega-3 fats.

- **A lowered homocysteine level**. Having a high level of this toxic amino acid in the blood can indicate a real vulnerability to many degenerative diseases, from strokes to Alzheimer's. The Holford Diet encourages the best defence: lots of green, leafy vegetables, beans and seeds plus supplementing B vitamins and crucial minerals in a high-strength multivitamin.

- **No more blues**. Being overweight can be depressing, and it's now known that overweight people have lower levels of the 'happy' brain chemical serotonin. A low-GL diet emphasising high-quality carbohydrates will help you beat the blues by raising serotonin levels – and, of course, helping you shift the weight.

- **A sharper mind**. A diet high in omega-3s, vitamins C and E and the nutrients that will help balance blood sugar – such as the Holford Diet – will banish mental 'fogs', poor concentration and memory, and significantly reduce the risk of developing Alzheimer's.

- **Freedom from stress**. Long-term stress causes too much of the hormone cortisol to circulate in the body, and cortisol can damage the brain. But cutting out sugar and stimulants can swiftly lower stress levels, and give your brain a chance to recover and rebuild itself.

- **Lowered risk of disease**. The Holford Diet, with its emphasis on balancing blood sugar, can clearly reduce your risk of getting diabetes. But it can also significantly decrease your risk of developing heart disease or strokes, cancer and arthritis.

This is a diet where you don't only lose weight. You look great and feel great: clear-headed, calm, glowing and knowing that you are getting healthier as each week passes. The first benefit you are going to experience is a big increase in your energy levels. As one Holford dieter, Dawn V, told me:

❝ *My only problem is coping with the extra energy!* ❞

Increase your energy

Newton's Third Law of Thermodynamics, applied to what you eat, says that all the energy you consume as calories must go somewhere. You've been putting some of it down into storage as fat. But, as we've now amply seen, on the Holford Diet three things are going to happen: you'll start to burn off fat, you'll find yourself eating less without even trying, and your energy levels will shoot up.

When I first came into the field of nutrition, I was deeply impressed by the work of a then maverick called Dr Roy Walford, professor of pathology at the UCLA School of Medicine in Los Angeles, who claimed he had discovered the secret of eternal youth. Dr Walford (who sadly died of a rare genetic neurological disease called ALS) is now respected as one of the truly pioneering gerontologists of our time. Walford had proved how to increase the lifespan of any animal by up to 30 per cent! He fed laboratory animals food that had slightly fewer calories, but was of very high quality, with high levels of vitamins and minerals and a low glycemic load. These lucky animals clocked the equivalent of 130 human years! But what really impressed me was seeing them. His diet hadn't just added years to their life; it had clearly added life to their years. Compared with the 'normal' animals, they looked healthy and lean, and were very active and inquisitive.

I started following the human equivalent of his diet – which was very close to today's Holford Diet – and I've stayed lean and physically and mentally active ever since. The research Dr Walford started is now being tested on humans in a long-term study, and so far all the signs are good. His lucky volunteers have all the same positive characteristics that the animals displayed on his diet and are bang on course for reaching 100 with the health of a 60-year-old. It's looking more and more as if you really can turn back the clock.

Energy, or the lack of it, is the bane of the twenty-first century. When the Institute for Optimum Nutrition (ION) conducted Britain's biggest ever 'ONUK' health survey in 2002, a staggering 80 per cent of people reported low energy. We also found that the more overweight a person was, the more likely they were to complain of fatigue. It's ironic that overweight people should feel tired when their bodies are a storehouse packed full of energy-giving fat.

As I've shown, the trouble is that food is being converted straight to fat rather than straight to energy. When you change your body's metabolism to use the energy in your food more efficiently, you'll be off and running.

But don't take my word for it. Here's what people say:

John G:

> ❛ *I lost 13lb [5.9kg] in a month and, amazingly, I lost my craving for sweets! My energy also increased so much.* ❜

Rebecca C:

> ❛ *I lost 22lbs [10kg] in eight weeks. My energy is amazing.* ❜

Carol P:

> ❛ *I lost 30lb [13.6kg]. I have more energy. I feel happy and my mood is more even.* ❜

Marianne B:

> ❛ *It's as if someone has given me a magic pill and said, "You'll have more energy, you'll feel calm and you'll feel less stressed." It's worked better than I would have believed. I am full of energy, my skin has improved dramatically, my cholesterol level has dropped by a third in seven weeks and I've lost 14lb [6.3kg], especially around my middle.* ❜

She magazine selected 10 volunteers. This is what the magazine reported: 'Increased alertness was a significant benefit. By the third day, everybody felt well – alert on rising, and three of us (including me) were bounding about, full of the joys of spring. Two out of ten felt hungry, but the rest said that, as far as hunger was concerned, it was a comparatively easy diet to stick to. Mrs Kilby noted by day four that her concentration had improved, and this was backed up by comments from other testers. Nobody had that weak and wobbly feeling associated with dieting. By the end of the week, everyone had stayed the course. Weight loss over the week varied from 3lb to 7lb, 4–5lb being the average.'

The *Sunday Times* selected one volunteer. This is what she said:

> ❛ *After the first few days I began to feel wonderful – alert and fit and thoroughly detoxified with no more puffy eyes staring back from the bathroom mirror. There's no shortage of recipe ideas. I lost 10lb in a month.* ❜

In the early days, when we put people on this diet, 86 per cent reported a definite improvement in energy. Using our checklist, the average 'low energy' score was 7, and, three to six months later, the average score was 3.

Now it's your turn to check your score. Energy levels are intimately linked to insulin resistance and blood sugar balance, as we've seen throughout this book. So, to figure out your score, go back to the Are you insulin-resistant? questionnaire on page 61.

If you answer yes to seven or more questions, you are struggling to keep your blood sugar level even, and you probably have serious energy slumps or feel exhausted much of the time.

If you answer yes to between seven and ten questions, you are beginning to show signs of a sugar sensitivity, which needs to be addressed. You may have several dips in energy a day.

If you answer yes to fewer than four questions, you are unlikely to have a blood sugar problem, and your energy level is on the up and up or consistently high.

Make a note of your score, then retest yourself in three months.

It's not all right to feel just 'all right'. I want you to feel full of energy, however old you are. Are you ready for it?

8

Look Better, Live Longer

Did you know your skin renews itself every 20 days? We are literally making new skin cells every day, and the healthier your diet, the healthier your skin. I know because, as I mentioned at the start of this book, I suffered for seven years with bad acne, and saw numerous specialists whose advice ranged from special cleansing routines to creams and antibiotics. Some of these substances made a mild difference, but none really worked. Then I discovered optimum nutrition and within one month the spots were gone. Within three months, the scarring was visibly reduced. Why?

There are six secrets to having great skin, and all of them are fulfilled by following the Holford Diet. If you suffer from skin problems you may just find that they clear up quickly on this diet, as Pieter, Linda and Marianne did.

Pieter L:

❛I was suffering from recurring eczema on my hands. The standard treatment for eczema was cortisone, which made my skin go thin for months on end. My cholesterol was high and I was overweight. Within three months of following the advice in your book, I reached my ideal weight and my cholesterol dropped dramatically. I have maintained these levels for two years now. I have also solved my eczema problem. ❜

Linda H, who lost 5.9kg (13lb) in four weeks, also found her skin transformed:

❛An unexpected benefit was that the redness, or rosacea, I'd always noticed on my face and which I thought was a result of ageing, disappeared. My

energy also increased, so much that I realised I hadn't understood how tired and rundown I was before. I thought being tired was just a normal part of life! ❯

Marianne B, a volunteer in our weight-loss trial:

❮ *I used to have a skin condition called acne rosacea where you get swelling and redness on the face. That has diminished so considerably over eight weeks I'm astonished. Nothing has done that before. No medication supplied by the dermatologist, no cream that you can buy over the counter has ever produced an effect like eating on the Holford Diet has.* ❯

She also lost 6.4kg (14lb) in seven weeks.

Inner balance

The first, and most important step, is to keep your blood sugar level even. When your blood sugar level peaks too high, which is the fate of the insulin-resistant, the skin also receives excess sugar. Bacteria in the skin feed off sugar, which is what causes spots. When the blood sugar level dips too low, the body produces adrenalin. This increases the production of sebum, an oily secretion in the skin, which in excess can block pores and cause an isolated pocket of infection to grow.

The reason excess sebum can block pores, as well as make the skin oily, is that the sebum gets oxidised, making it hard. The skin is always being bombarded with free radicals, rogue molecules that are sometimes called oxidants.

Major baddies as far as your skin and your health are concerned, oxidants originate from anything burned, especially fats. So they're in cigarette smoke (there are a trillion in each puff), fried food, burned meat and exhaust fumes, as well as the air itself, since particles become damaged by the sun's burning rays. In truth, you are exposed to something like a bucketful of oxidants each year. These are damaging your skin every day and that is why people who live near the equator, or at high altitudes, and are therefore exposed to stronger sunlight, have much older-looking skin.

There are only two things you can do to minimise oxidant skin damage: either limit your exposure to strong sunlight or rub on a sunscreen when you do, and take in more antioxidant nutrients through diet and supplements.

Top Tip

You can feed the skin with antioxidants from the outside. The best skin product I know is Environ. The antioxidant-rich cream is applied directly to your skin. The results are amazing. (See page 434 for details.)

Essential antioxidants

The Holford Diet is naturally full of antioxidants, partly by luck and partly by design. Some of the all-time best, low-GL fruits and vegetables also have the highest levels of antioxidants. To stay young and healthy you need to eat antioxidant-rich foods every day.

When I first came into the field of nutrition we used to measure the amount of antioxidant nutrients in food, including vitamin A, betacarotene, vitamin C, vitamin E, selenium, zinc, glutathione and co-enzyme Q10. We then started to discover more and more plant-based antioxidants. An example of these phytonutrients is anthocyanidins in berries and allicin in garlic.

A method for measuring a food's total anti-ageing antioxidant power was then invented, called the 'ORAC score' of a food ('ORAC' stands for 'oxygen radical absorption capacity'). The ORAC score of a food is the single best measure of a food's anti-ageing potential. To give you some examples I've listed below some of the top common fruits and vegetables, starting with those with the highest ORAC scores.[2] I've also listed their GL for a 100g (3½oz) serving.

Top anti-ageing fruits

	ORAC per 100g (3½oz)	ⒼⓁ per 100g (3½oz)
Plums	7,581	5
Blueberries	6,552	1
Prunes	6,552	17
Blackberries	5,347	1
Raspberries	4,882	1
Strawberries	3,577	1
Cherries	3,365	2

	ORAC per 100g (3½oz)	ⒼⓁ per 100g (3½oz)
Raisins	3,037	46
Apple	**2,210–4,275**	**5**
Oranges	**1,819**	**5**
Peach	**1,814**	**4**
Grapefruit, pink	**1,548**	**3**
Grapes, red	1,260	7
Kiwi fruit	**1,210**	**5**
Apricot	**1,115**	**4**
Banana	879	10
Cantaloupe melon	315	4

Although raisins and prunes have a high ORAC rating, they also send your blood sugar soaring. Remember, the GL limit for a snack on the Holford Diet is five points. I've put the best all-rounders in this list – berries, plums, oranges, cherries and pink grapefruit – in bold, because these fruits will both help you lose weight and keep your skin healthy.

Be aware, however, that these are the scores for the whole fruit, not the juice. Although an orange is the equivalent of 5 ⒼⓁ, and therefore a perfect snack for the diet, a 250ml (9fl oz) glass of orange juice, which normally contains the juice and the sugar of between two and three oranges, has a GL of 13 points. That's too much.

In the chart below I've picked out the best vegetables, both for their ORAC score and their GL, highlighted in bold

Top anti-ageing vegetables

	ORAC per 100g (3½oz)	ⒼⓁ per serving
Garlic clove, raw	**5,346**	**1**
Broccoli, boiled	**2,386**	**2**
Sweet potato	2,115	12.5
Avocado	**1,933**	**1**
Beetroot	1,767	5
Asparagus, cooked	**1,644**	**2**
Spinach	**1,515**	**1**
Onion	**1,220**	**2**
Potato	1,138	16

	ORAC per 100g (3½oz)	ⓖⓛ per serving
Brussels sprouts	980	2
Carrot, raw	666	3
Peas, frozen	600	3
Pumpkin	483	3
Corn	413	9
Tomato	367	3
Carrot, boiled	317	3

As you can see in the chart above, some of the best antioxidant vegetables are also the best fatburning vegetables, with a low GL score. I recommend you have a serving of one of these top scorers every day, with the exception of avocado – don't have more than three a week.

Of all the antioxidant nutrients, the two most important for the skin are vitamins A and C. Vitamin A is what protects your skin from sun damage. Vitamin C makes collagen, a substance that's a bit like 'glue' holding your cells together. When you lack vitamin C, your skin loses its tone and wrinkles develop. On the Holford Diet I not only recommend you to eat foods naturally rich in these nutrients but I also recommend that you supplement with a multivitamin containing at least 1,500mcg of vitamin A, plus 1,000g (or even 2,000g) of vitamin C, which is the optimal amount for fatburning, anti-ageing and boosting your immune system.

Fats and flexibility

The third secret for healthy skin is to eat the right fats. Essential fats, found in seeds and fish, are vital for your skin and, without them, it can look dry and old. Skin cells contain these essential fats, which not only keep skin looking young and flexible but are also needed to reduce skin inflammation. Omega-3 fats are very powerful anti-inflammatory agents that can reduce redness and swelling in conditions such as eczema.

The Holford Diet recommends that you eat foods naturally high in essential fats, such as oily fish, seeds and nuts. These essential fats not only help your skin but they also help you to burn fat. You may also choose to use them as supplements, as I do every day. I take a supplement that contains a combination of EPA and DHA, which are the most powerful omega-3 fats, and GLA, the most powerful omega-6 fat. (See also Chapter 27.)

Liquid loveliness

The final secret for healthy skin is to drink enough water – and that means eight glasses a day (approximately 2 litres). The body is 66 per cent water and you need to keep it topped up with water to function properly, from the cellular and chemical levels up. Here, essential fats are invaluable, helping to maintain perfect water balance in the body by keeping the right amount of it inside your cells.

Drinking enough water to stay hydrated is not only good for your health, it also helps to reduce your appetite, as we often mistake thirst for hunger.

The calorie connection

Skin cells are not much different from other cells in your body and, for this reason, those four secrets for healthy skin – balance your blood sugar, eat an antioxidant-rich diet, get enough essential fats and drink eight glasses of water a day – are also the top tips for staying young and slowing down the ageing process. And there are two more.

In the last chapter I told you about the excellent research of Dr Roy Walford, who proved that if you cut down on calories you live longer. Calorie restriction, however, is not the same as malnutrition. It is about giving the body exactly what it needs and no more.

That's exactly what the Holford Diet is all about. Many foods in today's diet provide 'empty' calories. That is, they provide sugar or saturated fat, but none of the micronutrients needed to process them. These foods are out if you want to lose weight and extend your lifespan. Nutrient-dense foods such as fish, beans, nuts or seeds provide as many nutrients as calories, plus, in the case of fresh fruit and vegetables, plenty of essential and calorie-free water.

Since the first animal experiments in 1935, studies on several species have shown that animals eating 30 to 40 per cent fewer calories extend their lifespan by a third to (in the case of fish) a half. However, it isn't just about limiting calories. These animals were given optimum nutrition as well as fewer calories, with good intakes of antioxidants.

There's every reason to assume the same principle applies to humans. Consider the islanders of Okinawa in Japan. They eat 17 to 40 per cent fewer calories than other Japanese and have more centenarians than any other population. According to Dr Walford, 'You can extend longevity by restricting food even after full adulthood and middle age.'

Having a high-quality diet with minimal calories also means minimal oxidative stress on the body. You are giving yourself exactly what you need and no more. But how much is that? Dr Walford said that you can extend lifespan by cutting calories by 10 to 25 per cent. He ate between 1,500 and 2,000 calories a day, compared with the average intake of 2,500 to 3,000 calories. And that is exactly what I recommend you do. The recipes in the Holford Diet, and the menus based on them, are designed to be less calorific, yet fill you up and satisfy your appetite in the healthiest way possible.

Life insurance companies know well the correlation between weight and longevity. Based on these statistics, weight charts give an ideal weight range for your height. You can see one of these in Appendix 1. Generally, the ideal weight for increased life expectancy is the low end of this range. Even more important, as we've seen in this book, is keeping your body fat percentage down, which can also be greatly helped by a regular exercise regime. Appendix 1 also shows you how to calculate this percentage.

The homocysteine factor

Homocysteine is a toxic amino acid (a building block of protein) found in the blood. You may not have heard of it yet, but you certainly will.

Your homocysteine level is a stronger predictor of your risk of having a heart attack or stroke than your cholesterol level. This is quite literally the most important medical breakthrough of the twenty-first century and I can't do it justice here – which is why I've written a book, *The H Factor* (Piatkus), with Dr James Braly, an expert on this subject. Over 10,000 medical studies have linked high levels of this amino acid to about 100 medical conditions, including obesity.

A comprehensive research study at the University of Bergen in Norway, published in 2001 in the *American Journal of Clinical Nutrition*,[3] measured the homocysteine levels of 4,766 men and women aged 65 to 67 in 1992, and then recorded any deaths over the next five years. During this time, 162 men and 97 women died. The researchers then looked at the risk of death in relation to their homocysteine levels. This is what they found: 'A strong relation was found between homocysteine and *all* causes of mortality.' They discovered that the chances of a 65–67-year-old dying from any cause increased by almost 50 per cent for every five-unit increase in homocysteine!

So, how can you lower levels of this toxic amino acid? It all hinges on something called SAMe.

Put simply, if you have a high homocysteine level, it means you've got a blockage in your body's ability to turn protein into one of the most important anti-ageing nutrients of all, s-adenosyl methionine. SAMe is what's called a methyl donor. Every single second of your life there are a billion chemical reactions in your body, in which one chemical is turned into another by adding on what's called a methyl group. The regulation of insulin, adrenalin and serotonin – three body chemicals that are vital to weight control – all depend on methyl reactions.

If you've got fully functional methyl reactions, you will be very healthy, happy and 'connected'. I call this having a high 'methyl IQ', and this is indicated by a low homocysteine level in your blood. If you have a high homocysteine level that means you have a poor methyl IQ and are likely to gain weight easily, have insulin resistance, have depression and are at greater risk of developing diabetes, heart disease, strokes and Alzheimer's later in life.

The average 'H' score is 10–11 units. The ideal is 6. I often see patients with levels of 20 or more. With every 5-unit drop in your H score, you almost halve your risk of dying prematurely. If, for example, your H score was 16, and you drop it to six or less and maintain it there, you can probably add around 10 years to your life!

High-homocysteine and methylation problems, on the other hand, literally age your cells faster, drain vitality from you and make you feel old far beyond your years. Homocysteine ages the body directly. If, for example, you expose the cells that line arteries throughout your body to homocysteine, the cells get older much more quickly.[4]

So, finally, we are discovering that the reason we age is twofold. Cells, and their replacement 'instructions', get increasingly damaged by poor methylation and excessive oxidation, both of which are reflected by your homocysteine score.

This is great news because it's easily remedied. The right diet and supplements can rapidly reverse both poor methylation and excessive oxidation, bringing your homocysteine level into the superhealthy range below 6 units. This is important because it means you really can measure where you are regarding homocysteine, and adjust your diet and supplements accordingly. By the way, you can measure your own homocysteine level using a home test kit (see www.thehfactor.com or the Resources section on page 435).

The key homocysteine-busting nutrients are vitamins B_2, B_6, folic acid, B_{12}, zinc and magnesium. The high-strength multivitamin I recommend taking, along with the Holford Diet, provides optimum amounts of these. In fact, the diet is the perfect way to lower your homocysteine level and improve your health.

9

Improve Your Mood and Memory

Being overweight and feeling blue are connected in more ways than one. Being overweight can be depressing in its own right – you don't look as good as you could, you may be tired, it may be harder to walk up stairs or run for the bus. However, scientists are discovering a much closer connection between these two conditions after looking at what happens in the brains of those prone to depression and weight gain.

A consistent finding is that both overweight people and depressed people have low levels of serotonin in the brain. This is the brain's 'happy' chemical and it also controls your appetite. SSRI anti-depressants help promote serotonin in the brain and not only relieve depression in up to 50 per cent of people but they also reduce appetite.

However, the side effects of SSRIs are in themselves depressing, so much so that most SSRI drugs are now banned in children up to the age of 18 and are under review for adults. Although there are more than 25 reported side effects, the main concern is that something like one in ten adolescents was found to develop suicidal tendencies as a result of taking these drugs. Of course, these problems are not restricted to children. Adults on SSRIs more than double their risk of suicide, according to a review in the *British Medical Journal*.[5]

Protein and serotonin

Serotonin is made directly from a nutrient that you and I eat every day. It's an amino acid called tryptophan, found in protein foods. If you take tryptophan out of a person's diet, two things will happen: first, they'll become depressed, and, second, they'll crave carbohydrates.

When you eat protein foods such as chicken or fish, you will raise blood levels of tryptophan. Tryptophan then turns into 5-hydroxytryptophan (5-HTP), small amounts of which are also present in beans, fish and other protein foods, and then into serotonin. The body stores 5-HTP in the platelets in the blood before passing it to the brain.

Now, you might logically think that a high-protein diet, for example bacon and eggs for breakfast rather than a high-carbohydrate choice such as a croissant, toast or cereal, would increase the brain's levels of serotonin best. It doesn't. Research by Professor Richard Wurtman and Judith Wurtman at the Massachusetts Institute of Technology (MIT) has consistently shown that meals containing carbohydrate, rather than protein, raise serotonin best.[6]

The reason for this apparent anomaly is that tryptophan in the bloodstream competes very badly with all the other amino acids in protein, so little gets across into the brain. However, when you eat a carbohydrate food such as an apple, this causes some insulin to be released into the bloodstream, which carries the tryptophan and 5-HTP into the brain, and causes serotonin levels to rise.

This may be why many depressed people crave sweet foods to give them a lift.

So, if you find sugar makes you feel happier, you are probably low in serotonin. The trouble is, a vicious cycle lies this way: most carbohydrate snacks are high in refined sugar and fat, and make you fat, which is depressing. The alternative is to follow my low-GL diet. It worked for Asa N:

> ❛ I have suffered from low blood sugar, mood swings and serious sugar cravings most of my adult life, so for me the main aim of wanting to try the GL programme was not to lose weight, but to gain some control of my life. And the results have been fantastic! I have followed the GL programme for nearly two months now and not only are the recipes fabulously tasty, they are also remarkably quick and easy to prepare. And my cravings have more or less gone (even in the days leading up to my period!). I really enjoy planning the meals a few days in advance and by now I have been through most of the recipes, including the cakes, which are fabulous (I do always make sure I have a supply of xylitol at home). I have also lost about 5lb [2.25kg] and feel much more energetic than I have in ages. ❜

Judith Wurtman, who directs the Program in Women's Health at the MIT Clinical Research Center, says that when you stop eating carbohydrates on a high-protein diet, your brain stops regulating serotonin, leading to low mood and food cravings: 'When serotonin is made and becomes active in your brain, its effect on your appetite is to make you feel full before your stomach is stuffed and stretched. Serotonin is crucial not only to control your appetite and stop you from overeating; it's essential to keep your moods regulated.'

Carbohydrate cravings

This explains the common craving of high-protein dieters (especially women) for carbohydrates. Women have much less serotonin in their brains than men, so a serotonin-depleting diet will make women feel irritable. Some people feel down in the afternoon or early evening and crave carbohydrate.

According to Wurtman's clinical studies, if the carbohydrate craver eats protein instead, he or she will become grumpy, irritable or restless. Furthermore, filling up on fatty foods such as bacon or cheese makes you tired, lethargic and apathetic. This is another reason why I don't favour high-protein, low-carbohydrate diets.

One way to guarantee healthy serotonin levels is to supplement with 5-HTP. This not only improves your mood, but will also reduce your appetite, especially for sugary foods.

Another nutrient that controls carb cravings, boosts your mood and assists weight loss is the mineral chromium. As well as stabilising your blood sugar and helping you lose weight (we'll look at this a little later in this chapter), it's also an excellent antidepressant if you suffer from what's called 'atypical' depression. 'Atypical' depression is so called because it differs markedly from 'classic' depression, where sufferers have little appetite, don't eat enough, lose weight and can't sleep. Let's look at some of the symptoms of atypical depression; if you answer yes to five or more of these questions, you might be suffering from it:

- Do you crave sweets or other carbohydrates?

- Do you tend to gain weight?

- Are you tired for no obvious reason?

- Do your arms or legs feel heavy?

- Do you tend to feel sleepy or groggy much of the time?

- Are your feelings easily hurt by the rejection of others?

- Did your depression begin before the age of 30?

Atypical depression is estimated to affect anywhere from 25 to 42 per cent of the depressed population, and an even higher percentage among depressed women, so it's actually extremely common (and misnamed).

A chance discovery by Dr Malcolm McLeod, clinical professor of psychiatry at the University of North Carolina in the US, suggested that people who suffer from atypical depression might benefit from chromium supplementation.[7] In a small double-blind study published in 2003, McLeod gave 10 patients suffering from atypical depression chromium supplements of 600mcg a day, and five others a placebo, for eight weeks.[8]

The results were dramatic. Seven out of the ten taking the supplements showed a big improvement, as opposed to none on the placebo. Their HRS (Hamilton Rating Score of Depression) dropped by an unheard-of 83 per cent: that is, from 29 – major depression – to 5, which is classed as not depressed. A larger trial at Cornell University in the US, involving 113 participants, confirmed the finding in 2005. After eight weeks, 65 per cent of the people taking chromium had had a major improvement, compared to 33 per cent on placebos.[9] Chromium has no toxicity or side effects at these levels of intake (10,000mcg is toxic), other than better energy and weight control.

Sugar, as you are no doubt beginning to understand, lies at the heart of numerous problems such as unstable blood sugar, exhaustion and weight gain – it has also been implicated in aggressive behaviour,[10] anxiety,[11] hyperactivity and attention deficit,[12] depression,[13] eating disorders,[14] fatigue,[15] learning difficulties[16] and PMS. So it's a good idea to ditch the stuff – and the best way of doing that is by following the Holford Diet.

A sharper mind

The effect of nutrition on the brain is a matter of keen interest these days. We now know that memory and concentration, as well as mood, depend hugely on what we put in our digestive systems. Keeping an even blood sugar level is key, as is an optimal intake of essential fats and antioxidants.

To illustrate just how vital these essential nutrients are, consider these studies. One study measured the amount of DHA, an omega-3 fat, in the umbilical cord of newborn babies and found that those with higher levels were faster thinkers eight years later. Another study gave infants extra DHA for the first four months and found that they thought faster six years later. These benefits of essential fats are seen at both ends of the age spectrum. A person's risk of developing Alzheimer's falls by 60 per cent if they eat a diet high in omega-3 fats, especially DHA, according to recent research by Dr Martha Morris at Chicago's Rush Institute for Healthy Aging. Vitamins E and C, both in diet and supplements, have also been shown to cut the risk of age-related memory problems by more than 60 per cent![17] Eating a more Mediterranean-style diet with more fruit, vegetables, fish, legumes and whole-grain cereals, all regular foods in the Holford Diet, is associated with a 40 per cent decreased risk of developing Alzheimer's.[18]

Then there's the homocysteine factor (see page 106). Dropping your homocysteine level by five points halves the risk of Alzheimer's, according to a study published in the *New England Journal of Medicine*.[19]

You'll be getting all of the nutrients essential for a sharper mind on the Holford Diet.

Staying cool

We had a look at the effect stress has on mind and body in Chapter 3. A mild dose of stress can actually stimulate memory and mental alertness, but long-term stress is definitely bad news: it causes too much of the hormone cortisol to circulate in the body, and this literally damages the brain. Another factor that causes too much of the stress hormone cortisol is blood sugar peaks and troughs. When your blood sugar level crashes, the body produces more cortisol. It thinks you are being starved and goes into panic mode.

Raised levels of cortisol have been linked to poorer memory and a shrinking of the brain's memory-sorting centre. This is probably why either high stress or high sugar worsens memory and concentration. After only two weeks of the raised cortisol levels of stress, the dendrite 'arms' of brain cells, which reach out to connect with other brain cells, start to shrivel up, according to research carried out at Stanford University in California by Robert Sapolsky, professor of neuroscience.[20]

The good news is that such damage isn't permanent. Stop the stress and the dendrites grow back. And one way to reduce your stress levels is to reduce your intake of sugar and stimulants. The more dependent on stimulants you are, and the more your blood sugar levels fluctuate, the more you are likely to react stressfully to life's inevitable challenges.

With the right nutrition and the right attitude, age-related memory loss doesn't need to happen to you. You can build new brain cells at any age. Research clearly shows that healthy, well-educated elderly people can show no decline in mental function right up to death, and no increased rate of brain shrinkage even after 65. It's a 'use it or lose it' situation.

People on the Holford Diet often report big improvements in mood, concentration and memory. In an eight-week trial we ran on volunteers on the Holford Diet almost all (94 per cent) reported greater energy, two-thirds had greater concentration, memory or alertness and half reported fewer feelings of depression and more stable moods.[21]

10

Prevent and Reverse Diabetes

The Holford Diet is the diet par excellence for both preventing and reversing diabetes. Professional diabetes associations around the world are adopting GL counting as an essential part of managing diabetes. Hundreds of studies now prove that a low-GL diet helps to improve blood sugar balance and hence reduce the need for medication. These are well summarised in a review article in the *Journal of the American Medical Association* for those who want the science.[22]

The fact that eating a low-GL diet is the ultimate solution to weight control – by stabilising your blood sugar balance – is proven by its extraordinary ability to reverse diabetes. Once a person is obese their risk of developing diabetes is 77 times greater – again clear proof that weight gain is about losing blood sugar control.

The worldwide incidence of diabetes is running out of control. Every 5 minutes in Britain someone is diagnosed with the condition. By 2010 approximately 3 million people in Britain will have diabetes. But it's the same the world over: India, Africa, China, America, Australia. If you are of Asian or African origin your risk is even higher. In Australia 275 people develop diabetes every single day. The older you are, and the more overweight you are, the higher your risk. In Britain, one in seven people over 40 develop diabetes and our drug bill for diabetes is close to £1 billion a year and rising. In America, $174 billion, that's one tenth of the entire US health budget, is spent on diabetes treatment and care.[23]

The scandal is that we already know the solution and it's not drugs – it's a low-GL diet. Eating a low-GL diet doesn't just prevent diabetes, it reverses it. Before I show you the proof, it's worth understanding a little about the nature of the beast.

What is diabetes?

Basically, diabetes is what happens when you have too much sugar in your blood. This happens because a person eats too much sugar or too many high-GL foods, and because their insulin isn't working properly. As soon as your blood sugar goes too high the body pumps insulin into the bloodstream, which gets the excess out as fast as possible, converting much of it into fat.

This conversion of excess sugar into fat happens in the liver. It is well established in animal studies that if you feed them high-GL diets rather than low-GL diets they literally make twice as much fat – and suffer from a 'fatty liver' as a result.[24]

If you don't make enough insulin, or you are insulin resistant, your blood sugar level stays too high. This is bad news because glucose – blood sugar, which fuels our brain and body – is highly toxic in large amounts, damaging arteries, brain cells, kidneys and the eyes. Glucose also feeds infections, chronic inflammation and promotes the formation of blood clots; some 80 per cent of people with diabetes die from cardiovascular disease. Every year, a thousand people with diabetes start kidney dialysis; others go blind. Half of all diabetics have one or more of these complications. So the human cost is very high. Much of this damage happens because sugar sticks to and damages protein, producing what are called 'advanced glycation end-products', nicknamed AGEs – and that's what they do: age you rapidly.

There are two kinds of diabetes: insulin-dependent diabetes (type 1) and non-insulin-dependent diabetes (type 2). Type-1 diabetes is rare. It usually develops in children whose immune systems mistakenly attack cells in the pancreas that make insulin. It's called an 'autoimmune' disease and is linked with food allergy (more on this in Chapter 15). Without insulin you can't control blood sugar. These people therefore need to inject insulin. The next best thing is following my low-GL diet, plus certain supplements, because this decreases the need for insulin. Type-1 diabetes is not, however, reversible.

By far the most common type of diabetes is type-2 diabetes. This is a direct consequence of diet and lifestyle, the single greatest factor being weight gain. With the right diet and supplements type-2 diabetes is completely reversible or controllable to the point where no insulin or medication is necessary.

The diagnosis of diabetes is based on testing your blood sugar level in one of three ways. First, if your 'fasting' blood glucose level is too high (above 7.8 mmol/l) that means your insulin isn't working. Second, if you eat something sweet – the equivalent of the sugar in a can of fizzy drink – and two hours later your blood glucose is above 11 mmol/l, then you're diagnosed with diabetes. But the most sensitive test of all is a measure of your 'long-term' blood sugar levels. Every time your blood sugar levels go too high, creating blood sugar 'spikes', your red blood cells get a little more sugar coated. This is measured as glycosylated haemoglobin, meaning sugar-coated red blood cells. This is also called HbA1c and is an example of an AGE – a messed-up molecule that can cause immense damage. If your blood level is above 7 per cent you'll be diagnosed with diabetes.

Ideally, you want your 'fasting' blood sugar level to be below 6, your 'after a meal' blood sugar level to be below 7 and your glycosylated haemoglobin to be as low as possible, and certainly below 6.3 per cent.[25] The healthiest people have a glycosylated haemoglobin of between 4 per cent and 5 per cent. You can test your own glycosylated haemoglobin – which is the most sensitive indicator of where you are at on the road to diabetes – using a simple home-test kit (see Resources).

A tale of two diabetics

To make all this real let's look at the case of a recently diagnosed diabetic on standard diabetic medication, and a long-term diabetic, injecting insulin.

Kyra, aged 37, was diagnosed with diabetes in January 2007. Kyra's fasting glucose level was 11 (it should be below 6), and her glycosylated haemoglobin level was 7.8 (it should be below 6.3). She was overweight, weighing in at 114kg (18st.). She was prescribed the drug Metformin, 500mg, twice a day, by her GP who told her she would remain on the drug for the rest of her life. Metformin improves your sensitivity to insulin.

Kyra was referred to a diabetes specialist, and a dietician who recommended a low-fat, low-sugar, low-calorie diet, limiting fruit to no more than five portions per day. The dietician told her to stop eating pumpkin seeds because they are 'high in fat' (in animal studies pumpkin extracts help to stabilise insulin levels[26]) and to drink diet cola instead of cola.

Kyra didn't like the idea of being on drugs for the rest of her life. Her diabetes specialist told her that diabetes was reversible with diet and exercise and, if she did manage to get her blood sugar below 6 for a week, she could halve her Metformin drug dose, and if it was then consistently below 6 she could stop the medication. (Metformin, also called Glucophage, is one of the best anti-diabetes drugs, but many people do get side effects and it can knock out vitamin B_{12} and raise homocysteine levels.[27] This, in turn, increases the risk of heart disease.) The drug did help lower her blood sugar to an average of 7 and she followed the conventional low-fat, low-calorie diet, cutting down her sugar intake, and started walking every day.

She came to see me in April and had done well, losing 6.3kg (1st.) in under three months, but she still suffered from low energy, dizziness, mood swings and digestive complaints. She went on my low-GL diet, and started supplementing chromium, 600mcg, cinnamon, vitamin C and a high-potency multivitamin. Within days her blood sugar was normal and, three weeks later she didn't need medication. Six weeks after starting my low-GL diet her blood sugar level was normal (averaging 5.5), and glycosylated haemoglobin was normal (6.2 per cent), without medication, and she had lost another 6.3kg (1st.) in weight. Kyra was delighted:

(*My doctor told me I'd be on medication for the rest of my life. I am really thrilled to have been able to come off medication and still have a stable blood sugar. My energy is much better. My skin is clearer, mood more stable and I've lost 14lb. I feel in control of food instead of it being in control of me.*)

One year later she's lost another 6.3kg (1st.), so she's 19kg (3st.) lighter since her diagnosis. Her glycosylated haemoglobin is 5.2 per cent, which is perfect, and blood glucose now averages 5. She still has no sugar cravings, but enjoys good energy and mood. She's cut back on the chromium and now takes 200mcg. Her doctor is delighted.

But what if you've suffered from diabetes for years, and need insulin to control it? Can a low-GL diet still reverse it? Hannemor, a nurse in Norway, is a case in point.

Hannemor started gaining weight in her thirties, from 60kg (9st. 6lb) to 75kg (11st. 11lb). She followed official nutritional recommendations and did not overeat but, year on year, continued to gain weight. In 1992, at the age of 61, she was diagnosed with type-2 diabetes, hypertension and low thyroid, and weighed 120kg (18¾st.). Her blood sugar was out of control and her glycosylated haemoglobin was 8.9 per cent. She was treated with a cocktail of drugs and ended up injecting 150 units of insulin a day. But, despite all this, her weight continued to increase, so she decided she had to do something different. She sought the advice of diabetes expert Dr Fedon Lindberg in Norway, who put her on a strict low-GL diet and exercise regime. To cut a long story short, today she needs no insulin, takes no medication, has a normal blood sugar and glycosylated haemoglobin and her weight has stabilised below 80kg (12½st.). Her story was published in the *Norwegian Journal of Medicine*.[28]

The dangers of insulin

The likely reason why Hannemor's weight continued to increase on insulin is that insulin's job is to store excess sugar in the blood as fat. So, having too much insulin actually promotes weight gain. The antidote is a low-GL diet. The higher your insulin the more effective a low-GL diet is.[29] By following my low-GL diet your blood sugar level is naturally more even, so your body doesn't have to produce so much insulin.

There's another problem with making, or injecting, too much insulin: it increases cholesterol production in the liver, it constricts blood vessels making your blood pressure go up and it stimulates the release of dangerous fats called triglycerides. So it's bad news for heart disease. Eating a low-GL diet lowers both insulin levels and cholesterol in diabetics.[30]

Some diabetes drugs, called sulfonylureas (brands include Amaryl, Euglucon and Diamicron), are designed to stimulate the beta cells in the pancreas to produce more insulin. Most type-2 diabetics produce too much insulin already – the problem is that the insulin that's produced just does not function properly. It makes little sense, stimulating the pancreas to produce even more in order to accommodate the very same poor dietary choices that lead to the development of diabetes in the first place. These drugs also increase the risk of death from cardiovascular disease, according to a five-year study of 5,500 diabetics, published in 2006 in the *Canadian Medical Association Journal*. The higher the drug dose and the more consistently the patients took the drugs, the greater the risk of cardiovascular death.[31] When you get your diet right, these drugs often become unnecessary.

In fact, a major government-funded study in the US, testing the effects of aggressive drug strategies to lower blood sugar levels in more than 10,000 diabetics, had to be abandoned due to much higher cardiovascular deaths.[32] The newspapers were full of medical experts who were 'shocked' by these results. But actually, they're nothing new.

Back in 1970 a similar study on diabetic drugs versus placebos had to be abandoned early due to more than double the cardiovascular deaths in those on the drugs.[33]

Instead of trying to cheat the system by stimulating more insulin release, the solution for weight gain, diabetes and heart disease is to eat a low-GL diet. As a result you'll need less insulin to keep your blood sugar level stable, and you'll improve your sensitivity to insulin naturally so that you need less to get the job done (more on how to do this in a minute). One study testing the effects of a low-GL, versus a high-GL and a high-fat diet, of equal calories, found that the low-GL diet improved insulin sensitivity much better than the other diets.

Diabetes can be controlled, reversed and prevented by following my low-GL diet. If you've been told that diet doesn't make that big a difference to diabetes that's because most of the studies in the past have been putting people on the wrong kind of diets: low in fat, rather than specifically low GL.

Even so, the combination of diet improvement and exercise outperforms drug treatment alone. Persuading a large number of people to change their diet, and to exercise, isn't easy but a good attempt was made by researchers at George Washington University in Washington DC, who published their findings in 2005. The team selected volunteers who had signs of glucose intolerance and were therefore at high risk of developing diabetes, then split them into three groups. One received placebos, the next 850mg of Metformin twice a day, and the third began to make lifestyle changes designed to lower weight by 7 per cent, including 2½ hours of exercise a week (20 minutes a day). At the end of three years, among those who made the lifestyle changes, 41 per cent were no longer glucose intolerant. Among those who took Metformin, 17 per cent were no longer glucose intolerant, compared to the placebo. So the lifestyle change was more than twice as effective.[34] And you don't have to wait long. One trial found significant changes, consistent with reversing diabetes, in three weeks with an improved diet and exercise.[35]

What's more, despite the prevailing medical view, the dietary approach is likely to be more cost-effective. Based on the data from a massive diabetes prevention programme launched in the US in 2002, Dr William Herman, professor of internal medicine at the University of Michigan School of Medicine, built a computer simulation to estimate the cost-effectiveness of changing one's lifestyle versus taking diabetes drugs.[36] He showed that taking Metformin might delay the onset of diabetes by three years, whereas a change in diet and exercise delays it by 11 years. His team estimated that the drug would cost $29,000 per year of healthy life saved, while the diet and exercise regime would cost $8,800. 'The bottom line,' says Herman, 'is that lifestyle intervention is more cost-effective than a pill.'

Exercise is a vital piece of the prevention equation. A review of 14 good-quality trials found that, although exercise alone did not decrease weight, it did lower glycosylated haemoglobin by the kind of amount one might expect from a drug.[37] As your energy goes up on my low-GL diet you'll find that so too does your desire to exercise.

Low-fat diets don't work as well as low-GL diets for diabetes

According to diabetes expert Professor Charles Clark, author of *Diabetes Revolution* (Vermilion): 'There is a simple cure for the obesity and diabetes epidemic but everyone is looking in the wrong place. We blame overeating or fat consumption, but the real villain in both diabetes and obesity is the large amount of refined carbohydrates we eat. It's this that pushes up our blood sugar levels and leads to diabetes. Meanwhile, our bodies store the extra blood sugar as fat and so we put on weight.'

Not only does this make sense but also it's supported by so much science that it's time to bury the low-fat, low-calorie diet myth once and for all. Before we look at the evidence, there are two kinds of studies to consider. First there are 'prospective' surveys, where people's diets are analysed over a period of years, and the incidents of diabetes are recorded and then compared to various dietary factors. Then there are 'intervention' studies where people are put on specific diets and their risk of developing diabetes, or perhaps their blood sugar or glycosylated haemoglobin levels are measured, to see which diet works the best.

For example, two recent prospective studies found that following a low-fat diet didn't decrease the risk of diabetes, but having a high intake of sugar increased risk.[38] And in China, a study involving over 64,000 people, found that the higher the GL of a person's diet the higher was their risk of diabetes.[39] In Japan, it was found that the higher the GL the higher were markers for diabetes risk, such as glucose and glycosylated haemoglobin levels.[40] And in Australia it was found that eating more vegetables and low-GL foods cuts diabetes risk by a quarter.[41]

What is more, in the US 85,059 women were monitored over 20 years and it was concluded that those who ate less carbohydrate and got most of their fat and protein from vegetable sources were at less risk of developing diabetes. The low-carbohydrate diets were better than low-fat diets in preventing diabetes. The low-carbohydrate diet is the equivalent of my low-GL diet and is yet more evidence that this is the best choice for preventing diabetes.[42]

An interesting comparison of different diets was investigated and published in 2008 in the *New England Journal of Medicine*. Volunteers were put on to one of three diets: a conventional low-calorie, low-fat diet; a Mediterranean diet, restricted in calories and high in fibre and monounsaturated fats; and a high-protein, high-fat, low-carb diet, similar to the Atkins Diet, but emphasising vegetarian sources of protein rather than meat and dairy products.[43] The low-fat diet was the least effective for weight loss. The Mediterranean diet was the most effective for diabetes, and significantly lowered glucose levels in diabetics.

As we've discussed before, there are two ways of lowering the sugar load on your body. One is a low-carb diet, high in protein and fat. This is more akin to the Atkins Diet. While there are dangers with this extreme kind of diet (see page 402) it is, technically, a low-GL diet because it is very low in carbohydrate. It also works for reducing diabetes indicators and risk.[44]

The other is a more Mediterranean-style diet rich in olive oil, grains, fruits, nuts, vegetables and fish, but low in meat, dairy products and alcohol. This is also low GL because the kind of carbohydrates eaten release their sugar content slowly. Again, there are plenty of studies showing the health benefits of a Mediterranean diet on diabetes, heart disease, health and weight. For example, a study in Spain tracked the diets of 13,000 people over four and a half years. Those who most closely followed the principles of the Mediterranean diet cut their risk of developing diabetes by 83 per cent.[45] But weight loss isn't always that spectacular, partly because, even though the foods eaten are all low-GL you can still eat too many of them. As I pointed out previously, one of the key factors in the healthy Mediterranean lifestyle of old was walking, so eating large quantities of food wasn't a problem. The average citizen of Crete would walk seven miles a day. Today, Greece is one of five countries in Europe who have a greater percentage of obese men than America. The quantity of food may not have changed so much, but the amount of exercise certainly has.

My low-GL diet offers the best of both worlds, because it gives you a simple way to control the total GL of your diet (by limiting the amount of carbohydrates you eat and making sure you eat the kind of foods that contain slow-releasing carbohydrates) and it incorporates all the key principles that will help you stabilise your blood sugar, lose sugar cravings and increase your energy. And it has none of the downsides of diets high in animal protein.

A recent issue of the *British Medical Journal* stated that 'taking prescription drugs (glitazones) to prevent diabetes cannot be justified',[46] favouring instead a diet-and-lifestyle approach. With close to £1 billion spent on diabetes drugs per year, this inexpensive, natural approach might help save a lot of lives and money. By 2010 one in six people over 40 are expected to have diabetes, at a cost of 10 per cent of the UK's National Health budget.

Supplements that work

As well as following my low-GL diet, I recommend supplementing your diet with the essential mineral chromium, vitamin C and the spice cinnamon. In fact, these all help to keep your blood sugar level even, and assist weight control even if you don't have diabetes. I'll tell you more about supplements that assist weight loss in Chapter 16.

Chromium helps stabilise your blood sugar

Over a dozen studies now confirm that 400mcg to 600mcg of chromium a day, which is more than ten times the average intake in the British diet, helps stabilise blood sugar. In some studies this non-toxic mineral, which is widely available in health-food shops, has reversed diabetes. Chromium works by improving the sensitivity to insulin, the hormone that controls blood sugar levels. Insulin resistance is the first indication of pre-diabetes, and is thought to affect one in four people in Britain, and over 90 per cent of obese people.

Studies have shown that low chromium intake in the diet is associated with an increased prevalence of type-2 (adult onset) diabetes. The average diet provides about 30mcg from wholefoods. The more refined foods and sugar you eat the worse your chromium intake.

A landmark study in 1997 looked at 120 Chinese patients with type-2 diabetes, 60 of whom were given 200µg chromium per day and 60 of whom were given 1,000µg/day. After just two months, significant improvements were seen in glucose control, in both groups. After four months, there was almost a 30 per cent reduction in glucose levels in the higher dosage group.[47] In fact chromium has been shown to dramatically decrease the need for medication in many diabetics and in some cases to eliminate the need for drugs completely.[48]

A larger study in 1999 followed over 800 diabetics who were taking insulin or anti-hyperglycemic drugs.[49] The patients were given 500mcg chromium per day for ten months, and, as you can see from the chart below, there was a major improvement in both fasting blood sugar levels and blood sugar levels after meals. It also decreased the incidence of diabetes symptoms, including fatigue, thirst and frequent urination in 90 per cent of patients.

A 2007 review of over 40 randomised controlled trials found that giving type-2 diabetics chromium improves their fasting blood sugar levels and also decreases glycosylated haemoglobin levels. The study, published in *Diabetes Care*, found that the best effects were seen with chromium in doses of 400–1,000mcg per day.[50] Despite being about ten times higher than you would get from a so-called well-balanced diet there are no known adverse effects of supplementation below 10,000mcg a day, according the UK's Committee on Toxicity.[51]

The time taken for the effects of chromium supplementation to be seen is not so clear, although a study of elderly patients with diabetes reported decreased fasting glucose levels after just three weeks.[52]

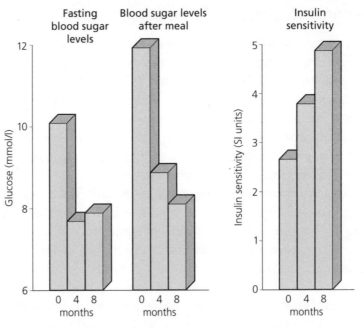

The effects of chromium on blood sugar and insulin resistance

Another point of consideration is the dosage of chromium required to see significant results. The majority of studies showing improvements in glucose control have used quantities of over 400μg per day, although improvements in insulin sensitivity were seen in patients taking just 200μg per day in two studies.[53] Most available chromium supplements are 200μg, but in relation to diabetes, a daily intake of 400 to 600mcg is most likely to be effective. I've not found it necessary to have more than this. I recommend taking chromium in the morning and at lunch. It can be overstimulating if taken in the evening – not so good if you have difficulty sleeping.

There is some debate about the best form of chromium. Is it chromium picolinate, or chromium polynicotinate? (Chromium polynicotinate contains vitamin B_3, which works in synergy with chromium.) Both appear to be effective and better than chromium chloride, used in some cheaper supplements.

High levels of vitamin C more than halves diabetes risk

Another important vitamin for people with diabetes is vitamin C. Having a high level of vitamin C in your blood, consistent with that achieved by supplementation *and* eating a diet high in fruit and vegetables, reduces your risk of diabetes by 62 per cent. That's the conclusion of a study of over 21,000 people over a 12-year period, published in the *Archives of Internal Medicine*.[54] Those in the top fifth of plasma vitamin C levels were 62 per cent less likely to develop diabetes, compared to those in the bottom fifth. The greater a person's vitamin C levels the lesser was their risk. This relationship was much stronger than the relationship between their intake of fruit and vegetables – those eating the highest amount of fruit and vegetables alone (i.e. no supplementation) reduced their diabetes risk by 22 per cent. The lead author, Anne-Helen Harding from Addenbrooke's Hospital in Cambridge, said, 'The strong independent association observed in this prospective study, together with biological plausibility, provides persuasive evidence of a beneficial effect of vitamin C and fruit and vegetable intake on diabetes risk.' The researchers state that vitamin C's antioxidant properties may be specifically protective against diabetes.

The plasma level of vitamin C needed to induce this risk reduction was above 1.1mg/dl for men and 1.29mg/dl for women. Those who supplement 1g a day have, on average, a level of 1.62mg/dl, whereas those who take a basic multivitamin, usually containing 60–80mg of vitamin C, have a level of 0.94mg/dl, compared to those who do not take supplements, who average 0.66mg/dl.

One study in India gave diabetics either 500mg or 1,000mg of vitamin C. Only those taking 1,000mg of vitamin C a day had a significant decrease in both their blood sugar levels, and glycosylated haemoglobin.[55]

Therefore, my advice is to cover all bases and eat plenty of fruit and vegetables, which are a cornerstone of my low-GL diet, and also supplement 1g (1,000mg) of vitamin C every day.

A spoonful of cinnamon

Cinnamon is a safe and inexpensive aromatic spice, which has been used for many years in traditional herbal medicine for treatment of type-2 diabetes. The active ingredient in cinnamon, MCHP, mimics the action of the hormone insulin, which removes excess sugar from the bloodstream.

Animal studies have found that there is a positive effect on blood sugar levels when treated with cinnamon. A study in 2005 found that following a high-sugar meal, cinnamon reduced blood sugar and increased insulin levels for up to 30 minutes.[56]

Another animal study found that after just two weeks of cinnamon administration, there were positive effects on fat levels and blood sugar levels, and after six weeks insulin levels and 'good' HDL cholesterol had also increased.[57]

There have also been positive findings in human studies. For example, a research group found that when pre-diabetics were given a cinnamon extract called Cinnulin® for 12 weeks, there were improvements in several features of the metabolic syndrome (blood sugar levels, blood pressure and body fat percentage).[58] Another recent study on people with diabetes found similar results. Thirty-nine patients who were given cinnamon extract for four months showed a substantial reduction in blood sugar levels taken after a meal and a 10 per cent reduction in blood sugar levels taken after fasting. Interestingly, diabetics with the poorest blood glucose control showed the biggest improvements with cinnamon.

Another study in 2003 gave people with diabetes 1g, 3g or 6g of cinnamon per day.[59] (One gram is about half a teaspoon.) All responded to the cinnamon within weeks, with blood sugar levels 20 per cent lower on average than those of a control group. Some of the volunteers taking cinnamon even achieved normal blood sugar levels. Tellingly, blood sugar started creeping up again after the diabetics stopped taking cinnamon. Not all studies, however, have shown a positive result. The jury is still out.

Based on these results you might want to add half a teaspoon of cinnamon, which is also an excellent antioxidant, to your diet. Alternatively, supplement a cinnamon extract such as Cinnulin, which has a high concentration of MHCP, the active ingredient. In this case 500mg is sufficient.

Daily exercise is vital too

Exercise is a vital piece of the equation for reversing diabetes.[60] Exercising daily stabilises your blood sugar levels, lowering glycosylated haemoglobin, even if you don't lose weight, and cutting your risk of both diabetes and heart disease. The combination of exercise and a low-GL diet is a winning formula. But many people don't exercise because they feel too tired. The good news is that following my low-GL diet gives you the energy to get you going on a regular exercise routine. See Chapter 17 for more on exercise. For diabetes reversal I recommend the equivalent of 30 minutes exercise every day.

In summary, whether you have type-1 (insulin-dependent) or type-2 diabetes, by following a low-GL diet you minimise your body's need to produce insulin. Remember:

- Follow my low-GL diet strictly.

- Supplement 400–600mcg of chromium daily.

- Supplement 1g of vitamin C daily.

- Have half a teaspoon of cinnamon daily.

- Exercise daily.

Bear in mind that your need for medication may decrease, so it is important to monitor your blood sugar levels and inform your primary care practitioner accordingly. If you have type-2 diabetes, there's a good chance you'll end up not needing any medication. If you have type-1 (insulin-dependent) diabetes, the same recommendations apply, but you'll still need insulin, although possibly less of it.

I recommend you start the diet first, together with 1g of vitamin C and a good multivitamin (usually taken twice a day). Then, three days later add a supplement of 200mcg of chromium. Then, three days later increase this to 400mcg, and three days later increase it to 600mcg while monitoring your blood sugar levels.

Linda B and Adrian L are cases that illustrate this point. Linda's whole family started the Holford Diet.

❝ *When we first started I thought it would be difficult. The thought of cooking three meals a day with all these new foods was daunting. But it's been so easy. We used to be total chocoholics, eating sweets and chocolate every day. None of us have eaten any chocolate or sweets since the diet. It's a miracle. We've had no cravings. I would never have believed this is possible. It's quite unbelievable. My daughter, who loses weight very slowly, has lost between 5kg [11lb] and 6kg [13¼lb], I've lost 7.5kg [16½lb]; my husband has lost 8kg [1¼st.] and my son, who is not so overweight, has lost 5kg [11lb] all in the last six weeks. The other thing is the energy. I was permanently tired. I could have spent the whole day in bed. Now my energy level is incredible. My blood sugar is well under control (I'm diabetic) and I've been able to halve my medication. It's been so easy.* ❞

Linda was taking a sulfonylurea drug and Metformin. Within days of following the diet the sulfonylurea drug, which lowers blood sugar, became unnecessary. In fact, the drug lowered her now-stable blood sugar too much, so her doctor advised her to stop taking it.

Adrian, a chef, had followed every diet that's ever come out and, year after year, he gained weight – until he reached a little over 145kg (22st. 11lb). A medical check-up identified that he had diabetes with a glucose level of 19.8. His doctor advised the Holford Diet and, six weeks later, he had normal blood sugar levels.

❝ *My doctor advised the Holford Diet. I am a totally changed person. I feel incredible … I've lost 38kg [6st.] in six months and 10in [25cm] off my belly. I'm meant to take Metformin every day, but most of the time I forget to take it. After a month on the diet my blood sugar was stable – never above 6. Generally, it ranges from a normal 4.2–5.5. It's amazing. It's totally changed my life.* ❞

Adrian then started taking cinnamon and chromium and now no longer needs any medication.

Diabetes (type-2) is not only controllable but it is also reversible by following my low-GL diet.

11

Lower your Cholesterol and Blood Pressure and Prevent Heart Disease

You may be surprised to discover that the best way to lower your risk of heart disease is to eat a low-GL diet. One of the most enduring myths about heart disease is that it is caused by eating too much fat and cholesterol, and the way to reverse it is to eat a low-fat, low-cholesterol diet, and take cholesterol-lowering drugs. This is wrong.

Although it is true that having a very high cholesterol level increases your risk of heart disease, this has nothing to do with eating cholesterol. The body makes its own. Eggs are one of the richest sources of cholesterol and, for the past 30 years I've hunted for studies to show that eating eggs increases either your blood cholesterol or your risk for heart disease. I can't find any. For example, a recent study involving over 21,000 participants concludes, 'Egg consumption was not associated with incident MI [Myocardial Infarct = heart attack] or stroke.' This was true even in those with already high cholesterol levels. There was a hint of an increased risk in diabetics eating seven or more eggs a week.[61] Many other studies show the same thing: eggs neither raise your risk for heart disease nor raise blood cholesterol.[62] In contrast, another study shows that having two eggs for breakfast, which is one of the low-GL breakfasts in this diet, promotes weight loss compared to eating a carbohydrate-based breakfast such as a bagel or toast.[63] I recommend you eat four to six eggs a week on the Holford Diet. They are positively good for you.

What many scientists are starting to realise is that a high blood cholesterol level is a marker, not the cause, of heart disease.[64] One of the best ways to lower your risk of heart disease, and to normalise cholesterol and high blood pressure, is to follow my low-GL diet. Another is to reduce your stress level.

Andrew, from Dublin, is a case in point. His cholesterol measured 8.8 mmol/l. (It's apparently meant to be below 5 mmol/l, although many heart experts think that this cut-off point is too low.) He was put on cholesterol-lowering drugs called statins and, six months later, his cholesterol was 8.7. The lack of response plus unpleasant side effects – which are experienced by many people on statins – led him to stop. He described himself as very stressed and tired. He had five coffees a day to keep himself going and found it hard to relax in the evening and would have a couple of drinks. He was also gaining weight and not sleeping well.

He heard me on television asking for a volunteer with high cholesterol for a three-week experiment and rang up the television station. I put him on my low-GL diet and recommended certain supplements. Three weeks later we met at the TV station for the 'reveal'. He had lost 4.5kg (10lb), his energy levels were great, he no longer felt stressed and he was sleeping much better. We then tested his cholesterol and it had dropped to a healthy 4.9!

Keeping your blood sugar level even not only helps you lose weight but it also gives you more energy and makes you less stressed. That's because blood sugar peaks and troughs trigger adrenal hormones. These make you more likely to react stressfully, and also promote the body's equivalent of stress, which is called inflammation. Inflammation, in turn, leads to heart disease.

The rapid transformation in Andrew might sound amazing, but I hear it all the time. Like the lady I met recently who went to her doctor for a check-up and was told she had high blood pressure and cholesterol and would need to take cholesterol-lowering statins and blood pressure drugs. She didn't want to take drugs for the rest of her life.

> *My doctor told me that if it wasn't reduced within about eight weeks, I would have to go on statins and blood-pressure tablets. After going to the nurse for six weeks, nothing was happening and I decided to take control and to go on a diet. So I joined Zest4Life [which is our low-GL weight-loss club – see www.zest4life.eu]. Within ten weeks I lost 26lb [10.4kg]. I returned to the doctor who tested my blood pressure and sent me for a cholesterol test, both of which were lowered, and the result is that I do not need to go on the statins!*

Before I show you the evidence that proves why my low-GL diet is the perfect way to prevent and reverse heart disease, let's examine the whole cholesterol story in more detail.

The great cholesterol swindle

It all started in 1913 when a Russian scientist called Anitischkov fed rabbits a high-cholesterol diet and they developed arterial blockages full of cholesterol and died. Rabbits eat grass, not cholesterol, and have no way to process it. The same does not apply to humans. However, thus began almost 100 years of misinformation about cholesterol.

Here are some facts that may surprise you:

- Eating cholesterol doesn't raise cholesterol.

- Eating fat doesn't raise cholesterol.

- Eating cholesterol and fat don't increase heart-disease risk.

- Having too low a cholesterol level (below 4 mmol/l) is as dangerous as being too high (above 6 mmol/l).

- The current guideline that deems a person with a cholesterol level above 5 as worthy of a lifetime of taking statin drugs is more to do with money than science.

- Statin drugs, designed to lower cholesterol, generated $20 billion in sales last year.

- Statins don't reduce mortality if given to healthy people.

- They do reduce the risk of another heart attack in men who have had a heart attack.

- They don't significantly reduce risk in women who haven't had a cardiovascular event.

- Stroke risk isn't predicted by a high cholesterol level. In fact, having a low cholesterol level is more predictive.

'I think we have been sold a pup. A rather large pup – more of a full-grown blue whale, in fact,' says Dr Malcolm Kendrick, cardiology expert and author of *The Cholesterol Con*, an eloquent exposé of the cholesterol myth.

Although statin drugs do reduce the risk of a second heart attack, Dr Kendrick doesn't think it has anything to do with their cholesterol-lowering effect. They probably reduce inflammation, which is what really causes heart disease. The fact that statin drugs will lower your cholesterol is a no-brainer because they block its normal production in the liver. Since cholesterol is a vital substance – for example, for the brain and nerves, and for making hormones – if the liver can't make it, it will suck whatever cholesterol there is out of the blood.

Statins lower cholesterol by blocking an enzyme vital for its production. The trouble is that that enzyme also makes a vital antioxidant called co-enzyme Q_{10} (CoQ_{10}), inducing deficiency. This results in a whole host of side effects, especially muscle weakness and heart-muscle problems, experienced by one in two people. The risk of inducing CoQ_{10} deficiency is now a mandatory warning on packets of statins in Canada. Supplementing CoQ_{10} at a daily dose of 90mg does mitigate some of the side effects. In any event, taking statins is a red herring. It's a bit like covering up the red light that's flashing in your car to tell you something is wrong. Instead, you have to find out what's causing the red light to flash – or the high cholesterol.

So what *does* reduce heart-disease risk? Reducing stress, increasing omega-3 fats, a low-GL diet, more magnesium (itself depleted by stress), less nicotine and probably less caffeine, taking B vitamins (which lower homocysteine), vitamin C and high-dose niacin, plus stress-reducing exercise. That's it in a nutshell and most of these are part of my Holford Diet recommendations.

Niacin (B_3) is particularly useful if you have high cholesterol. Niacin, at 1,000mg a day, will normalise excessively high cholesterol and raise HDL (the 'good' kind of cholesterol) levels much more effectively than statins, but, like statins, may reduce heart-disease risk by other mechanisms. (I think high cholesterol and low HDL is an indicator of risk, but probably not the cause of the risk. Low-GL diets also tend to normalise these.) The other key factor that lowers heart-disease risk is omega-3 fish oils (see Chapter 14 for more on this).

The whole cholesterol scenario is quite fascinating, because having a high cholesterol level has become a 'disease' in its own right. In other words, you could be perfectly healthy, visit your doctor for a check-up, and leave with a disease you never knew you had, and a prescription for a statin drug. The doctor benefits financially from testing and treating you, the drug company obviously benefits, but whether *you* do is dubious. The latest recommendation from the American Academy of Pediatrics is to test all eight-year-old children, and prescribe statins accordingly![65]

Why a low-GL diet is good for your heart

As we saw with Andrew, you can lower your cholesterol quickly, and cut your risk of heart disease, simply by following my low-GL-diet principles. That's what researchers at the Harvard School of Public Health found in a massive survey of the dietary habits and health risks of 82,802 women and during 20 years of follow up. Their study showed that a high-GL diet almost doubles (to 95 per cent) the risk of heart disease compared to a low-GL diet.[66] They also found that diets that provide more protein from vegetable sources – as does the Holford Diet – lower cardiovascular risk. This confirms an earlier study involving 75,000 nurses in which those with a high-GL diet doubled their risk of heart disease.[67]

When you go for a check-up you're likely to get your blood pressure measured and, if you have a blood test, it'll test your triglycerides, which is the fat level in your blood, and your cholesterol. You may get a score for your total cholesterol, as well as your HDL and LDL cholesterol. HDL is nicknamed 'good' cholesterol and LDL 'bad' cholesterol. So, you want low triglycerides, low total cholesterol with a high HDL and low LDL. One of the best indicators of low heart-disease risk is having a low total cholesterol/HDL ratio. For example, if your cholesterol is 5 and your HDL is 2.5 that's 5/2.5 = 2. If your cholesterol/HDL ratio is 3 or less, meaning one third or more of your total cholesterol is HDL cholesterol, this equates to low risk. You also want low blood pressure.

By 2002 there were ten good-quality trials showing that eating low-GL foods alone will lower your cholesterol, especially the 'bad' LDL cholesterol, and triglycerides.[68] More recently, a comprehensive review, published by the Cochrane Library in 2007, concluded that, 'Overweight or obese people lost more weight on a low Glycaemic Load diet and had more improvement in lipid profiles than those receiving conventional (low-fat, low-calorie) diets.' [69] Bad, LDL, cholesterol went down, and good, HDL, cholesterol went up.

This is a consistent finding in every study testing the effects of low-GL diets. For example, a study testing the effects of a low-GL diet versus a conventional low-calorie, low-fat diet on cardiovascular risk factors in obese young adults over a year reported that those on the low-GL diet had a significant decrease in their triglyceride levels, and the greatest decrease in LDL cholesterol, and increase in HDL cholesterol.[70]

Contrary to perceived wisdom, Atkins-style high-protein, high-fat, low-carb diets (which are also low-GL) do also lower cholesterol and heart-disease risk more than conventional low-fat diets. But not as well as low-GL diets that contain more carbohydrates, provided those carbs are the right slow-releasing kind. One study compared this kind of diet with a high-protein, low-carb diet and it significantly lowered total cholesterol and the undesirable LDL cholesterol more than the high-protein, low-carb diets. It also produced the greatest fat loss.[71]

One of the hidden benefits of my low-GL diet is that it's naturally high in soluble fibres found in foods such as oats and vegetables, as well as plant sterols, which are found in beans, lentils, nuts and seeds. Both soluble fibres[72] and plant sterols[73] are known to lower cholesterol. David Jenkins, who invented the Glycemic Index, devised an interesting study, published in the *American Journal of Clinical Nutrition*, to test which works better – diet or drugs.

He put 34 patients with high cholesterol on three types of diet, each one for a month, although they were assigned in random order. The diets were: a low-fat diet; a low-fat diet plus statins; and a diet high in plant sterols. On the high-plant-sterol diet, the participants ate the equivalent of 2.5g of plant sterols, in:

- 50g of soya (a glass of soya milk, or a small serving of tofu, or a small soya burger)

- 35g of almonds (a small handful of almonds)

- 25g of soluble fibre from oats and vegetables (the equivalent of five oatcakes, plus a bowl of oats and three servings of vegetables).

Both the statins diet and the plant-sterol diet significantly lowered LDL cholesterol to the same degree, but nine of the volunteers (26 per cent), achieved their lowest LDL cholesterol while on the plant-sterol diet, not the statins.[74]

In the words of Professor David Jenkins, 'People interested in lowering their cholesterol should probably acquire a taste for tofu and oatmeal.' My low-GL diet contains these and other foods rich in soluble fibres and plant sterols.

Lower your blood pressure

High blood pressure is one of the top risk factors for heart disease and stroke. It has been linked with 50 per cent of coronary artery disease, 75 per cent of strokes, and it kills over 110,000 people in England every year. A high-GL diet raises insulin levels, which then stimulate the sympathetic nervous system, the one that primes you for action, which in turn releases chemicals that tighten the arteries. Too much insulin also encourages the body to hold on to salt and water, which also raises blood pressure.[75] To avoid the blood-pressure-raising potential of sugar and other refined carbohydrates, the best option is a low-GL diet. In a trial we ran on 16 volunteers, blood pressure dropped by six points in eight weeks on my low-GL diet.[76] There's also evidence that plant sterols in soya, also found in other beans, lentils, nuts and seeds, lower your blood pressure.[77]

So, if it's a low-cholesterol, low blood pressure and low-heart-disease risk you are after, you can do no better than my low-GL diet. It's also high in antioxidants and essential omega-3 fats. The National Heart Forum estimate that if you could normalise your cholesterol and blood pressure, do some exercise on a regular basis, quit smoking and lose weight, that alone would reduce your risk by almost a third. [78] Couple this with the many benefits of my low-GL diet, plus supplementing with a multivitamin containing antioxidants including vitamin E, homocysteine-lowering B vitamins, plus an extra 1g of vitamin C and daily exercise, and there's a good chance you could eradicate your risk completely.

12

Other Benefits

A healthy diet and lifestyle helps the body fight disease. The Holford Diet is rich in antioxidants and essential fats, and low in damaging fats and meat, making it the ideal diet for protection against diet-related illnesses such as some forms of cancer and arthritis.

Cancer – the link to diet and lifestyle

Most people are still not aware that the primary risk factor for cancer is diet. When the World Cancer Research Fund examined more than 5,000 studies on diet and cancer, they concluded that you could halve the risk of cancer by changing your diet.[79]

Many people mistakenly think that cancer is largely genetic. It isn't, and the following study, which involved 45,000 pairs of twins, will show you why I can say this with confidence.

This study, published in the *New England Journal of Medicine*, looked at whether people with the same genes had the same risk of cancer. What they found was that cancer is more likely to be caused by diet and lifestyle choices than by genes. Identical twins, who are genetically the same, had no more than 15 per cent chance of developing the same cancer. This suggests that the cause of most cancers is about 85 per cent environmental – that is, down to factors such as diet, lifestyle and exposure to toxic chemicals. This study concluded that an unhealthy diet, smoking and a lack of exercise accounted for up to 82 per cent of cancers studied.[80]

But what's emerging is that the best kind of diet for minimising cancer risk is a low-GL diet, high in antioxidants, with more vegetarian sources of protein and less meat and dairy products. To understand why, we need to understand a little bit about cancer.

To some extent you can divide cancer into two kinds. First, there are cancers of the lungs and digestive tract – oesophagus, stomach, colorectal cancer. These are strongly linked to diet, with alcohol, smoking, hot drinks and meat being the major culprits. Burnt meat is by far the worst offender. Anyone eating burned or browned meat every day is significantly increasing their risk.

The other kind are hormonal cancers, most notably breast and prostate cancer as well as ovarian cancer. All of these, and especially breast cancer, are linked to 'oestrogen dominance' and to high-GL diets, and also diets high in animal protein and dairy products. Oestrogen is the hormone that encourages the growth of hormone-sensitive tissue, including breast and uterine cells, and an excess of oestrogen signals (or a lack of progesterone, which counters the effects of oestrogen) can promote breast cancer.

Ten years ago I went public with my views on HRT, saying that it was an unacceptable risk factor for breast cancer, a view that is finally being accepted by government bodies around the world. But many women's diets are also to blame. The reason is twofold.

First, as you start to lose blood sugar balance, and become overweight and insulin-resistant, the resulting excess insulin, and what are called insulin-like growth factors (IGF), promote cancer cell growth. Then the excess body fat produces oestrogen. Yes, fat cells – not just the ovaries – produce oestrogen. This leads to a lifetime of extra exposure to oestrogen. Among postmenopausal women, both weight gain and high insulin levels are strongly associated with an increased risk of breast cancer, whereas weight loss is associated with a reduced risk.[81] That's risk number one.

Here's risk number two. Increased consumption of high-GL foods leads, as we've seen, to insulin resistance, present in the vast majority of overweight people and 25 per cent of those who are not overweight. Insulin resistance, and eating a high-GL diet, is strongly linked to polycystic ovary syndrome (PCOS). With this condition, women have more and more cycles in which they don't ovulate, and only if a woman ovulates is progesterone produced. So, oestrogen, unopposed by progesterone, can then trigger breast cancer. If you want to go deeper into this subject read my book *Say No to Cancer*, by Piatkus.

Generally, the higher your intake of sugar and high-GL foods, the higher your risk of cancer. But this is especially true for hormone-related cancers, including breast cancer,[82] especially in pre- and post-menopausal women,[83] ovarian cancer,[84] endometrial cancer,[85] thyroid cancer,[86] and prostate cancer.[87] There is also an association with colorectal cancer,[88] although not all studies agree about this.[89] Colorectal cancer is more strongly associated with a diet high in meat and alcohol, and low in vegetables. Hormonal cancers are also linked to diets high in meat and dairy, so you can see why I'm seriously concerned about the long-term consequences of millions of people following high-protein diets based on these foods as a means to lose weight.

The Holford Diet, on the other hand, is a perfect diet in all respects, not only for losing weight, but also for preventing both digestive cancers and hormonal cancers. Once again, the low-GL foods – high in antioxidants, essential fats and B vitamins – all help to keep your body fighting fit. The emphasis on fresh, organic foods wherever possible is important here, too. In fact, in all its essentials this diet matches the recommendations of the World Cancer Research Fund for reducing cancer risk. Supplementing with a good high-strength multivitamin, plus 1g or 2g of vitamin C, further boosts your body's natural immunity.

I have seen this approach not only keep thousands of women free from breast cancer, but even help to reverse the cancer in women who have it. That's what happened to Betty, who first consulted me in 1986. Here's what she says:

> ❛ *I feel moved to tell you I consulted you in 1986 with a recurrence of breast cancer. Now, 13 years later, I am pleased to tell you I have just celebrated my seventy-fifth birthday and am fit and well, taking no medication and attending no clinics. I am sure this is in large part due to the advice I received from you.* ❜

Say no to arthritis

If you've got aching joints, welcome to the club. Nine out of ten people have arthritis by the time they're 60. I want to make sure you're one of the one in ten who don't. It's a vicious circle, because once you develop aching joints you don't want to exercise, and then weight gain is just around the corner.

However, you will be pleased to hear that the principles of the Holford Diet work extremely well at repairing arthritic joints. That is because the five main causes of inflammation and damage to joints are all reversible. These are:

- Glycation, which means damage caused by sugar
- Inflammation caused by a lack of essential fats

- Too much oxidation, and not enough antioxidants

- Allergy

- Lack of joint-building minerals and nutrients such as glucosamine

Glycation is inflammation caused by glucose imbalance and insulin resistance. Glucose can damage joints in the same way that it damages arteries. That's why there is a strong link between diabetes and arthritis. Whereas ordinarily the adrenal hormone cortisol – the body's best anti-inflammatory agent – can handle such problems, out-of-control blood sugar results in adrenal exhaustion. So it's far better to restore blood sugar balance to avoid the damage in the first place. Reducing your use of stimulants such as caffeine and nicotine also helps.

The next cause of inflammation is a lack of what are called prostaglandins, the hormone-like substances made from essential fats, especially omega-3 fats. A diet high in meat and dairy, which are high in saturated fats, promotes pain and inflammation, whereas a diet high in fish and seeds, and therefore high in essential fats, reduces it. That's what the Holford Diet achieves.

Then there are free radicals, or oxidants. In much the same way that oxidants from exhaust fumes or cigarettes damage your skin, oxidants in the bloodstream damage joints. That's why a diet high in antioxidants, backed up by supplements, helps to reduce inflammation.

The final common cause of arthritis is having unidentified food allergies. John is a case in point. He could barely walk 100 yards without pain and had to go up the stairs on his hands and knees, despite being on a lot of medication. He took Yorktest's IgG allergy test and discovered he was allergic to certain foods. Once he eliminated these from his diet he began to feel less pain. He gradually reduced his medication and now needs none. He no longer experiences pain and he has regained his mobility.

Once inflammation is under control, joints can and do repair themselves. This, of course, requires a good supply of bone-building minerals such as calcium, magnesium and zinc, all abundant in wholefoods, which I recommend you eat on the Holford Diet. Seeds are an especially good source of these nutrients, as well as an excellent source of essential fats. When you put all this together with appropriate supplements, you have an incredibly powerful anti-arthritis strategy.

Take Ed. I met him after he had retired from a highly successful business career. He had the money, he had the time, but he could barely walk without experiencing pain, let alone pursue his passion for golf. I advised him on how to change his diet and what supplements to take. It took him three months to become pain-free. Here's what he said:

> ❝ *I used to have constant pain in my knees and joints, could not play golf or walk more than ten minutes without resting my legs. Since following your advice my discomfort has decreased 95–100 per cent. It is a different life when you can travel and play golf every day. I never would have believed my pain could be reduced by such a large degree, and no return, no matter how much activity in a day or week.* ❞

If you would like to find out more specifically about arthritis, I recommend you read my book *Say No to Arthritis* (Piatkus).

I know you just want to lose weight – and you will. But I hope I have convinced you that the diet you are about to start will change your life for the better. You will not only feel the benefits in the next few weeks but you will also *live* the benefits for years to come. The Holford Diet is a diet for living your life to the full. Here are the benefits:

- If you choose to eat low-GL foods that are also high in antioxidants you will improve your skin. These include berries, plums, grapefruit and oranges, as well as kale, spinach, tenderstem broccoli, beetroot, Brussels sprouts and avocados.

- You need some carbohydrate to make serotonin in the brain, which keeps you happy and reduces your appetite.

- By controlling your blood sugar and providing brain-friendly nutrients, the Holford Diet helps sharpen your memory and concentration.

- You can slow down the ageing process and extend your lifespan by following the Holford Diet because you'll be eating less quantity (calories) and more quality (optimum nutrition).

- The Holford Diet also helps to lower many vital statistics that mean a greater risk of disease, including your cholesterol, triglycerides, homocysteine and blood pressure.

- The Holford Diet helps to prevent heart disease, cancer, diabetes, Alzheimer's and arthritis and is consistent with the cutting-edge science of disease prevention through nutrition.

PART THREE

Five Simple Principles

13

Step 1: Balance Your Blood Sugar

We've seen how the key to losing weight and increasing energy is stabilising your blood sugar and insulin response to food. Now I'm going to explain the dynamics of this process so that it's crystal-clear why you are following the rules of this diet. The principles are remarkably simple, and this way of eating will become part of your daily routine very quickly.

There are four ways to stabilise your blood sugar:

1 Reduce the total amount of carbohydrates in your diet.

2 Choose low-glycemic-load (GL) carbohydrates.

3 Combine carbohydrates with protein.

4 Cut back on stimulants and stress.

Sounds great, you're thinking, but how do I put it all into practice?

The lowdown on carbohydrates

I'm going to make it really easy. As far as carbohydrates are concerned there are only two rules:

Rule 1: Eat no more than 40 Ⓖ a day.

Rule 2: At main meals, eat low-GL carbohydrates with protein-rich foods.

We've had a look at GL in Part One. If a food is high-GL, such as white bread, it will contain a lot of fast-releasing carbohydrate that will contribute to seesawing blood sugar and all the ills that leads to, such as weight gain, lethargy and insulin resistance. (Note that the figure of 40 ⓖ a day refers to what we *eat*; there's an extra of allowance of 5 ⓖ for drinks – or the occasional dessert or sweet – as discussed in Chapter 23.)

Everything I'm going to tell you in this chapter is designed to reverse this process, stabilise your blood sugar, lower your insulin release, make you more responsive to the insulin you produce and turn you into a high-energy fatburner. You'll feel better and the weight will fall away. It's a win–win situation for you and your body.

So low-GL eating is vital for health. Now we need to find out more about this crucial scoring system.

What determines GL?

How a food is processed, prepared or cooked is a key element in the GL of a food, and therefore in what it will do to your blood sugar.

In the diagram below, you can see how blood sugar levels, followed by insulin, rise and fall after eating spaghetti. As the blood glucose level rises the body produces insulin, and down it comes again.

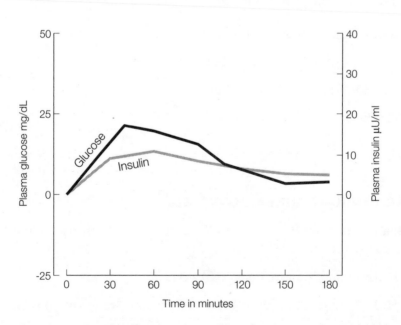

Glycemic response: spaghetti Within 40 minutes of eating spaghetti, blood sugar levels are at a maximum. The body releases insulin to help get the glucose out of the blood and into body cells. Two hours later both blood glucose and insulin levels have returned to normal.

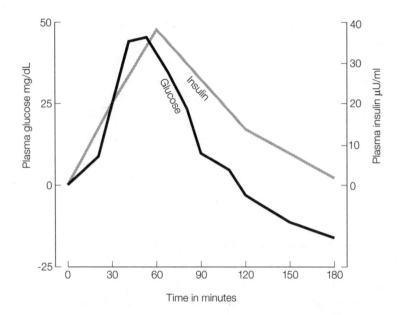

Time in minutes

Glycemic response: bread Within 40 minutes of eating bread, blood sugar levels are almost double those seen with spaghetti. The body produces more than three times as much insulin to bring blood glucose levels under control. The body overreacts and blood glucose goes too low, leading to strong cravings for something sweet or a stimulant such as caffeine.

The diagram above shows what happens when you eat white bread. Notice that the blood sugar level not only peaks twice as high when compared with the pasta, but it also dips much lower. It's the peaks that damage your arteries, making them less responsive to insulin, and the troughs that leave you tired, sleepy and craving carbohydrates or stimulants. Again, you can see a massive increase in insulin release. In fact, compared with levels for spaghetti, four times as much insulin was produced in the first two hours after eating that bread!

What's fascinating is that this particular bread and spaghetti were made from the same flour, using the same amount.[1] So the only difference is in the processing. Bread rises when you feed yeast with sugar, and it is then baked for some time. Pasta is just wheat, and perhaps some egg. It has no yeast or sugar and it isn't cooked for so long.

It's obvious that this small difference in preparation makes a big difference in blood sugar response, and hence in how much weight you put on. That's why I recommend that you eat very little bread, but you certainly don't need to give up pasta, especially if it's wholewheat as opposed to refined.

Harking back to Rule 2, it's also important *how* you eat your low-GL carbs. I'm going to recommend that you eat some fat and protein with your carbohydrate because this will lessen its low-GL score even further.

We'll be looking at the kinds of combinations that work best to lower your blood sugar in a while. But, for now, let's stick to the GL scenario, exploring which carbohydrates you can eat lots of and which you should probably avoid.

Enter the GI

It was the discovery that even quite similar foods could have very different effects on blood sugar that led to classifying foods as slow- or fast-releasing carbohydrates. The fast-releasing foods include white bread, which as we saw above are like rocket fuel, releasing their glucose in a sudden burst. They give a quick shot of energy with a rapid burnout. Slow-releasing carbohydrates such as wholewheat spaghetti supply steadier energy over a longer period of time, and thus help in balancing blood sugar levels.

But how do you know what is fast- and what is slow-releasing? This is where the GI – the glycemic index – comes in. I've already described GI in general terms but it's important to understand how the GI of a food is determined. The GI is a scale that compares the levels to which different foods raise your blood sugar with the effect of pure glucose (see the diagram opposite). It is also key in determining a food's GL.

To discover a food's GI, a portion of it providing 50g (1¾oz) of carbohydrate is eaten, and the effect on the person's blood sugar over a three-hour period is compared to the effect of eating 50g of glucose. Glucose is used for comparison as the 'reference' food, because it requires no digestion and is the fastest-releasing carbohydrate.

In the diagram opposite you can see that the curve created by eating 50g (1¾oz) of glucose is given a value of 100. If another food raises blood sugar level significantly, and for some time, the area under the curve made by glucose is bigger. Conversely, if a food hardly raises blood glucose levels at all, and only for a short time, the area under the curve is smaller. The diagram shows a comparison of an apple, which is a slow-releasing carbohydrate, with glucose. You can see that the area created by the apple's curve is valued at 39, inside the 'normal' range, whereas the curve for glucose, at 100, is well above. The amount of food tested obviously affects how high the blood sugar level will go.

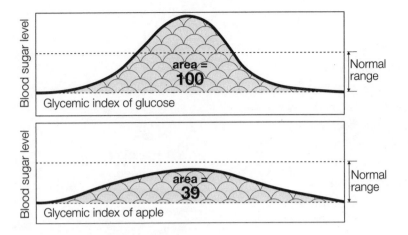

Measuring the glycemic index of a food

Below you can see the GI for a variety of foods. As I pointed out on page 73, there are some important exceptions but as a general rule, a high-GI score indicates the ones to avoid; a low-GI score, the ones to eat. As you can see, apples and oats are slow-releasing, whereas raisins and puffed-rice cereal are fast.

Glycemic index of common foods

Sugars			
Maltose	105	Grapes	46
Glucose	100	Orange	42
Sucrose (sugar)	68	Strawberries	40
Honey	55	Raspberries	40
Lactose	46	Plum	39
Fructose (fruit sugar)	19	Apple	38
Xylitol	8	Pear	38
		Grapefruit	25
		Cherries	22

Fruit			
Dates	103	**Grains and grain products**	
Watermelon	72	French baguette	95
Pineapple	59	White rice	72
Melon	65	Bagel	72
Raisins	64	Wholemeal bread	71
Kiwi fruit	53	White bread	70
Banana	52	Crumpet	69

Ryvita	64	**Dairy products**	
Pastry	59	Ice cream	61
Basmati rice	58	Yoghurt	36
Wholegrain rye bread	58	Skimmed milk	32
Brown rice	55	Whole milk	27
Brown basmati long-grain rice	47		
Instant noodles	47		
Wholegrain wheat bread	46	**Vegetables**	
White spaghetti	40	Parsnips (cooked)	97
Wholemeal spaghetti	37	Potato (baked)	85
Barley	26	French fries	75
		Beetroot (cooked)	64
Cereals		Sweet potato	61
Puffed rice	82	Potato (new, boiled)	57
Cornflakes	81	Sweetcorn	54
Shredded wheat	75	Peas	48
Weetabix	70	Carrot	47
Kellogg's Special K	69		
Porridge oats	58	**Snacks and drinks**	
Muesli	55	Lucozade	95
Kellogg's All-Bran	42	Jellybeans	80
		Fanta	68
Pulses		Squash (diluted)	66
Baked beans	48	Corn chips	63
Chickpeas	42	Muesli bar	61
Black-eyed beans	42	Potato crisps	54
Haricot beans	38	Orange juice	50
Butter beans	36	Mars Bar	49
Lentils	29	Chocolate bar	49
Kidney beans	28	Apple juice	40
Soya beans	14	Peanuts	14

So much for GI. But what's the inside story on what makes one food fast-releasing and another slow? There are two main factors.

The first is how 'complex' the carbohydrate is. The diagram opposite illustrates the chemical structure of glucose, regular white sugar and oats. You don't need to be a scientist to see that oats are more complex than sugar and sugar is more complex than glucose. All it means is that there's more *to* them.

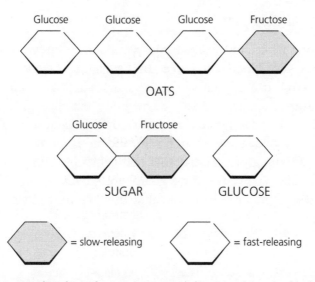

Oats are more complex than glucose Oats need digesting into single glucose units, which takes time and slows down the release of its sugars. This sugar, which is a molecule of glucose and fructose, is slower in turn than a glucose molecule, which needs no digesting and directly enters the bloodstream.

Since the body can use only glucose for fuel, the sugar pictured – sucrose – has to be chopped in two to release the glucose. When you eat sugar, an enzyme released in the gut does this job for you and before long the glucose is whizzing around your bloodstream.

The carbohydrate in oats, however, needs a lot of digesting into smaller and smaller units in the digestive tract before the glucose is released into the blood. This takes longer, so you don't get such a massive and immediate blood sugar rise. Oats are a veritable superfood, proven to be helpful in the treatment of diabetes and cardiovascular disease.[2]

Cooking some foods affects the release rate by 'pre-digesting' the carbs they contain. That's why the more you cook a carbohydrate food the faster-releasing it gets. Take potatoes. A baked potato, with a GI score of 85, is worse than a boiled potato, which has a GI of 57. Oats, however, are an exception. There's little difference between porridge and oat flakes eaten raw. This is largely because the cooking time is very short – you are really rehydrating rather than cooking.

Another factor that slows down the release of carbohydrate in food is fibre. Fibre is an indigestible carbohydrate, and generally the more fibre a food contains, the slower is the breakdown of carbohydrate. This is doubly true for foods that contain soluble fibre such as oats. (Fibre is examined in more depth on page 153.)

Sugars – and sugars

There's one more important thing you need to know. Not all simple sugars raise your blood sugar level. In the diagram below you can see the chemical structure of lactose (milk sugar), sucrose (white sugar) and maltose (grain sugar or malt). The body can use only glucose for energy. So, once the glucose is removed from lactose you're left with galactose, and once the glucose is removed from sucrose you're left with fructose. What happens to fructose and galactose, shown in grey in the diagram? The answer is they go to your liver, where they can be converted into glucose. But this takes time, so they're classed as slow-releasing.

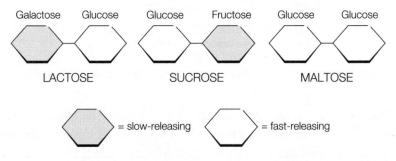

Lactose (milk sugar) vs. sucrose (white sugar) vs. maltose (grain sugar or malt)
Galactose and fructose (shown in grey) are slow-releasing sugars whereas glucose is fast. Hence lactose and sucrose are much more slow-releasing than maltose, a grain sugar (malt), which is quickly digested into two glucose molecules.

Now look at the GI score of glucose, sucrose and fructose on page 147. As you would expect, glucose is the fastest (100), fructose the slowest (19) and sucrose – a combination of glucose and fructose – is in the middle (68). You'll also notice that maltose is as fast as glucose, and honey isn't far off, at 55. That's because 'malt', the sugar, is naturally present in grains and artificially added to things such as cereals and breads – as malted wheat, for example. As you can see from the diagram above, malt is just two glucose molecules. It needs virtually no digestion. Most honey is basically glucose (also called dextrose, or grape sugar since it's also found in grapes), especially commercial honey which is heated to clean out impurities and make it easier to pack into jars.

Now have a look at dairy products. You'd expect things such as ice cream to be high-GI. But it isn't that high. It scores 61. This is because lactose is quite slow-releasing. (Be aware, though, that poor-quality ice creams have added glucose.) Milk or yoghurt score lower still (27–36).

Looking at fruits, even these can be fast- or slow-releasing. Not all contain fructose. Dates, for example, contain mainly glucose. Grapes and bananas are also high, whereas apples and berries are mainly fructose. Even better than fructose is a natural sugar called xylitol, which is found in particularly high amounts in plums. This is the reason why plums have a low GI score. Xylitol has less than half the GI score of fructose and a tenth of the GI score of sugar, and is highly preferable to any artificial sweetener. Hence 10 teaspoons of xylitol, which tastes just as good, has the same effect on your blood sugar as one teaspoon of regular sugar. I use only xylitol as a sweetener and never use sugar.

The GI score of a food is very useful, but there's one problem. Compare carrots with chocolate, or watermelon with French fries. Why do they have such similar scores? Aren't carrots supposed to be good for you? You'd be absolutely right. Aside from the vitamins and other important nutrients they contain, a carrot or a slice of watermelon contains comparatively little carbohydrate. In fact, you'd have to eat two large carrots to get the same amount of carbohydrate, and the same effect on your weight, as four pieces of chocolate. The chances are you'll eat a lot more than four pieces of chocolate and a lot less than two carrots. This kind of inconsistency is why the GI is a bit misleading.

It's the GL that counts

This is where GL comes in – it's the best way of telling to what extent a food is likely to contribute to weight gain. I touched on this earlier in the book but let's look at it in detail.

GL is a simple calculation, taking into account both the amount of carbohydrate in a food (the quantity) and its GI (the quality). To get a food's GL, you just multiply its GI by the amount of carbohydrate it contains (the exact formula is given in Appendix 1). The result will tell you exactly what a given serving of a food does to your blood sugar. I've worked out the GL of literally hundreds of foods for you and you can find my GL in Appendix 2.

The chart below shows a number of high- and low-GL foods. The GL of the quantities listed is 10 Ⓖ – so, for example, two entire punnets of strawberries have the same GL as two dates.

10 ⒼⓁ of common foods compared

10 ⒼⓁ of low-GL foods	10 ⒼⓁ of high-GL foods
4 small cans tomato juice	1 small can cranberry juice drink
2 slices wholegrain rye bread	1 slice white bread
2 large punnets of strawberries	2 dates
Large bowl peanuts	Packet of crisps
Carton orange juice	Glass of Lucozade
3 bowls muesli (sugar-free)	1 bowl cornflakes

As the golden rule of the Holford Diet is to eat no more than 40 ⒼⓁ a day, it's obvious that if you choose high-GL foods you won't be eating much. You could lose weight this way, but that's not what I want you to do.

It's infinitely more satisfying for you to eat low-GL carbohydrates. You'll be able to eat more, experiment with the recipes more and generally enjoy your food (remember how that feels?). Let me make this real for you by showing you a typical day in a Holford dieter's diet versus a typical diet. ⒼⓁ are shown for each food.

Holford daily diet		Average daily diet	
Breakfast	ⒼⓁ	*Breakfast*	ⒼⓁ
A bowl of porridge 30g (1oz)	2	A bowl of cornflakes	21
Half a grated apple	3	Banana	12
Small tub of natural yoghurt	2	Milk	2
And some milk	2		35
	9		
Morning snack		*Morning snack*	
Punnet of strawberries	1	Mars Bar	26
Lunch		*Lunch*	
Substantial tuna salad, 3 oatcakes	11	Tuna salad baguette	15
Afternoon snack		*Afternoon snack*	
Pear + handful of peanuts	4	Packet of crisps	11
Dinner		*Dinner*	
Tomato soup, salmon, sweetcorn and green beans	12	Pizza with Parmesan cheese and tomato sauce, plus salad	23
Good day total ⒼⓁ	37	**Bad day total** ⒼⓁ	110

Take a good look at the food on the left. Imagine you ate that breakfast, rather than the one on the right. It would definitely be more filling, wouldn't it? But it's not just that: by eating it, you'd have cut your propensity to turn glucose into fat by a third! The great news about eating the GL way is that you can actually eat more food *and* lose weight. And it's all delicious.

I'm going to give you many mouthwatering recipes and menus ranging from the simple to the elegant, all designed to keep you going within the 45 Ⓖ a day limit. Between these and your own 'freestyle' choices using the complete GL food chart on page 383, you'll soon learn which carbohydrates to go for, while your body unlearns how to store glucose as fat.

Before we run through the best low-GL foods, I'd like to explain in depth the two important qualities of food that lower GL: fibre and combining protein with carbohydrate.

The fibre factor

There's one kind of carbohydrate that's neither slow- nor fast-releasing. This is fibre – all the parts of plants that digestive enzymes cannot break down (although some is digested by bacteria in the colon). Although it can't be digested, it does serve a purpose. When you eat a food high in fibre, it tends to slow down the release of sugars in the food. And that, as far as weight control is concerned, is good news.

High-fibre diets are definitely recommended for a variety of general health reasons. People who eat more fibre don't usually suffer from constipation, and have a lower risk of getting bowel cancer, diabetes or certain kinds of bowel disease. As it is a natural constituent of fruits, vegetables, lentils, beans and wholegrains, there should be no need to add extra fibre if you're eating these foods. Fibre is calorie-free and there is little doubt that a diet high in naturally occurring fibre is more filling. After all, which would you find most filling to eat: two biscuits or a pound of carrots?

One of the main reasons why high-fibre foods are more satisfying is that fibre absorbs water, so it becomes bulkier in the gut. About 10 litres (17½ pints) of digestive juices are released every day into the digestive tract, so a food's capability for absorbing this water would make a big difference to how bulky the food would become. Wheat fibre, as in bran, is not very absorbent compared with some vegetable fibres. Placed in water, it will swell to ten times its original volume. The fibre from the Japanese konjac plant, however, swells to 100 times its volume! Konjac fibre is given to people with diabetes in Japan because it helps stabilise blood sugar by 'slow-releasing' any eaten carbohydrates.

Soluble or insoluble?

There are two primary kinds of fibre in food: soluble and insoluble. Many foods contain both. Insoluble fibre bulks up faecal content and can 'brush' the gut like a broom, preventing constipation. Soluble fibre is different, dissolving in the gut to form a jellylike substance. This kind of fibre slows down the release of glucose into the bloodstream.

Whole cereal grains contain both kinds of fibre and will slow down glucose release the most, whereas ground fibre (as is found in wholemeal bread) has little effect. Fruit and vegetable juices are devoid of fibre, and that's why the sugars they contain are so fast-releasing.

The soluble fibre found in beans, lentils and oats is particularly effective at slowing down the digestion of food and thus the blood sugar response. Insoluble fibre makes you feel full immediately after eating, whereas soluble fibre reduces appetite nine or more hours later. This could be down to its effect on glucose in the bloodstream, but, whatever the case, it makes food more satisfying in the longer term.[3] There are quite a few different kinds of fibre in these two categories, but suffice to say that it's important to eat unprocessed wholefoods to get the most fibre you possibly can.

King of fibres

Of the fibres in grains, oat fibre is the best at controlling blood sugar and is therefore included in the Holford Diet.[4] Some sources of soluble fibre used therapeutically to help with digestion, diabetes and weight loss are even better, however. These include psyllium husks (available from health-food shops) and konjac fibre, which I mentioned above (available by mail order – see Resources on page 432). The konjac plant is rich in a soluble fibre called glucomannan, and this has been found to be the most effective at controlling blood sugar.

As such, it's a brilliant aid for healthy weight loss. Two studies, one in Japan[5] and one in the US,[6] reported an additional 450g (1lb) weight loss a week when patients took 3g of glucomannan a day. At the Institute for Optimum Nutrition (ION), we decided to put glucomannan to the test by giving 3g a day to 10 overweight people over a three-month period.[7] None made any apparent change to their diet or exercise regime. Nine completed the trial, with an average weight loss of 2.9kg (6lb 6oz) each, thus confirming the usefulness of this unique fibre.

> **Top Tip**
>
> Taking 5g (5 capsules) of konjac extract before each meal can halve the GL score and fill you up so that you eat less. Always take the capsules with a large glass of water. The glucomannan they contain is at least 50 times more effective than bran.

Be aware that, thanks to a quirk in a new food law, glucomannan is no longer allowed to be sold in the UK. However, konjac root extract is. Konjac extract contains about 60 per cent glucomannan, so a daily intake of 5g would be equivalent to 3g of glucomannan (see Resources on page 432).

The power of protein

We've concentrated primarily on carbohydrates so far. But you'll be eating proteins and fats as well, and the balance of these with carbohydrates in each meal makes a big difference to blood sugar balance and fatburning efficiency.

Barry Sears, author of *Enter the Zone*, first made it widely known that combining protein-rich foods with slow-releasing carbohydrates helps to programme you to burn fat. Remember how high insulin is bad news, and high glucagon (see page 64) is good news as far as fatburning is concerned? Well, protein foods tend to trigger a small and equal release of both insulin and glucagons – which happens to be the ideal. Carbohydrates, especially fast-releasing carbohydrates such as cakes and sweets, trigger a substantial release of insulin with little or no glucagon response. Eating fat has little direct effect on either insulin or glucagon. The relative effects of each combination are shown below (the lower and more equal the number of '+', the better the combination):

Effects of protein, carbohydrate and fat on insulin and glucagon

Food eaten	Insulin level	Glucagon level
Carbohydrate only	+++++	no change
Protein only	++	++
Fat only	no change	no change
Carbohydrate and fat	++++	no change
Protein and fat	++	++
High protein and low-GL carbohydrate	++	+
High-GL carbohydrate and low protein	++++++++	+
Low-GL carbohydrate and medium protein	+++	++

From this research, you can see that the best three combinations are either protein only, protein and fat, or low-GL carbohydrates and medium protein. As we've seen, the trouble with a high protein and fat diet is that it isn't good for your health. It's also very restrictive. That's why the best all-round diet for consistent and easily maintained weight loss, with the lowest boredom factor, is to eat low-GL carbohydrates, plus protein. It's great for your health and equally effective for your waistline.

How much protein?

Very high protein diets have proved effective in weight control, partly because they help to hinder the body in its turning of food into fat and also because you eat less on them. But a lot of the weight loss is water. This is partly because when you starve the body of glucose it breaks down stores of glucose called glycogen, which is stored with water. The other reason is that, when you eat too much protein without enough carbohydrates, ketones are produced. These are toxic, and the body tries hard to get rid of them in urine, which contributes to the fluid weight loss. But any pounds of water lost will come back.

Although we all need something in the region of 40g (1½oz) of protein a day, eating above 80g (3oz) a day over the long term will boost your risk of developing osteoporosis, because protein is acidic and can deplete the bones of calcium. It also stresses the kidneys. If the protein source is beef or dairy produce, this may increase risk of breast or prostate cancer. Also, if a person chooses meat as their main source of protein, their diet will inevitably become high in saturated fat, increasing the risk of heart disease and even weight gain. There's not much point in being thin and dead!

Best ratio for fatburning

On a short-term basis, such as 30 days up to three months, increasing your protein intake to between 60g (2¼oz) and 75g (2¾oz) a day and focusing on fish, chicken and vegetarian sources can help restore blood sugar control[8] and boost fatburning. For this reason the Holford Diet provides a greater proportion of calories from protein than the average diet – 25 per cent over a norm of 17 – to control blood sugar balance and reduce insulin resistance. After that period, the protein percentage drops to 20 per cent of calories to maintain fatburning. Once you've reached your goal and need only to maintain your weight and blood sugar balance over the long term, the ideal amount of protein would be 15 to 20 per cent of calories.

But you won't have to mess about with calorie counting, as this isn't that kind of diet. So exactly what all this means in terms of the food you eat is explained simply and clearly in Part Four. I'll tell you exactly what to do. For now, check out the table below showing the ideal balance of proteins, carbs and fats.

The Perfect Balance

	Protein	Carbohydrate	Fat
Average diet	17%	48%	35%
Holford Diet (for the first 30 days up to three months)	25%	50%	25%
Holford Diet (for maintenance)	15–20%	55–60%	25%

Since we all need to eat some protein, some carbohydrates and the right kind of fats, the best combination is to eat low-GL carbohydrate foods that are also rich in protein. Beans and lentils are an example. People who live in countries whose diets contain these are consistently thinner and healthier.

The easiest and healthiest way to achieve this perfect balance is to eat the equivalent of 60g (2¼oz) of protein and 120g (4¼oz) of low-GL carbohydrate in a day, and to divide it evenly between each meal, that is, 20g (¾oz) of protein and roughly 40g (1½oz) of carbohydrate, at breakfast, lunch and dinner. You needn't worry too much about the maths: the recipes will do this for you. (Details on the quantity and quality of fats to be eaten are given in the next chapter.) Roughly two-thirds of your carbohydrates need to come from vegetables and fruit, and one-third from things such as grains and more 'starchy' vegetables.

The simplest way to visualise your meals, as far as lunch and dinner are concerned, is to eat any one of the protein-rich foods shown below, with an equivalent-sized serving of any carbohydrate-rich food, plus two servings of vegetables. Remember the plate model from page 89?

To maximise fatburning, you will probably be eating more protein-rich foods in relation to carbohydrate-rich foods than you are used to, as well as more fresh fruit and veg. The amount of carbohydrate or protein provided by non-starchy vegetables (broccoli, kale, cabbage, peas, spinach, carrots and so on) is small, so these can be eaten relatively freely on the Holford Diet. Aim, too, for two pieces of low-GL fruit a day.

Fatburning food combinations

(Note: a more comprehensive list of foods is given on pages 302–310.)
Here are a few examples:

Protein	Carbohydrate	Vegetables
Poached salmon	on brown basmati rice	with a green salad
Marinated tofu	on wholewheat pasta	with steam-fried vegetables
Grilled chicken breast	with boiled new potatoes	and steamed runner beans
Cottage cheese	on oatcakes/rye bread	with broccoli and tomato salad

The Holford Diet snacks are also great protein-and-carb combinations. For instance, eating a few almonds or pumpkin seeds, which are high in essential fats and protein, at the same time as some low-GL fruit can further slow the effect of fruit sugar on your blood sugar. But remember: fruits such as apples and strawberries have a low-GL, so you are already doing brilliantly by choosing these.

For breakfast, you can achieve the right balance and amount of protein and low-GL carbohydrate by, for example, eating a cup of oat flakes with some seeds, some berries and either skimmed milk or soya milk, if you're allergic to milk.

Above all, don't worry about having to calculate all this – the lowdown later in this part and the menus and recipes in Part Five make it remarkably easy.

We've now looked in depth at how to pinpoint the best carbohydrates, and how to combine them with protein for the most efficient fatburning. But what if you, like millions of others, are in the grip of caffeine and chocolate? Dealing with these very twenty-first-century addictions is essential to balancing your blood sugar – and, as you'll see, surprisingly painless.

Are you addicted to sugar or stimulants?

Ever had an 'I'd kill for a muffin' moment? Or perhaps it was a double espresso, a bar of chocolate or even a piece of toast? Whatever the object of your desire, the urge to get at it probably felt overwhelming at the time. Yet, this is a perfectly normal reaction to a blood sugar low.

It is virtually impossible to resist temptation when you're in the middle of a blood sugar crash. One of the reasons why sugar is so addictive is that it can cause a release of the body's own 'feel-good' chemicals, opioids and dopamine.

Animals can become addicted to sugar and show all the telltale withdrawal symptoms, including the shakes, when deprived, according to research by Dr Bartley Hoebel at Princeton University in the US. This is because the more you overstimulate the release of dopamine, the more insensitive you become to its effects. In a sense you are becoming 'dopamine-resistant' or addicted to your body's own natural highs. This, in turn, upsets your blood sugar levels and your ability to control your weight.

Dr Candace Pert, research professor in the physiology and biophysics department at Georgetown University Medical Center in Washington DC, says, 'I consider sugar to be a drug, a highly purified plant product that can become addictive. Relying on an artificial form of glucose – sugar – to give us a quick pick-me-up is analogous to, if not as dangerous as, shooting heroin.'[9] Dr Pert is among the chief scientists who discovered the central role endorphins play in addiction. There's certainly plenty of research out there to support her view.[10]

Sugar and high-GL carbs aren't the only culprits in the case. Stimulants, too, promote the brain's 'feelgood' chemicals. Remember the effect of our inbuilt fight-or-flight mechanism? It's as if we humans have a 'fifth gear' for emergencies.

In times of stress, the adrenal glands release a combination of hormones, including dopamine and adrenalin, that break down stores of glucose and raise your blood sugar levels, tapping into your energy reserves to provide instant fuel to deal with the apparent danger. Of course, today's 'emergencies' have nothing to do with woolly mammoths on the rampage but take place mainly inside our heads: overdrafts, relationships, parking tickets, and so on. But we still produce adrenalin, and that still raises blood sugar levels.

Stimulants have the same effect, stirring up adrenalin and dopamine. So, consuming nicotine or caffeine in colas, coffee, tea, cigarettes and chocolate, added to the stresses of twenty-first-century life, can seriously mess with your blood sugar.

So why do we do it? It's simply because millions of us are caught in the vicious cycle of blood sugar highs and lows already, and feel exhausted much of the time. Stimulants seem to promise instant energy – while, of course, making the problem worse.

We may be eating fast-releasing carbohydrates, devoid of vitamins and minerals. We may be drinking two or three coffees before noon just to deal with our morning weariness. We 'learn' how to cope with the rebound blood sugar low after a meal by having a coffee. If we haven't eaten for two hours, we go for another coffee. And, when we drag ourselves home after a hard day's work, we may be drinking still more just to stay awake.

You may feel that coffee, which speeds up the metabolism, is not only keeping you going but helping with weight loss. The irony is that in the not-so-long term it contributes to weight gain by fuelling blood sugar imbalance. According to research from Holland by Dr Paul Smits and colleagues at the University of Nijmegen, a single shot of caffeine can raise adrenalin fivefold, thus raising blood glucose, and decrease insulin sensitivity by 15 per cent. This means you become more resistant to insulin and more likely to turn glucose into fat.[11]

A cup of chaos

Stimulants are addictive. That's why you need more and more to keep you going. Before long, one cup of coffee and the odd cigarette becomes six or more lattes, mochaccinos or filter coffees and a pack of cigarettes. By the time you reach this stage, you can't even get going in the morning without a stimulant. The combination of coffee, tea or nicotine with stress, high-GI foods and sugar means you lose your blood sugar control and wake up each morning with low blood sugar levels and not enough adrenalin to kick-start your day. So you adopt one of two strategies:

- You reluctantly crawl out of bed on remote control and head for the kettle, make yourself a strong cup of tea or coffee, light up a cigarette or have some fast-releasing sugar in the form of toast, with some sugar on it called jam. Up go your blood sugar and adrenalin levels and you start to feel normal.

Or ...

- You lie in bed and start to think about all the things that have gone wrong, could go wrong, will go wrong. You start to worry about everything you've got to do, haven't done and should have done. About 10 minutes of this gets enough adrenalin pumping to get you out of bed.

One of the most seductive aspects of coffee is that it actually seems to make you feel better, more energised and alert. But, wondered Dr Peter Rogers, a psychologist at Bristol University, does coffee actually increase your energy and mental performance, or just relieve the symptoms of withdrawal? When he researched this he found that, after that sacred morning cup of coffee, coffee drinkers don't feel any better than people who never drink coffee. Coffee drinkers just feel better than they did when they woke up.[12] In other words, drinking coffee relieves the symptoms of withdrawal from coffee. And in the middle sits Starbucks, and all the other coffee franchises, making a buck or two! It's addictive.

Caffeine blocks the receptors for a brain chemical called *adenosine*, whose function is to stop the release of the motivating neurotransmitters dopamine and adrenalin. With less adenosine activity, levels of dopamine and adrenalin increase, as does alertness and motivation. Peak concentration occurs 30 to 60 minutes after you down that cup.

The more caffeine you consume, the more your body and brain become insensitive to their own natural stimulants, dopamine and adrenalin, as well as insulin. You then need more stimulants to feel normal, and keep pushing the body to produce more dopamine and adrenalin. The net result is adrenal exhaustion – an inability to produce these important chemicals of motivation and communication. Apathy, depression, exhaustion and an inability to cope set in.

Coffee, of course, isn't the only source of caffeine. There's as much in a strong cup of tea as a regular cup of coffee. Caffeine is also the active ingredient in most colas and energy drinks such as Red Bull, which sold more than 3.5 billion cans worldwide in 2007. Chocolate and green tea also contain caffeine, although in much smaller amounts. Have a look at the chart below.

How much caffeine?

Product	Caffeine content
Coca-Cola Classic 350ml (12fl oz)	46mg
Diet Coke 350ml (12fl oz)	46mg
Red Bull	80mg
Hot cocoa 150ml (5fl oz)	10mg
Coffee, instant 150ml (5fl oz)	40–105mg
Coffee, espresso, cappuccino, latte	30–50mg
Coffee, filter 150ml (5fl oz)	110–150mg

continued

Product	Caffeine content
Coffee, Starbucks (grande)	500mg
Decaffeinated coffee 150ml (5fl oz)	0.3mg
Tea 150ml (5fl oz)	20–100mg
Green tea 150ml (5fl oz)	20–30mg
Chocolate cake (1 slice)	20–30mg
Bittersweet chocolate 28g (1oz)	5–35mg
Pro Plus	50mg
PEP	30mg

And, if you add sugar to your coffee, or drink it while eating a sweet food, such as toast and jam, or drink a lot of cola with added sugar, you'll exacerbate the effect of the caffeine on your blood sugar balance, and end up piling on even more weight. In a study by researchers at the Department of Human Health and Nutritional Sciences, University of Guelph in Canada, volunteers were given a high-GL or a low-GL cereal with a coffee or decaf. When they were given coffee, their blood sugar rose more than twice as much, they produced much more insulin (the fat-storing hormone), and also their sensitivity to the insulin substantially reduced compared to those given decaf. There was not much difference in this effect whether they were given a high- or low-GL cereal.[13] The moral of this story is: don't have coffee with carbohydrate food – and ideally, don't consume caffeine anyway.

The dangers of diet drinks

Many people turn to sugar-free caffeinated drinks instead of coffee. Is Coke Zero zero nutrition, zero natural ingredients or zero good for you? Of course, the idea is, that by containing no actual sugar it's meant to be good for you. 'The stag night without the wedding' says one ad. Here are the typical ingredients:

water
aspartame
acesulfame k
phosphoric acid
citric acid
caffeine
sodium benzoate (E211)
sulphate ammonia caramel (E150d)

Water You can't knock water, but when it's cooked up with this family of chemicals?

Aspartame is widely used as a sweetener in snacks, sweets, desserts and 'diet' foods. It may adversely affect people with PKU (phenylketonuria). Recent reports show the possibility of headaches, blindness and seizures with long-term, high-dose aspartame. Another study reports a raised risk of a rare kind of brain tumour, called lymphoma. The EU has given it a clean bill of health, but clearly some people react badly.

Acesulfame K is another sweetener that causes cancer in animals. Acetoacetamide, which is a breakdown product, causes thyroid problems in animals. It's commonly mixed with aspartame but no one really knows how safe this is.

Phosphoric acid High intakes of phosphoric acid erode teeth enamel and bones. Hence the link with a high consumption of fizzy drinks and low bone density in children. A child consuming 1.5 litres (2¾ pints) of phosphorated drinks a day has five times the chance of having low calcium levels.

Citric acid is found in fruit and is quite harmless on its own. However, combined with sodium benzoate (see below), especially at high temperatures, citric acid could produce carcinogenic benzene.

Caffeine is an addictive stimulant with all kinds of downsides when consumed in excess. There's about 10mg per 100ml (3½fl oz), so a 330ml can is 30mg, and a 1.5 litre bottle is 150mg. That's the equivalent of two coffees.

Sodium benzoate is widely used as a preservative in many foods, including drinks, low-sugar products, cereals and meat products. It can temporarily inhibit the function of digestive enzymes and may deplete glycine levels. Sodium benzoate should be avoided by those with allergic conditions such as hay fever, hives and asthma.

Sulphite ammonia caramel is a colouring made by heating sugar, but it is not 'technically' sugar. This colouring has not been fully evaluated for its potential carcinogenicity or reproductive toxicity, but ammonia is highly toxic.

That's it. Of course, these drinks are addictive, and doubly bad news if consumed with a carbohydrate meal or snack. I recommend anyone with half a brain to avoid these drinks like the plague.

That's why I recommend you cut right back on stimulants, including sugar, right at the start of the diet. If the very thought fills you with dread, and leaves you wondering how you'll ever get to work without that morning cup, it's pretty certain you're addicted. But by quitting you'll be trading a dispiriting round of fatigue and sudden jolts to the system for feeling energetic all day, every day.

Before you panic, let me say that this is not for life. What I'm asking you to do is go cold turkey: give up stimulants and sugar when you start on the diet and supplement programme, and stay off them for at least two weeks to a month.

Of course, the reason we react to the thought of stopping stimulants is that we 'know' we'll feel terrible without them. We know this for a fact because it's the very symptoms of withdrawal – feeling tired, grumpy and foggy-headed – that makes that cup of tea or cappuccino seem like manna from heaven. But, ten minutes later, you want another one.

Once your blood sugar and adrenalin levels are back to normal, however, you can take or leave these stimulants.

So, if you follow the Holford Diet and take the supplements I recommend, going cold turkey may well turn out to be much easier than you thought. Nine out of ten people say, two weeks later, that they feel so good they just don't need stimulants any more. With their energy levels soaring, they just don't need the endless jolts to the system that used to punctuate their days.

The first step is to get real about your use of stimulants. This means completing the 'stimulant inventory' opposite, for a week. Write down what you consume every day, and then add up your total at the end of the week. Be honest!

	1 Unit	Sun	Mon	Tue	Wed	Thu	Fri	Sat
Green tea	2 cups							
Tea	1 cup							
Coffee	1 cup							
Cola or caffeinated drinks	1 can							
Caffeine pills such as No-Doz, Excedrin, Dexatrim	1 pill							
Chocolate	2oz/57g							
Alcohol Wine Beer or lager (ordinary strength) Spirits	Small glass ½ pint Single shot							
Added sugar	1 tsp/5g							
Hidden sugar (see sugar contents on ingredients lists)	1 tsp/5g							
Cigarettes	1 cigarette							

Add up your total number of 'units'. The ideal is 5 or fewer per week. If you are having more than 10 stimulant units a week, this is going to have an effect on your energy and weight.

Eating slow-releasing energy foods and taking energy-stabilising vitamins and minerals, which we'll be investigating in Part Four, will give you even energy levels, and the need for stimulants will evaporate. You'll look back on those bleary-eyed mornings and exhausted afternoons with wonder. As one Holford Diet volunteer quoted earlier said, 'One of the hardest, but best things about it was the insistence on giving up coffee and stimulants.' (She also lost 4.5kg/10lb in a month.)

Kicking the habit

How does the Holford Diet help you quit? Since all stimulants affect blood sugar levels, you can keep yours even by always having something substantial for breakfast, such as an oat-based, not too refined cereal; or unsweetened live yogurt with apple, ground sesame seeds and wheatgerm; or an egg. You can snack frequently on fresh fruit, and twice a day you can add a small handful of nuts or seeds.

Eating a highly alkaline-forming diet can reduce cravings for cigarettes and alcohol, so eat plenty of low-GL fruit and fresh vegetables (fruit and veg are alkaline-forming whereas meat and dairy are acid-forming). These high-fibre foods also help to keep your blood sugar levels even, and keep you on an even keel. The worst thing you can do is go for hours without eating – but this isn't something I would ever recommend, anyway.

There are also supplements that help. These include extra doses of the amino acid tyrosine to support your own ability to make dopamine and adrenalin, as well as extra chromium to help increase your sensitivity to insulin, plus adaptogens such as ginseng and Siberian ginseng, which help with fatigue.[14] If you'd like to find out more about this read my book *How To Quit Without Feeling S**t*, or visit the website www.how2quit.co.uk.

In this way, going cold turkey at the same time as starting the diet will simply not be the nightmare you imagine. I realise that giving up cigarettes might be a little more difficult than tossing out the beer, wine or coffee, but even that process will be significantly smoothed once your blood sugar steadies.

My diet will help stabilise your blood sugar and reduce your cravings. Here are the main stimulants that are affecting your health and your ability to lose weight:

Coffee contains three stimulants: caffeine, theobromine and theophylline. Although caffeine is the strongest, theophylline is known to disturb normal sleep patterns and theobromine has an effect similar to caffeine's, although it is present in much smaller amounts in coffee. So decaffeinated coffee isn't exactly stimulant-free.

As a nutritionist, I have seen many people cleared of minor health problems such as tiredness and headaches just from cutting out their two or three coffees a day. After you quit, you may get withdrawal symptoms for up to three days. These reflect how addicted you've become. If you begin to feel perky and your health improves afterwards, that's a good indication that you're better off without coffee – and, in any case, I recommend having it only as a very occasional treat. The most popular alternatives are Teecino, Caro Extra or Bambu (made with roasted chicory and malted barley), dandelion coffee (from Symingtons or Lanes) or herbal teas.

Tea is the great British addiction. As we've seen, a strong cup of tea contains as much caffeine as a weak cup of coffee and it is certainly addictive. Tea also contains tannin, which interferes with the absorption of vital minerals such as iron and zinc. Particularly addictive is Earl Grey tea, which contains an extra stimulant, bergamot. If you find you drink more than the occasional weak cuppa, it's time to stop. The best-tasting alternatives are rooibos tea (red bush tea) with milk, and herbal or fruit teas.

Chocolate bars are usually full of sugar, and cocoa, the active ingredient, provides significant quantities of the stimulant theobromine, also found in coffee. The action of theobromine is similar to caffeine's, though not as strong. Chocolate also contains small amounts of caffeine. So with an array of stimulants, plenty of sugar and a truly delicious taste and 'mouth feel', it's all too easy to become a chocoholic. If you stop eating it for a couple of weeks, and substitute fruit, and healthy 'sweets' from health-food shops that are sugar-free and the like, you will find yourself losing the craving.

Cola and 'energy' drinks contain anything from 46 to 80mg of caffeine per can, as we saw in the chart on pages 161–2. These drinks are also often high in sugar and colourings and their net stimulant effect can be considerable. Check the ingredients list and stay away from drinks containing caffeine and chemical additives or colourings.

Cigarettes raise blood sugar levels by acting as a mild stimulant to the central nervous system. There is also evidence that smoking is linked to an increase in insulin resistance. In addition to disturbing blood sugar balance, cigarette smoking drains the body of vital nutrients and contributes to numerous other diseases such as cancer and heart disease. So, needless to say, cigarettes are a big no-no. If you are addicted to smoking, I can't recommend highly enough the benefits of quitting. Not only will it lower your risk of getting certain kinds of cancer and other diseases but it will also keep you looking younger and feeling much better overall.

For confirmed smokers, I generally recommend stabilising blood sugar first with the diet. This will make stopping easier. Also, you will not get the rebound weight gain that often happens if you haven't solved the underlying issue for every smoker, which is blood sugar imbalance. I also recommend increasing your daily exercise during the time you stop smoking, which further boosts your metabolism and stops any rebound weight gain.

There are now a number of successful methods for quitting, however. One of the largely ignored keys is rebalancing your body's chemistry away from addiction. In relation to quitting smoking this is explained in detail in my book *How To Quit Without Feeling S**t* – visit www.how2quit.co.uk for details. Following this plan will dramatically decrease your symptoms of withdrawal and increase your chances of success.

Alcohol is not strictly a stimulant, but is chemically similar to sugar, and potentially very addictive. It's also high in calories. Drinking can suppress appetite but lead to cravings for more alcohol, so you can end up quaffing empty calories with no nutritional value. Worse, alcohol destroys or prevents the absorption of many nutrients, including vitamin C, B complex, calcium, magnesium and zinc.

Alcohol can also make you fat. It's the most rapidly absorbed sugar, with one-fifth being absorbed directly through the stomach. It takes almost two hours to use up 10g of alcohol – the amount in half a pint of beer. It can be rapidly turned to fat by the action of insulin. With chronic use it converts into fat rather than glucose or glycogen and is stored in the liver. Alcohol also interferes with the liver's ability to break down amino acids and turn them into glucose when blood sugar levels are too low.

So, in this sense, alcohol messes up blood sugar and fat control, and regular drinkers tend to put on weight. Habitual drinking can damage the liver, leading to even further inability to control both blood sugar levels and weight. You'll achieve the best results on the Holford Diet by having no more than three small drinks a week, and preferably none for two weeks to a month. In Chapter 23 on drinks and desserts I'll explain how different drinks count towards your daily 5 ⑮ allowance. A dry white wine, for example, is much better than a beer.

The stress connection

Sugar and stimulants may not be the only factors playing merry hell with your blood sugar. Serious stress has a very similar effect. If you think you are suffering from it, you're not alone. Many people wake up in a state of anxiety, arrive at work stressed out from commuting, have to contend with a lot of stress at work and go home in a state of near collapse. Unfortunately, a life of non-stop twenty-first-century stress takes its toll on your body's chemistry.

We've seen how stimulants trigger the release of adrenalin and cortisol, which prepare the body for action. Stress does this too. The flood of glucose this then releases for our use stimulates, in its turn, yet more hormones to take the glucose out of circulation. Whereas adrenalin works fast and is gone fast, cortisol lingers. If you're stressed for weeks at a time, your cortisol level stays high, and this is bad news. High cortisol levels, the hallmark of the overstressed, make you even more insulin-resistant and even more prone to put on weight. Let me explain why.

Insulin puts glucose into storage, whereas adrenalin and cortisol rapidly raise the glucose supply to cells for fight or flight – partly by blocking insulin's fat-storing effect. That sounds like good news, at least in the short term. And it is. That's why high stress and stimulants, such as coffee, can keep you thin. But when the effect of insulin is blocked, the body simply produces more – and the more it produces, the more insulin-resistant you become. So, over the long term, stress can actually lead to weight gain.

How stressed are you?

Take a look at the symptoms below. If they sound familiar to you, then you know what I'm talking about. They suggest adrenal stress overload.

- Hard to get up in the morning
- Tired all the time
- Craving certain foods
- Anger, irritability, aggressiveness
- Mood swings

- Restlessness

- Energy slump during the day

- Regular feelings of weakness

- Apathy

- Depression

- Feeling cold all the time

In our ONUK survey on 37,000 people, 71 per cent had a high stress rating.[15] If you're frequently stressed, you are not alone. In a survey of patients visiting ION most halved their stress scores after six months of improved nutrition, substituting slow-releasing carbohydrates for sugar and stimulants.

The amazing thing is that if you balance your blood sugar, it not only affects your weight but also has wide-reaching benefits for your health, your mood and your ability to deal with the inevitable challenges of life. When you're stressed, even molehills seem like mountains. When your energy levels are good and your mind is clear, life immediately smoothes out and calms down. As fatburner diet volunteers from *She* magazine agreed, 'Increased alertness was a significant benefit. By the third day, everybody felt well – alert on rising, and three of us (including me) were bounding about, full of the joys of spring.'

The only way out of the prison of stress, sugar and stimulants is to reduce or avoid all forms of concentrated sweetness, tea, coffee, alcohol and cigarettes, and start eating foods that help to keep your blood sugar level stable. By changing to the right foods, backed up with specific nutritional supplements, most people feel an amazing improvement in energy within days.

That's why I recommend that you:

- avoid regular tea and coffee

- stop eating chocolate (you can have some after two weeks to a month!)

- quit smoking

- avoid regular alcohol and reduce your overall intake to three small glasses a week

- do what you can to avoid continuously high stress levels

Remember, the very best way is to have *nothing* stimulating when you start the diet. That includes decaf coffee (the continuing taste of coffee doesn't help you break the habit).

After that, but *only if you have to*, you can drink the occasional cup of weak tea. But coffee, as I've indicated, pretty much has to go. Soon you'll find you can sail past coffee bars with not even a twinge of longing – and with a lot more energy than in the days you were chained to a cup.

As far as sugar is concerned, you'll have to be on the lookout. It comes in many disguises. Peruse food labels for glucose, dextrose and sucrose. Honey is also best avoided for those first two weeks. Fructose (fruit sugar) is somewhat better, but, even so, the emphasis over these two weeks is to get the sweetness you need from whole foods, such as fruit, instead of sugar on cereals or in desserts.

It's also a good idea to start cutting down the overall sweetness of what you eat. For example, you can add water to fruit juice. Three oranges may have gone into a glass of the juice. Would you eat that many whole fruits at one go? Even though oranges contain mainly fructose, there's a lot of it in pure juice. Dilute it by a third. You'll soon get used to it. After two weeks, you'll find your craving for sweetness is fading – and overall, you'll be more than ready to get going with the Holford Diet.

Summary

- Avoid sugar in its many disguises and foods that contain fast-releasing carbohydrates with a high-GL score (above 10 per serving).

- Eat foods that contain low-GL carbohydrates (below 10 per serving).

- Eat no more than 40 Ⓖ a day.

- Eat low-GL carbohydrates *with* protein-rich foods.

- Eat whole, unadulterated foods high in soluble fibre (beans, lentils, oats).

- Consider supplementing with konjac extract for the glucomannan it contains.

- Cut back on stimulants right at the start of the diet.

- Do what you can to avoid continuously high stress levels.

Part Four shows you how to do all this.

14

Step 2: Eat Good Fats and Avoid Bad Fats

It may seem counterintuitive, but some kinds of fats boost fatburning. These are the essential fatty acids, or EFAs. So entrenched have we become in fat phobia and the promotion of low-fat diets that the role of EFAs in helping you to burn fat has gone largely unnoticed.

The original idea was that, since 1 gram of fat gives more calories (9 calories) than 1 gram of protein or carbohydrate (approximately 4 calories), the quickest way to cut calories was to cut fat. Theoretically, this should have been the best way to lose weight, if you believe conventional calorie theory. We now know, however, that this isn't true. Low-GL diets work better than low-fat diets, and the GL of your diet predicts weight gain much more accurately than the fat content of your diet.[16]

Go fish

What is more, we discovered there were essential fats (polyunsaturates) and nonessential fats (saturates). When you eat 100g (3½oz) of saturated fat, all your body can do is burn it for energy or store it as fat. On the other hand, when you eat 100g (3½oz) of the essential polyunsaturated fats from seeds, their oils or fatty fish, the brain and nerves use them, and they boost immunity, balance hormones, reduce inflammation and promote healthy skin. Only if there's any left will the body use EFAs for energy or to store as fat. In other words, one calorie of saturated fat has an entirely different effect on the body in terms of weight control and health than one calorie of polyunsaturated fat.

And it gets even better. Since you need essential fats, it should come as no surprise to find out that we have 'fat receptors' in the mouth.

These register whether or not you've eaten what you need. We humans crave fat in the same way we crave sugar or protein. However, only when you eat the right fat – the essential kind – does your body stop craving that smooth, creamy texture. Not only are you satisfied, but you've just consumed a very special substance.

The omega-3 EFAs – found in flaxseeds and pumpkin seeds and oily cold-water fish such as mackerel, herring, salmon and tuna – keep extra weight at bay in a number of ways. They help make hormone-like substances called *prostaglandins*, which help to control metabolism and fatburning. They also help to control and limit the potential damage of insulin resistance, by calming down the inflammatory effects of bursts of high glucose in the blood, which damages the arteries.

Inflammation is the core imbalance that underlies so many diseases, and omega-3 EFAs help to reverse the process. Increasing your intake of omega-3 fats helps beat depression,[17] heart disease[18] and arthritis,[19] as well as helping to keep your memory and concentration sharp as you age.

The omega-6 EFAs, found in hot-climate seeds such as sunflower and sesame, have similar benefits to the omega-3s, and are especially good for the skin and maintaining hormone balance, for example in combating PMS, but not so important for the brain.

The fat in meat and dairy produce, which it is saturated, simply doesn't come near EFAs in the health stakes. (Luckily, the Holford Diet helps you reduce the amount of protein – and fat – you get from meat and dairy foods.) Worst of all fats, however, are the kind you find in processed and junk food or in deep-fried foods. These are called trans fats and hydrogenated fats (we look at these on page 177).

There is, however, an 'in-between' fat: monounsaturated, or omega-9, fat. Olive oil is a particularly rich source. Although this is nowhere near as good for you as food sources of the omega-3 fats, it is also nowhere near as bad for you as saturated fat or trans fats. A number of studies have found that if people switch from saturated to mono-unsaturated fats, this helps to stabilise blood sugar levels, improve insulin resistance and control diabetes.[20] This is good news, and a step in the right direction for fatburning.

My diet emphasises omega-rich foods and avoids trans, hydrogenated and saturated fats as much as possible. Below you'll see the common food sources of these different kinds of fats. (Please note that most foods contain a mixture of fats, so some appear more than once, as they're rich in several kinds.)

Fat family	Good dietary sources
Omega-3 family	Fish, especially salmon, mackerel, herring, tuna and sardines; flaxseeds, pumpkin seeds and walnuts and their oils
Omega-6 family	Sunflower, sesame and pumpkin seeds and their oils; also safflower oil, corn oil, soya oil
Omega-9 family	Olive oil, almonds, walnuts
Saturated fat	Meat, dairy produce and most eggs (chickens fed flaxseeds have more omega-3 fats in their eggs)
Trans and hydrogenated fats	Deep-fried food, burned or browned fat, margarines, most processed meats (such as hamburgers, sausages), and most vegetarian meat substitutes (such as vege sausages)

As you can see from the diagram opposite, modern times have seen big changes in our fat intake. From 1900 to 2000 there was a massive increase in overall fat intake – although we have started to eat less since the late 1980s – as well as a big increase in saturated fat and a decrease in the best fat of all: omega-3s. Consumption of the essential omega-6 fat has gone up, reflecting the switch from butter to margarine. However, this is slightly misleading because a lot of this 'polyunsaturated vegetable oil', which is what you find on the label, has been processed or 'hydrogenated' in such a way that it's as bad for you as saturated fat, if not worse (see page 177).

Say no to saturated fat

To lose weight, it is definitely desirable to cut down on saturated fat. Nowadays even the average child consumes over 317kg (700lb) of saturated fat, the equivalent of 1,314 packets of lard, between the ages of 6 and 16. Eating excess fat is associated with obesity,[21] heart disease, cancer and diabetes, and it puts extra stress on the body's metabolism.

Despite all this evidence, the current craze for high-protein, low-carb diets often kicks off with 60 per cent of calories from fat! This is double the mainstream recommendations and almost three times what I'd recommend you to eat.

Why coconut oil is different

However, not all saturated fat is the same. Animal-based saturated fats are made of short-chain triglycerides. Coconut oil, on the other hand, is a

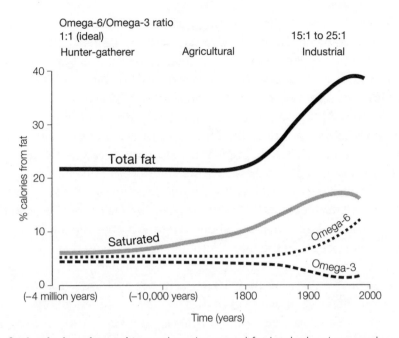

How fat intake has changed In modern times total fat intake has increased. Saturated fat intake has increased, although it is now levelling off. Omega-6 fat intake has increased but this is slightly misleading because much of it is 'hydrogenated' vegetable oils, which act like saturated fats. Omega-3 fats, in fish and seeds, have gone down, leading to widespread deficiency.
Leaf and Weber, *American Journal of Clinical Nutrition* 1987

medium-chain triglyceride (more on this in a moment). The thinking was that coconut oil, as a saturated fat, must be bad for you. But that's wrong. In fact, research indicates that coconut oil is likely to reduce your risk of heart disease, lower your cholesterol, help you lose weight and rejuvenate your skin. Furthermore, studies of populations with diets traditionally high in coconut show that the people are generally in good health, without many of the chronic diseases found in modern Western nations.

What makes coconut and its oil superior is that they contain these medium-chain triglycerides, known as MCTs. MCTs are digested more easily than other fats, and your body uses them differently. Whereas other fats are stored in your body's cells, the MCTs in coconut oil are sent directly to your liver and converted into energy. So when you eat coconut oil, your body uses it more quickly, rather than storing it as body fat. In this way, MCTs are thermogenic – meaning that they actually speed up metabolism, so your body will burn more calories in a day and have more energy.

Farmers in the 1940s unwittingly illustrated this benefit when they attempted to use coconut oil to fatten up their animals. They found it made the animals lean and active instead. Later, animal experiments in the laboratory compared diets that were low or high in total fat, and contained different types of fat. Results showed that animals with more unsaturated oil and less coconut oil in their diet were fatter. This was even more important than the total amount of fat consumed. In other words, the animals that ate just a little unsaturated oil were fat, and those that ate a lot of coconut oil were lean.

Many human studies have supported this finding, including a study of people in the Yucatan Peninsula of Mexico, where coconut is a staple food. It showed that their metabolic rate was an average of 25 per cent higher than people in the US.[22] Although it may seem that coconut can do no wrong, it's important to keep things in perspective. Your diet should contain no more than 10 per cent of its calories from saturated fat. If you already follow my optimum health recommendations, your fat intake is likely to be well within this limit, so it's no problem to replace some of your current sources of saturated fat with coconut oil, milk, butter or cream. Ideally, the fat in your diet should come from a variety of sources. This includes seeds, nuts, oily fish, avocados, eggs, lean meat and coconut products.

Top Tip

All authorities agree that our total fat intake should be less than 30 per cent of total calories, but how do you know what percentage of fat is in the food you buy? Here is a simple equation that tells you if packaged food is too high in fat:

Look at the number of calories per 100g (3½oz) on the label. Now look at the number of grams of fat per 100g (3½oz) and multiply it by 10. Is this more than a third of the number of calories per 100g (3½oz)? If so, it's more than 30 per cent fat.

For example, yoghurt may provide 60 calories per 100g (3½oz). The fat content per 100g (3½oz) is 3.5g. Multiply by 10, giving you 35. Divide 35 by 60 (0.58). This means that more than 50 per cent of the calories in this yoghurt come from fat.

Try this simple formula when you next go shopping.

Hydrogenated – the 'H' word

Just as bad for you as saturated fats are polyunsaturated fats that have been processed, fried or damaged. Remember, the essential fats are polyunsaturated fats, but once they are messed around with they're as bad for you as saturated fats, if not worse. When the molecules of these essential fats are altered by food processing (called hydrogenation) or frying, they can no longer benefit the body and are called trans fats. Frying or heating can also make them rancid or oxidised, which means they can set up a chain reaction of oxidation in the body, damaging body cells. Food rich in trans fats include:

● French fries

● hamburgers

● deep-fried fish burgers

● deep-fried chicken nuggets

● confectionery

● chocolate bars

● potato and corn chips/crisps

● biscuits

● doughnuts

● margarine

● mayonnaise

● most salad dressings

Unfortunately, many vegetarian processed foods are also high in these hydrogenated fats. Check the label of vege burgers or vegetarian sausages. If the list of ingredients includes 'partially hydrogenated vegetable oils', don't buy it.

Say yes to omega-3 fats

Most of us are deficient in omega-3s already. But, as we've seen, eating them is vital for health – hence the 'essential' in 'essential fatty acid'. And of course they carry a host of health benefits, not least of which is their ability to boost fatburning.

Let's take a closer look at how they help in this respect. In the diagram below you can see how the body can make three kinds of prostaglandin – PG 1, 2 and 3. PG 1 and 3 are good for fatburning. PG 2 is not. Whereas omega-3 fats can make only the good PG 3, the omega-6 fats can produce either the good PG 1 or the bad PG 2. People producing a lot of insulin because of blood sugar imbalance tend to produce more PG 2. But there's a way to counteract this. Eating more omega-3s, which provide eicosapentaenoic acid or EPA, will help in turning their omega-6 fats into PG 1.

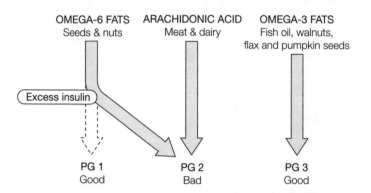

Too much insulin, a consequence of insulin resistance, encourages the formation of prostaglandins that promote inflammation, pain and swelling. Increased intake of omega-3 fats has the opposite effect, reducing pain and inflammation.

I've listed a few of the health benefits of eating omega-3 fats. But there are even more. They reduce the risk of heart disease and of dying from a sudden heart attack by 50 per cent,[23] and also halve your risk of ever suffering from Alzheimer's disease.[24] So omega-3s are one of your best friends, not just for fatburning but for all-over health. The Holford Diet specifically includes these essential fats in one of four ways:

Breakfast Two teaspoons of seeds (half pumpkin, half flax is excellent, or you can mix in some sesame and sunflower too) with your breakfast cereal, yoghurt or Get Up & Go (see page 436).

Snacks Two teaspoons of pumpkin seeds with fruit.

Main meals A small serving of oily fish or two teaspoons of pumpkin seeds on salad.

Salad dressings Two teaspoons of seed oil.

To achieve enough essential fats you need to pick *two* of any of the above options each day.

I realise that, if you've spent years avoiding fat like the plague, this routine might jar at first. Yet the truth is that these essential fats clear up dry skin, stimulate your metabolism, boost brain function, protect your heart and strengthen your immune system. So, in addition to losing weight more efficiently, you'll find that your skin and hair look better than ever, and that your mind and body are in great working order – with a little help from the omegas.

> **Top Tip**
>
> A great way to cut calories is to have a substantial breakfast and dinner and a light snack lunch, with two small snacks, mid-morning and mid-afternoon.

The amount of fat in the Holford Diet, which amounts to a quarter of the overall calories, is lower than that in the average diet, which provides about 35 per cent of calories as fat. But the biggest difference between the norm and the Holford Diet is not in the *quantity* but the *quality* of fat. Eating in this way means that less than a third of the fat you eat is saturated, compared with two-thirds in the average diet.

The recipes in Part Five will take care of all this for you. The way you cook foods is also important. The best method is actually leaving the food raw, but steaming, poaching, steam-frying, boiling, baking and grilling are all good too, in that order of preference. Avoid all deep-fried food and, as much as possible, anything fried.

Summary

- Eat foods high in the essential omega-3 and omega-6 fats, with an emphasis on omega-3 fats from fish, flax and pumpkin seeds and their oils.

- Avoid foods high in saturated, hydrogenated or processed fats.

- Avoid fried, burned or browned food.

Part Four shows you how you do all this.

15

Step 3: Eliminate Your Hidden Allergies

Not all the weight you want to lose is fat. You might be holding as much as 6.3kg (1st.) of extra fluid, or even more, without knowing it. And it could all be down to a food allergy.

One in three people has hidden food allergies, which cause the weight to pile on. If you are one of them, I'd like to help you find out what your 'bad' foods are and which foods to eat instead. I'd also like to show you how to desensitise yourself to foods you're allergic to so that you can eat them once more (though it's important to note this can't be done in all cases). This normally takes three months.

Rebecca S is a case in point. In her twenties Rebecca had stable weight and good skin, and exercised three or four times a week. But in her thirties she started to pile on the pounds. Over three years her weight drifted from 63kg (10st.) up to 82.5kg (13st.) and her dress size went up to 16. She also developed itchy patches on her face and had a lot of colds and sinus trouble. She didn't exercise because she didn't feel good.

❝ *I started feeling tired and lethargic and generally unwell. I didn't have the energy to go to the gym any more.* ❞

For breakfast she'd have toast, then a main meal of meat and potatoes with gravy for lunch, and a sandwich for dinner.

❝ *But it seemed like the foods I ate were blowing me up, which is why I thought I could have a food allergy.* ❞

She decided to test herself for a food allergy, which nowadays you can do from a home test kit, involving a pinprick of blood. The results showed that she was reacting to milk, egg white and gluten – the protein found in wheat, barley and rye. Within a week of excluding these foods she found that her skin and mood improved and the weight started to fall away. After six months she had lost 19kg (3st.).

After three months of strictly avoiding the foods she'd become allergic to, she reintroduced egg whites and then milk to see if there was a reaction. Now she's fine on both foods, but still reacts to wheat.

> ❝ *I can't tell you how much better I feel. I'm 100 per cent. It has transformed my health. Having the food intolerance test has been the best thing I've done. I wish I'd done it sooner.* ❞

In the end, she shed all the weight she'd gained during the previous three years.

But first, let's explore why losing water balance can cause considerable weight gain and see whether this may be part of your problem.

Water retention, allergies and bingeing

More than two-thirds of your body is water. If you dehydrate the body by not drinking enough water or by drinking lots of coffee or tea, which are diuretic and cause a loss of body fluid, you could lose weight. But this is neither healthy nor lasting weight loss.

Another way to lose water is to eat very few calories or very little carbohydrate. Then, as we've seen, the body will use up your glycogen, which is stored with water – thus you'll lose water too. However, this weight will come piling back on, unless you wish to live your entire life on a high-protein, low-carb diet, or a very low-calorie diet, guzzling coffee, dehydrating and ageing rapidly. It is excess body fat, not water, that is associated with the long-term problem of obesity.

Just in case you wondered, drinking plenty of water doesn't lead to weight gain (unless you were seriously dehydrated in the first place). In fact, the opposite is true. The more water you drink, the less likely you are to be overweight, according to the 'MyNutrition' survey we conducted on 30,000 people.

It's a good idea to drink, at the very least, 1 litre (1¾ pints) of water every day because it helps the body to eliminate toxins released from fatty tissue as you burn it up. It also helps to dilute the bloodstream to prevent an overconcentration of sugar or protein. (This is why you become thirsty after eating a large dinner or sweets.) Some people have reported tremendous weight loss and health improvements simply by drinking 2 litres (3½ pints) of water a day. I recommend you drink the equivalent of eight glasses of water every day, which includes any hot drinks such as herbal teas.

However, the body can sometimes retain too much water, creating unnecessary weight gain. This is not a consequence of drinking too much, but indicates instead a loss of the body's ability to control water balance, leading to oedema, or water retention.

Top Tip

Press the tip of your finger into the inside of your shinbone. Does your finger make a dent? If it does, you are probably waterlogged.

Breast tenderness, experienced by many women before their periods, is caused by water retention. In fact, women can easily gain 3.2–6.3kg (7–14lb) in body weight this way – and lose it in as little as 48 hours if the cause is eliminated.

Are you waterlogged?

1 Does your face look puffy, especially around the eyes?

2 Does your abdomen, on pressing, feel waterlogged and bloated?

3 Do your arms feel puffy rather than like pure fat and muscle?

4 Do your ankles ever swell up?

5 Do your fingers ever swell up so it's hard to get your rings off?

6 Do you have dry skin or dandruff?

7 Do you ever experience sudden fluctuations in your weight?

8 Do you suffer from breast tenderness?

9 Are you prone to allergies?

If you answer 'yes' to three or more of the questions above, the chances are that water retention is partly to blame for your weight problem. There are four reasons why retention of excess fluid in the body can occur, the most common of which is allergy. But let's look at the other three culprits first.

Are you fat deficient?

The first of these is fat deficiency. Of course, for many people 'fat' is a dirty word. Yet, as we learned in Chapter 14, you can't live without essential fats.

Have you ever wondered how the body could possibly be something like two-thirds water? How do we keep it all in? The answer is fat. The body holds its water within cells encased in a membrane that's made mainly of essential fats. If you lack them in your diet, you lose the ability to maintain the correct water balance. Your skin dries up and you may get dandruffy and sweaty. At the same time, your cells become waterlogged and you look puffy and gain weight.

As we've seen, essential fats are used in the body to make hormone-like substances called prostaglandins that help control the body's water balance. In women, these fats also balance hormones throughout the menstrual cycle. Without them, the body is more likely to retain excess fluid, especially premenstrually or during the menopause. So one way that consuming enough essential fats can help you to lose weight is through water loss, if you're suffering from water retention.

Are you sugarlogged?

You'll also retain excess fluid if your diet is full of sugar. There are two reasons for this. First, every molecule of sugar holds water wherever it is in the body and in whatever form it is in: glucose, glycogen or fat. If a person is 'sugarlogged' from eating too much sugar, they'll retain excess fluid. Although it is good to maintain proper glycogen stores, there is no need to have excess fat or excess circulating glucose. By balancing your blood sugar you also help to prevent excess weight being stored as water.

Secondly, too much sugar and too much insulin lead to sodium (salt) retention. Normally the kidneys remove the correct amount of sodium. However, when you lose control of your blood sugar, the kidneys don't filter out enough, so your body's sodium levels rise. Salt attracts water, and gradually your whole body becomes a little more waterlogged. In due course blood sugar problems can lead to kidney problems, including kidney stone formation. This is one of the reasons why high-protein diets, which also tax the kidneys, are not advisable for those with blood sugar problems.

How are your kidneys?

Your kidneys filter your blood and decide how much water to keep in your system and how much to excrete. This filtration happens through over a million clusters of tiny blood-vessel masses known as glomeruli, which collectively create a surface area about the size of your living room. Through the glomeruli you filter about 48 gallons (218 litres) of blood every day. Your ability to do this decreases with age so, especially if you are over 50, your kidneys may not be working 100 per cent. This needn't be a problem, but there is a point at which it becomes one.

One of the telltale signs of decreasing kidney function is swollen ankles, especially after drinking a lot. This means that the kidneys can't work fast enough to get rid of the excess fluid. One of the major reasons kidney function decreases is continual damage caused by peaks in blood sugar. The glucose damages the glomeruli. That's why people with diabetes are especially prone to kidney problems. If you do suspect you have poor kidney function it's best to get this checked by your doctor (and stay away from high-protein diets, as I indicated earlier).

Another way you can give your kidneys a break, and help reduce excess water retention, is to take in more potassium and magnesium and less sodium. On average, a person in Britain is eating at least 10g of sodium a day, which is at least ten times more than we need. The worst offending foods are meat and processed foods.

Potassium and the mineral magnesium, both very abundant in fruits and vegetables, help balance out sodium in the body. Potassium works together with sodium in maintaining water balance and proper nerve and muscle impulses. The more sodium you eat the more potassium you need, and few of us eat enough of the latter. Fruits, vegetables and wholegrains are rich in potassium. You need five servings of fruits and vegetables a day to get the right amount of it. Magnesium also helps balance hormones and helps solve premenstrual problems, especially breast tenderness.

A high-meat diet tends to be high in sodium, whereas a high plant-based diet, with more vegetarian food, tends to be high in potassium and low in sodium. The Holford Diet is therefore naturally low in salt.

Salt content of foods

Foods	Amount	Sodium contained (g)
Bacon	2 slices	2g
Typical pizza	1 large slice	1.5g
Sandwich	1 (ready made)	1.2g
Cornflakes	1 bowl	1g
Cheddar cheese	30g (a sandwich filling)	0.5g
Packet soups	1 serving	1g or more
Crisps	100g	2.7g
Bread	100g	1.3g
Burger and bun	1	1–2g
Sausages	100g (3)	5g

Not all salts are created equal

Much sodium is 'hidden' in the form of baking powder, brine or monosodium glutamate. As we've seen, the net result of too much sodium is water retention and weight gain, and possibly high blood pressure and muscle cramps. Although there is no 'need' to add salt as there's more than enough in natural foods, not all salts are created equal.

The different types of salt

	Sodium	Potassium	Magnesium	Other Trace minerals
Solo	41%	41%	17%	
LoSalt	33%	66%	0	0
Sea salt	<99%	0.2%	<1%	
Table salt	<100%	0	0	0

Table salt, the stuff you might sprinkle on your dinner, is pure sodium chloride. Sea salt isn't much better on the sodium front, although it does have tiny amounts of other beneficial minerals. LoSalt is OK on the sodium front, but doesn't taste great.

My favourite is Solo sea salt from Iceland, which has also been shown to actually lower high blood pressure, according to research published in the *British Medical Journal*.[25] Since blood pressure and water retention are caused by the same dynamics, it's a good bet that Solo salt will reduce the risk of water retention, and hence weight gain. This is because it has 60 per cent less sodium and much more of the beneficial minerals potassium and magnesium.

Also check the foods you buy. Most processed foods use sodium chloride, though you may be able to find some 'low sodium' foods that use Solo (these will have the company's logo – an 's' within a heart with the words 'low sodium sea salt co' encircling it).

The rundown on reducing water retention

In a nutshell, what you have to do to reduce the risk of excess water retention is:

● Balance your blood sugar.

● Eat five servings of fruits and vegetables every day.

● Eat seeds (rich in essential fats, plus magnesium and potassium).

● Eat wholefoods and wholegrains such as beans, lentils, brown rice and brown bread.

● Eat more oily fish (rich in essential fats) and less meat.

● Don't add salt to your food, unless it's Solo salt.

● Choose 'low sodium' processed foods.

● Drink the equivalent of eight glasses of water, including herbal teas, a day.

This alone may cause you to lose weight if water retention is part of your problem. But the real gold, in terms of weight loss, is to find out if you are allergic to any foods and, if so, to stay off them.

Is a hidden allergy leaving you waterlogged?

The most common reason for weight gain caused by fluid retention is allergy. The word 'allergy' simply means an intolerance that causes a reaction in the immune system.

Your body is like a tube. The digestive tract, which has a surface area the size of a small football field, is the gateway between the outside world and your body. It's guarded ferociously by your immune system. If a substance that isn't on the guest list, so to speak, tries to gatecrash and get through your digestive tract and into the bloodstream, your immune system goes haywire.

The reason why food intolerance can lead to weight gain, and difficulty losing it despite going on reduced-calorie diets, is complex but is starting to be unravelled. The most common kind of food intolerance leads to the production of IgG antibodies, which activate an immune reaction when you eat an offending food. This, in turn, increases inflammation in the body, raising certain known markers for inflammation such as TNF-a and C-reactive protein (CRP). Increased inflammation also increases water retention and bloating, as well other classic signs of food intolerance, including aching joints, headaches, blocked nose, irritable bowel syndrome and skin problems. However, these symptoms are often delayed by 24 to 48 hours, so it isn't easy to know what you react to just by observing how you feel after eating a particular food. Nor is it easy to work out what you're intolerant to just by observing how you feel by the short-term elimination of the food, because some people get withdrawal symptoms when they eliminate certain foods. To make matters worse, some potential offending foods, especially wheat and milk, have an immediate pay-off by producing opioid-like chemicals called gluteomorphins and caseomorphines that make you feel good. So, if anything, you are naturally drawn to these foods. The same is true with sugar, which, in the short term, promotes energy, but actually encourages inflammation and weight gain in the long term.

The more foods you eat that provoke an IgG antibody reaction (tested in a simple allergy test) the worse it is for your health and your weight. Your immune system should not produce large amounts of IgG antibodies and, if it does, you are likely to suffer from some degree of general malaise and symptoms that just don't seem to shift, as well as resistant weight loss.

For example, a recent study found that obese children had much higher IgG antibody levels than normal-weight children. 'Anti-food IgG antibodies are tightly associated with low grade systemic inflammation and with the thickness of carotid arteries', the study authors report. The researchers conclude that having IgG antibody reactions may be involved in the development of both obesity and atherosclerosis, and that a diet based on eliminating IgG-positive foods might be the way forward.[26] Inflammation also affects the gut, potentially making the gut wall more leaky or permeable, which, in turn, may increase food intolerances.

Take the case of Joanne M, who is 36. She didn't just have weight to lose, but girth.

❝ *I used to stand in front of the mirror, grab a handful of my tummy – and despair. After a big meal I looked five months pregnant! It wasn't just my weight, which hovered around 11st. [69.8kg], it was the bloating (I'd gone up to a size 16) and the physical symptoms. I'd have to undo my trousers every time I had a big meal and I was often constipated.*

When I was in my late teens, I was diagnosed with irritable bowel syndrome. Instead of looking for the cause, doctors simply prescribed drugs to ease the symptoms. Reading up about the problem, I got the impression that a high-fibre diet would help the constipation and stop my tummy bloating. But my health regime of wholemeal bread, baked potatoes and beans was actually making it worse.

I felt exhausted all the time and usually fell asleep by 9.30 in the evening. My husband Steve kept telling me I had to do something about it. So in September 2002 I sent away for a food intolerance blood test. The results told me I was sensitive to all dairy products, yeast, salmon, trout, haricot beans and string beans. Within a week I was going to the loo every two days (instead of weekly), my tummy was gone and I was down to a size 12. My lethargy was caused by the yeasty foods I ate. I've gone from 11st. 2lb [70.7kg] to 9st. 3lb [58.5kg] and look so much trimmer now. ❞

The more often you are reacting allergically, the more resistant you become to insulin. This is because the body releases masses of immune messengers called cytokines to deal with the allergy, and cytokines make you less responsive to insulin. Also, repeated allergic reactions mean that more garbage ends up in your bloodstream as your immune cells fight off the invaders.

As antibodies, cytokines and other immune cells move in to deal with allergic invaders, they make a lot of mess that has to be cleaned up by your liver, your body's detoxifying organ. Eventually, the liver's detox capacity gets overloaded. When this happens, your body dumps the toxins in the least harmful place: your fat cells. The more intoxicated your fat cells become, the more weight you gain and the harder it becomes to shift those extra pounds. This is why people with allergies find it harder and harder to lose weight. Also, this continual process of overintoxication can turn a mild allergy into something more severe.

Many people don't find out about their allergies until it's really obvious. Lori D, for instance, didn't think about testing herself for allergies until she nearly died at the age of 54 as a result of drinking a glass of pineapple juice.

I was 8½st. [54kg] until ten years ago when I suddenly went up to 15st. [95.2kg] and size 20. One fateful evening I had a sore throat and drank a litre [1¾ pints] of pineapple juice throughout the night. By morning my throat had closed up, I could hardly breathe and I'd turned purple. I drove to my GP, where I collapsed on the step.

Because of this I decided to have proper food tests done, which proved that not only was I intolerant to milk and yeast, but also to pineapple, cranberry and kidney beans. Now I've cut out those foods, I feel really good. My once stubby fingers are now slim and I've lost more than ½st. [3.2kg] in two weeks. Knowing I'm food intolerant helps as it makes me think about what I should be eating and helps me stick to my diet.

Discovering whether you're allergic

Allergies can be responsible for many symptoms, especially digestive problems, from bloating to constipation, and diarrhoea to abdominal cramps. These are almost always accompanied by mental and physical symptoms, such as mood changes, chronic tiredness, depression, increased appetite, sleepiness after meals, inability to concentrate and a host of minor ailments, from itches and rashes to asthma and sinus problems. Check yourself out with the questionnaire below.

Your instant allergy check

1   Can you gain weight in hours?

2   Do you get bloated after eating?

3   Do you suffer from diarrhoea or constipation?

4   Do you suffer from abdominal pain?

5   Do you sometimes get really sleepy after eating?

6   Do you suffer from hay fever?

7   Do you suffer from rashes, itches, asthma or shortness of breath?

8   Do you suffer from water retention (see the 'Are You Waterlogged?' questionnaire on page 182)?

9 Do you suffer from headaches?

10 Do you suffer from other aches or pains, from time to time, possibly after certain foods?

11 Do you get better on holidays abroad, when your diet is completely different?

If you have answered 'yes' to any of these questions, there's a real possibility that you have an allergy. If you answered 'yes' to four or more, it's pretty much guaranteed.

Top Tip

Do you get bloated after eating and have to undo a button or two? If so, it is very likely you are eating something you are allergic to.

As we've seen, bloating, pain, diarrhoea and constipation are often indicators of an allergy. Lisa M is a classic case. She had suffered for six years with abdominal bloating before she worked out it might be an allergy:

My bloating was so bad that my boyfriend David measured round my waist and found I'd ballooned by 5in [13cm] in one day. Anything I ate seemed to go straight through me – but despite that, I remained 5st. [31.7kg] overweight. My doctor reckoned my body had gone into starvation mode, making the most of anything I fed it because of my tummy upsets.

Lisa then took a food intolerance test, which revealed she was sensitive to eggs, milk, wheat, yeast, rye and beef:

I'd been practically living on these foods. I had eggs for breakfast most days, and for lunch I'd often choose cottage cheese and egg sandwiches, thinking they were a healthy option. Little did I know I was poisoning myself.

Within three days of dropping the culprit foods, Lisa began to feel much better:

I've now gone six months without a tummy upset and I've lost nearly 3st. [19kg]! I feel like I have my life back.

Pinpointing the allergen

It may seem odd, but more often than not the foods a person is allergic to are those they really crave. If you're craving and eating something frequently, as though you're mildly addicted, there is a chance you're allergic to that food. Through my work with a number of allergic and overweight clients, it became clear to me that they were bingeing only on certain food groups. When they were instructed to eat as much as they liked of anything *except* the suspected allergen (the food provoking an allergic reaction), they often ceased to binge. And, when they avoided the allergen completely, they often lost 1.3–1.8kg (3–4lb) and occasionally as much as 3.2kg (7lb), almost overnight.

This sort of short-term weight loss can only be the result of excess fluid retention, and nothing to do with fat. You can't burn 450g (1lb) of fat in 24 hours, even if you are starving – and much less, 3.2kg (7lb)!

One of the physical symptoms of an allergic reaction can be a sudden fluctuation in blood sugar level that, in turn, affects appetite. So could allergic reactions trigger bingeing? In honesty, nobody has a definite answer to this question, but my observations of a number of clients certainly show that sometimes allergies do play a role in overweight problems, and there's a one-in-three chance they play a role in yours.

There are two ways to find out what you are allergic to. The first we could call 'educated trial and error'. You need to avoid suspect foods for 14 days and note what happens by taking the pulse test, explained below.

The pulse test

Most people are free of symptoms within 14 days of avoiding an allergy-provoking food. And most will react on reintroducing the food within 48 hours, although some may have a reaction delayed by up to ten days. Delayed reactions are much harder to test. For some people, symptoms improve considerably when they leave out the offending foods. For others, noticeable changes are slight.

One simple way to help identify possible suspects is the pulse test. The pulse test demands that you avoid all suspect foods for 14 days, then reintroduce them one by one, with a 48-hour gap between each item to be tested. Take your resting pulse, sitting down, before you eat the food,

continued

then take it again after 10 minutes, 30 minutes and 60 minutes. Write all this down on a chart like the one opposite. If you have a marked increase in pulse rate of more than 10 points, or have any symptoms of ill health within 24 hours, including immediate weight gain, bloating, fatigue, headaches or joint aches, for example, avoid the food and wait 24 hours before testing the next food.

Although day-to-day changes in symptoms are hard to pin down to specific causes, avoidance of suspect foods for 14 days often lessens symptoms, which then increase significantly on reintroduction. So you'll be able to pinpoint which foods or drinks make you worse. It is very important to observe symptoms accurately, because you may have preconceived ideas about what you do or don't react to, perhaps because of what somebody told you, or because you dread being allergic to certain foods that you're addicted to.

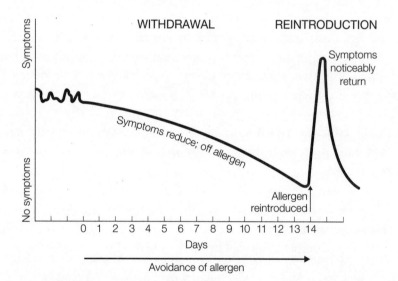

The avoidance/reintroduction test for allergies If you avoid a food you are allergic to you may notice an improvement in how you feel within 14 days. If you then reintroduce the food you may notice a return of symptoms.

(**Note:** if you have ever had a severe or life-threatening allergic reaction I recommend you to do this avoidance/reintroduction test *only* under the supervision of a suitably qualified practitioner.)

continued

Suspect food	Pulse	Pulse and symptoms	
	Before 10 mins	30 mins	60 mins
Egg	_____	_____	_____
Wheat	_____	_____	_____
Milk	_____	_____	_____
Yeast	_____	_____	_____
_____	_____	_____	_____
_____	_____	_____	_____

IgG allergy testing – the gold standard

Because the body sometimes delays its allergic reaction to a food, avoidance/reintroduction tests don't always pick the allergy up. This happens because you may not suspect the food, and so not test it. Or you may suspect only one food, yet be allergic to a range of them, so you'll continue to have a background of reactions and may thus have difficulty losing weight.

The best and truly accurate way to find out what you are allergic to is to have what's called a Quantitative IgG ELISA test. This is the gold standard of allergy testing. 'Quantitative' means the test shows not only whether you are allergic, but also how strong your allergic reaction is. Many of us live quite healthily with minor allergies. But stronger allergies can create all sorts of problems, including weight gain. 'ELISA' is the technology used. You don't need to know all the details but, trust me, it's the most accurate system. If it's done properly it is at least 93 per cent reproducible. It's used by almost all the best allergy laboratories in the world.

To convey why it's so good, I need to explain a bit about the human immune system.

Your immune system can produce tailor-made weapons that latch onto specific substances to help escort them out of your body. They are like bouncers on the lookout for troublemakers. The bouncers are called immunoglobulins, or Ig for short. There are different types. The real heavies are called IgE, although most allergies involve IgG reactions. IgE reactions tend to be more immediate and severe – like Lori's reaction to pineapple. However, most 'hidden' allergies that may be insidiously causing weight gain are IgG-based. In an ideal world you test for both, but I normally start by testing a person for IgG sensitivity to food. If you'd like to find out more about the science behind IgG-based food allergies and intolerances go to www.patrickholford.com/IgGfoodallergies.

All that's needed for testing is a pinprick of blood, which is absorbed into a tiny tube and sent to a laboratory. The lab then sends back an accurate readout of exactly what you are allergic to. Your body doesn't lie. You either have IgG bouncers tagged for wheat (for example) or you don't. Your diluted blood is introduced to a panel of liquid food 'testers' and, if you've got IgG for that food, a reaction takes place.

There are a number of laboratories who do IgG testing (see Resources on page 432), and one that offers a handy test kit you can use at home. Yorktest have devised a clever procedure that involves a painless pinprick device and an absorbent material that you place against the pinprick. This material is then sent to the laboratory for testing.

The good news about IgG-based allergies is that if you avoid the offending food strictly for three to six months, the body forgets that it is allergic to it. The reason is that there will no longer be any IgG antibodies in your system to that food. This doesn't hold for IgE-based reactions, however.

To give you an example, I have an IgE allergy to milk. I react within 15 minutes. Even if I avoid dairy products for a year, I still react if I consume some. I used to have an IgG to wheat. I avoided it for three months and now I no longer react. In my case, weight gain wasn't the problem: it was migraine headaches. I had them every other week from the ages of 6 to 20, until I discovered that wheat and milk were triggering them.

Fenton R, like myself, had regular headaches, sinusitis and fatigue and had been plagued by acid indigestion for 20 years. He was also gaining weight year on year. Doctors were unable to help him, suggesting he drank too much fizzy pop and should exercise more. And indigestion tablets helped for only about 20 minutes before the problem returned with redoubled force.

He decided to have a food intolerance test. The results came back showing he was intolerant of eggs, cow's milk, yeast and wheat. He took all the rogue foods out of his diet, for example by switching to soya milk, and within two days the indigestion began to ease. Now it has gone completely, along with all the other health problems that had dogged him – including an excess 12.7kg (2st.) in weight.

❝ It feels as though a shroud has been lifted from me. Not only have I lost the weight, but I also have 100 per cent more energy. It used to be an effort to go up the stairs. I used to get headaches most days, and they have gone. I used to get sinus twinges almost every day, and that has cleared up. I used to sweat a lot, and thought I was just a sweaty person. But now I can walk and run and just don't sweat. My skin used to be cold all the time but now it's nice and warm. I feel more relaxed as well. It had got to the stage where I couldn't even think clearly, but now I can do so again. ❞

The usual suspects

The most common foods or food groups that people are allergic or intolerant to are shown below, in order. Of all these foods, by far the most common allergy-provoking substances are dairy products, followed by yeast, eggs and wheat. This doesn't necessarily means that these foods are bad for you, it just depends on whether or not you are allergic or intolerant to them.

The most common food allergies are:

- cow's milk
- yeast
- eggs
- gliadin grains such as wheat (also rye and barley)
- nuts
- beans
- white fish
- shellfish

Cow's milk

The most common food allergy is to cow's milk. It's present in most cheeses, cream, yoghurt and butter and is hidden in all kinds of food; sometimes it's called 'casein', which is milk protein.

Logically, its status as an allergen isn't surprising, since it is a highly specific food, containing all kinds of hormones designed for the first few months of a calf's life. It's also a relatively recent addition to the human diet. Our ancestors, after all, weren't milking buffaloes. Approximately 75 per cent of people (25 per cent of people of Caucasian origin and 80 per cent of Asian, Native American or African origin) stop producing lactase, the enzyme that's needed to digest milk sugar, once they've been weaned. Is nature trying to tell us something? However, it's not the lactose – the sugar in milk – that causes the allergic reaction. It's the protein.

If you react to cow's milk, it doesn't necessarily mean you will react to goat's milk or sheep's milk. However, many people do. It's often best to eliminate all dairy food for the first three months, then try goat's milk or cheese or yoghurt.

As dairy is the most common allergen, it is used very little in the recipes in this book. If you do have difficulty tolerating it, you may find that you are all right with sheep's- or goat's-milk products. These are easier to digest though they have a distinctive, tangy flavour, much stronger than cow's milk. However, if you've had an allergy test and it's confirmed that you're allergic to all dairy, avoid all of it, including yoghurt and butter. In most cases, if you strictly avoid your allergy-provoking foods for three months, your body can 'unlearn' the allergy. So it doesn't have to be a life sentence.

There are many alternatives to dairy now, including soya and quinoa 'milks'. Try them out and find one you like. Use the GL chart on page 383 for your guide to quantity.

Yeast

After milk, yeast is the second most common culprit in allergies. Some people think they are allergic to wheat because they feel worse after eating bread. If you've noticed this – perhaps feeling sluggish, tired or blocked up – but feel fine after pasta, you may not be allergic to wheat, but to the yeast in the bread.

Take Janette B, who is 45. Noticing her weight creeping up, Janette didn't link it with food sensitivity.

> ❛ Over seven years my weight soared by 3st. [82.5kg] to 13½st. [85.7kg] and although I was a member of a slimming club, stuck strictly to a low-calorie diet, and took regular exercise, I could never lose more than about 1st. [6.3kg]. ❜

Not only was Janette heavier than before but she also felt constantly tired and uncomfortably bloated after meals, particularly when she'd eaten bread. 'I was so frustrated by my weight and so fed up with feeling exhausted that I decided to have a food intolerance test,' she said. The results showed she was intolerant of yeast and milk and also sensitive to corn and soya, as well as haricot and kidney beans. Simply by avoiding her 'bad' foods, Janette lost 15kg (2st. 5lb) in five months!

Yeast is not only in bread as baker's yeast but it's also in beer and, to a lesser extent, wine. Beer and lager are fermented with brewer's yeast. If you've noticed that you feel worse after beer or wine than after spirits – the 'cleanest' being vodka – then you may be yeast-sensitive. If you have been allergy-tested, you'll know whether you are allergic to brewer's or baker's yeast. Most people who are allergic to yeast at all are allergic to both. Wines are yeast-fermented. Champagne has very little yeast. However, the only guaranteed yeast-free alcoholic drinks are pure spirits. Since you won't be drinking much alcohol, it's best to stick to spirits for the first three months so that your body has a chance to unlearn your allergy.

If you're allergic to yeast, you've also got to be on the lookout for hidden yeast in stock cubes and processed food. As the Holford Diet features wholefoods and fresh ingredients, and avoids yeasted breads, this should be far less of a problem for you. I also recommend using yeast-free vegetable stock cubes by Marigold.

A word about alcohol: as well as causing allergies in some, alcohol irritates the digestive tract, making it more permeable to undigested food proteins. This increases your chances of developing an allergic reaction to anything, and it's why some people feel worse when they eat foods they are allergic to and drink alcohol at the same time. For example, you might be mildly allergic to wheat and milk and feel fine after either. But when you have both, plus alcohol, you don't feel great.

Wheat

This is the grain that more people react to than any other. It contains gluten, a sticky protein also found in rye and barley and oats. Gluten sensitivity occurs in about one in a hundred people,[27] but it is medically diagnosed in fewer than one in a thousand. However, there is something in gluten, called gliadin, which some people react to specifically. The only way to know for sure exactly what you are allergic or intolerant to is to have a food intolerance test. If you have had an allergy test you'll know whether you are sensitive to gluten, gliadin or wheat.

If you are gluten-sensitive, then you cannot eat wheat, rye, barley or oats. Excellent alternatives are rice, quinoa, buckwheat, millet and corn (although some gluten-sensitive people do react to corn). Quinoa and millet cook in much the same way as couscous. From the GL point of view, quinoa is the best. These days, you can find rice, corn and buckwheat breads and pastas in larger supermarkets and good health-food shops.

There's no gliadin in oats. If you are gliadin-sensitive, then you can eat oats, but not wheat, rye or barley. Oats also contain potent anti-inflammatory compounds.[28]

If you are only wheat-sensitive, it's relatively easy. Just eat rye, barley or oats. For example, you can eat rye bread, oatcakes and oat-flake cereals, but not Weetabix or wheat bread.

In the big scheme of things wheat's prominence as an allergen shouldn't be surprising. Grains are the second most recent addition to the human diet, and weren't eaten by hunter-gatherers. They were eaten by farmers for something like the last 10,000 years, but only in certain parts of the world. For example, no gluten grain naturally grows in North America, so Native Americans have been exposed to gluten for only about the last 200 years at most.

A worrying trend in the US, where 'low-carb' diets are the craze, is to remove the carbohydrates from wheat products so you're just eating the protein portion. As this is principally gluten, it's a recipe for disaster for anyone with a hidden gluten allergy.

Eggs

Some people are allergic to egg white, but not egg yolk. If you are sensitive to eggs, when you come to reintroduce them, it's best to start by reintroducing egg yolk. If you don't react within five days, then reintroduce egg white. Eggs are in quite a lot of processed foods and bakery items, so check the label carefully.

Nuts and beans

These are part of the same food family, along with fruit pips. In essence, they're all seeds. The most common individual allergens in this group are, in descending order, cashew nuts, Brazil nuts, almonds, peanuts, haricot beans and soya beans. You can react to one and not others, but if you do react to a member of this family there's a greater chance that you'll react to another member of the pip/bean/nut family. Coffee, from the coffee bean, and chocolate, from the cocoa bean, are also members of this family.

Fish

Another major allergen is fish, but most people who are allergic to it react to white fish, not the oily fish such as salmon, mackerel and herring that are so rich in omega-3s. If you're also allergic to those kinds, however, take a tablespoon of ground seeds with breakfast every day (see page 236), together with a good-quality supplement, to keep your essential fatty acids topped up.

Shellfish allergies are very common, with prawns and abalone two of the worst villains. You may be allergic to mussels, scallops, whelks, oysters and squid, which are molluscs – or to lobsters, crayfish, prawns and shrimps, which are crustaceans. Octopus is in a world of its own! Be careful here, though. If you're allergic to squid but not to octopus, be aware that some people sell squid labelled as octopus to make a bigger profit, because they can buy it more cheaply.

How the Holford Diet caters for you

If you suffer from food allergies, you don't have to feel deprived on the Holford Diet. It is always sensible to vary your diet as much as possible, and the menu plans and recipes in Chapters 26 and 27 are designed to include a wide range of ingredients. Such a varied diet, together with the introduction of exciting new foods such as quinoa, soya products and lesser-used legumes such as flageolet and cannellini beans, ensures that there is plenty to tempt your taste buds, even if you do have to avoid certain items.

When you have an allergy test, the best laboratories will give you clear instructions on what not to eat and what you can eat, as well as giving you the backup of a nutritionist to answer any of your questions. (See Resources, page 432.) By avoiding foods that cause symptoms, you will probably find improvements in your health that you didn't ever imagine. I can't count the times I've heard people say, 'I didn't even know I could feel this good.' The Holford Diet and supplements will also help to further reduce your allergic potential.

After three months of abstaining from the allergen, you may then find that you can tolerate it in small periodic 'doses'. For some people the allergy disappears completely. Others have to be careful about certain foods for life. Once you have more than a sneaking suspicion that you are allergic, it is best to have an allergy test.

Once you've identified what you are allergic to, and eliminated it, the next step is to improve your gut health. I recommend having a heaped teaspoon of glutamine powder in water last thing at night to help heal the gut, plus a probiotic supplement containing dairy and sugar-free acidophilus and bifido bacteria to help restore gut health. These are only necessary for a couple of weeks after eliminating your offending foods to restore gut health and reduce your allergic potential.

Summary

- Find out if you are allergic to something you're eating and avoid it. You can do an avoidance/reintroduction test but, quite frankly, it's better to have a proper 'quantitative IgG ELISA' test.

- After three months you can reintroduce the foods you tested positive for, although ideally not eating them every day.

- Even if you are not allergic to it, reduce the amount of cow's milk you eat and drink, substituting goat cheeses, soya produce and the like.

- Even if you are not allergic to it, reduce the amount of wheat you eat, substituting other grains such as oats, rye and rice.

- Limit alcohol. Ideally drink no more than three small glasses of wine, half-pints of beer or lager, or single spirits a week.

- Drink the equivalent of eight glasses of water a day.

Part Four shows you how you do all this.

16

Step 4: Take the Right Supplements

So far you've learned that by changing the quality of the big guys – fats, carbohydrates and proteins – you can lose weight because your body's metabolism finally starts working properly. Now, I'd like to take a look at the little guys: vitamins and minerals.

Your body's daily functions depend on myriad chemical reactions that, in turn, depend on vitamins and minerals. Your fatburning capability, for instance, relies on you getting optimal amounts of certain micronutrients. For example, to make insulin you need zinc and vitamin B_6. Insulin's ability to control blood sugar levels is helped by the mineral chromium. To turn glucose into energy, rather than fat, you need B vitamins, magnesium and vitamin C. And to burn fat you need all these, plus the B vitamin biotin.

No doubt you've heard the mantra 'As long as you eat a balanced diet you get all the vitamins and minerals you need' from someone, sometime. As I've said before, this is the greatest lie in nutrition today. Why? Because there's only a slim chance that your diet meets even the full range of RDAs – and also because it all hangs on your definition of 'need' as well as what you want from life.

RDAs, or recommended daily amounts of vitamins and minerals, are in any case misleading at best. Governments the world over have worked these out by starting from the bottom up – that is, looking merely at preventing the obvious vitamin-deficiency diseases. These range from scurvy (vitamin C deficiency) and beriberi (vitamin B_1) to pellagra (niacin). But, as we learn more and more about the health-promoting properties of vitamins and minerals, RDAs have crept up and up. In the UK, for instance, the RDA for vitamin C has moved up from 30mg to 45mg to 60mg, and in the US it's now 85mg.

The problems with RDAs go further than this, though. They are mere averages, and you are far from average. You are unique. According to Dr Roger Williams, a pioneer in nutrition who discovered vitamin B_5 (pantothenic acid) and helped discover folic acid, even twins with identical genes can have twentyfold differences in their nutritional needs![29] Where you live, how much exercise you get, your gender and your genes can easily alter your needs for various nutrients by a factor of ten. That's why I call the RDAs 'ridiculous dietary arbitraries'. So, if you are happy with average poor health, go for the RDAs.

Optimum nutrition, maximum weight loss

Let's say, though, that you want the most out of life. You want to be the right weight and stay there, and you see your health not just as an absence of ill health, but as total well-being. If this is you, you need *optimum* nutrition.

At ION, we worked out micronutrient needs by starting from the top down. We sought the intake of a vitamin that would promote optimal health, not prevent scurvy. We asked the question, 'What amount of vitamin X equates to the maximum possible well-being and the smallest possible risk of disease?' For the past 20 years, we've been investigating the effects of vitamins, minerals and essential fats on weight, IQ, memory, mood, energy, immunity, infections, lifespan, pregnancy and disease risk. From this we established the ODAs or *optimum daily amounts*. These are the amounts of nutrients that will tune up your body's metabolism, making it easier for you to lose weight, and keep it off for good.

Using vitamin C as an example, the RDA is 60mg. The average intake is 100mg. If you eat plenty of fruit and vegetables you could achieve 200mg. The optimal intake is somewhere between 1,000 and 3,000mg. The ODA is set at the mid-point of 2,000mg. The shortfall between a good diet (200mg) and the ODA (2,000mg) is 1,800mg. This is the kind of level worth supplementing.

Have a look at the chart opposite. You'll notice that the ODAs are often 10 times the RDAs. You'll also see what the average diet provides – and what you could be achieving if you eat a healthier diet, with plenty of wholefoods, fruit and vegetables. But there's still a shortfall between what we've researched as optimum and what you are likely to get in food.

NUTRIENTS	RDA	100% RDA	ODA
Vitamin A (mcg)	800	900▷ 1500▷ ◁Shortfall 1,000▷	2,500
Vitamin D (mcg)	5	4▷ 7▷ ◁Shortfall 4▷	11
Vitamin E (mg)	10	14▷ 50▷ ◁Shortfall 250▷	300
Vitamin C (mg)	60	100▷ 200▷ ◁Shortfall 1,800▷	2,000
Vitamin B₁ (mg)	1.4	2▷ 5▷ ◁Shortfall 30▷	35
Vitamin B₂ (mg)	1.6	2.18▷ 5▷ ◁Shortfall 30▷	35
Vitamin B₃ (mg)	18	39.6▷ 50▷ ◁Shortfall 35▷	85
Vitamin B₅ (mg)	6	2.175▷ 20▷ ◁Shortfall 80▷	100
Vitamin B₆ (mg)	2	3.1▷ 5▷ ◁Shortfall 70▷	75
Folic acid (mcg)	200	325.5▷ 400▷ ◁Shortfall 400▷	800
Vitamin B₁₂ (mcg)	1	5.95▷ 10▷ ◁Shortfall 15▷	25
Biotin (mcg)	150	36.50▷ 120▷ ◁Shortfall 105▷	225

GLA* (Omega-6) (mg)	–	20▷ 40▷ ◁Shortfall 110▷	150
EPA/DHA* (Omega-3) (mg)	–	60▷ 100▷ ◁Shortfall 600▷	700

Calcium (mg)	800	(800:good diet)▷ 912.5▷ ◁Shortfall 200▷	1,000
Iron (mg)	14	12.8▷ 15▷ ◁Shortfall 5▷	20
Magnesium (mg)	300	272▷ 350▷ ◁Shortfall 150▷	500
Zinc (mg)	15	9.3▷ 10▷ ◁Shortfall 10▷	20
Iodine (mcg)	150	193.5▷ 240▷ ◁Shortfall 60▷	300
Selenium (mcg)*	–	40▷ 50▷ ◁Shortfall 50▷	100
Chromium (mcg)*	–	50▷ 75▷ ◁Shortfall 50▷	125
Manganese (mcg)*	–	3▷ 6▷ ◁Shortfall 4▷	10

Key

■ Average diet
□ Good diet

RDA = Recommended daily allowance
ODA = Optimum daily allowance (diet plus supplements)
* items marked with an asterisk have no RDA

RDAs versus ODAs and dietary intakes This chart shows the differences between the RDA, our average intake, and our ideal intake. The grey amounts are the levels we could reach if we ate a good variety of fruit and vegetables daily – that is, a good diet.

And that's where supplements come in. They make up the difference – the difference between how you feel now and how you *could* feel if you were optimally nourished, losing weight steadily and feeling fantastic.

Turning glucose into fuel, not fat

To understand how vitamins and minerals help with the crucial job of fatburning, let's take a close look at what happens to glucose in the body.

The brain, muscles, liver, skin, immune system, heart and arteries are all simply a collection of cells that do different jobs for the body, whether it's digesting, thinking or moving. The fuel that keeps them going is, as we've found, glucose. So keeping an even level of blood sugar – the cells' fuel reserve – is the first step in making energy.

Within each of our 30 trillion or so cells exist tiny energy factories called mitochondria. These turn glucose into another chemical, pyruvic acid, a process that releases a small amount of energy, which can be used by the cell to carry out its work. If there isn't enough oxygen around while this is happening, a by-product called lactic acid builds up. That's why, when you do strenuous exercise after a relatively sedentary period, your muscles ache the next day. The more you exercise, developing larger muscles, the less strain you put on them and the more oxygen they can use. This is what aerobic exercise is all about: providing muscle cells with enough oxygen so that they can work properly.

Next, pyruvic acid is turned into acetyl-coenzyme A, or AcoA. This substance is perhaps the most vital in fuelling our body, because if you're starved of glucose, for example when a marathon runner 'hits the wall', you can break down fat or protein to make AcoA and use this for energy. But, because this method is relatively inefficient, your body prefers to rely on carbohydrates, and glucose, for fuel.

From this point on, oxygen is needed every step of the way. AcoA enters a series of chemical reactions known as the Krebs cycle (named after its discoverer, Ernst Krebs). During this, hydrogen molecules split off, meet oxygen – and *bang!* Energy is released. In fact over 90 per cent of all our energy is derived from this final stage. The waste products from this process are carbon dioxide (which we exhale), water (which goes to form urine) and heat. That's why you get hot when you exercise. Muscle cells make lots of energy, creating heat.

Best vitamins for fatburning

Complex carbohydrates and oxygen are only half the story. All these chemical reactions are carefully controlled by enzymes, which are themselves dependent on no fewer than nine vitamins and six minerals

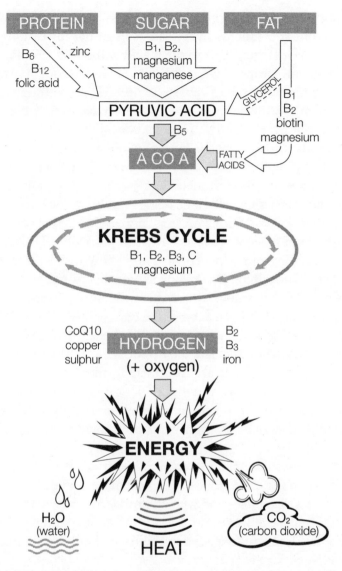

Turning food into energy The glucose we eat is converted within our cells to release and give us energy. This is done by enzymes that, in turn, depend on vitamins and minerals. Consuming enough vitamins and minerals helps turn food into energy instead of fat.

(see diagram above). If there is any shortage of these critical catalysts, your energy factories – the mitochondria – go out of tune. The result is inefficient energy production, a loss of stamina, highs and lows – or just lows. This leads to cravings. And whatever your body can't turn into energy easily it turns into fat. So part of the weight-control equation is making energy efficiently.

The important vitamins here are the B-complex vitamins, a family of eight different substances. Every one is essential for making energy. Glucose can't be turned into pyruvic acid without B_1 and B_2 (niacin). AcoA won't work properly without B_1, B_2, B_3 and, most important of all, B_5 (pantothenic acid). The Krebs cycle needs B_1, B_2 and B_3 to do its job properly, along with vitamin C. Fats and proteins can't be used to make energy without B_1, B_2, B_6, B_{12}, folic acid or biotin.

It used to be thought that as long as you ate a reasonable diet you'd get enough B vitamins. But studies have shown that, over the long term, slight deficiencies – which are all too easy to develop – result in depletion of these vitamins within cells. The results can be serious. Early warning signs are poor skin condition, anxiety, depression, mental confusion and irritability, fatigue and excessive weight in particular. Health and diet surveys, including our own, consistently show that people who take multivitamins containing B vitamins are less overweight.

Most people's diets fall short of the optimal requirements for these vital vitamins, and few even achieve the basic RDAs. In one ION study a group of 82 volunteers, many of whom already had a 'well-balanced diet', were assessed to calculate their optimal nutritional needs.[30] All 82 were given extra B vitamins in supplement form, often in doses 20 times that of the RDAs. After six months, 79 per cent of participants reported a definite improvement in energy, 61 per cent felt physically fitter and 60 per cent had noticed an improvement in their mental alertness and memory.

Being water-soluble and extremely sensitive to heat, B vitamins are easily lost when foods are boiled. The best natural sources are therefore fresh fruit, raw vegetables and wheatgerm. Seeds, nuts and wholegrains contain reasonable amounts, as do meat, fish, eggs and dairy produce. But these levels are reduced when the food is cooked or stored for a long time.

As well as eating these foods – and Part Four will give you the details – I strongly recommend that you use a high-strength multivitamin supplement to guarantee an optimal intake of all the B vitamins, plus 1,000mg of vitamin C.

Best minerals for fatburning

The minerals iron, calcium, magnesium, chromium and zinc are also vital for making energy. Calcium and magnesium are perhaps the most important, because all muscle cells need an adequate supply of these to be able to contract and relax. A shortage of magnesium, which is very common in people who don't eat a lot of fruit or vegetables, often results in cramps, as muscles are unable to relax. Magnesium is involved in 75 per cent of the enzymes in your body[31] – and it is absolutely vital for blood sugar control and burning carbohydrate for energy, rather than storing it as fat. Although most diets provide enough calcium, few provide enough magnesium. Good multivitamins will give you an additional 150mg of magnesium and calcium. It is well worth taking a supplement.

Zinc, together with vitamin B_6, is needed to make the enzymes that digest food.[32] They are also essential in the production of insulin. A lack of zinc disturbs appetite control and causes a loss of taste or smell, a combination that often leads to overeating of meat, cheese and other strong-tasting foods. Zinc deficiency is very widespread. The optimal intake is 20mg a day, whereas the average intake is 9mg.

It's well worth correcting this shortfall by taking a daily multivitamin/mineral that gives you 10mg of zinc, as well as eating zinc-rich foods such as seeds and 'seed' foods – meaning anything you could plant in the ground that would grow. This includes beans, peas and lentils. Broccoli, including the Tenderstem variety, are also good sources. The very best source of zinc, however, comes from oysters. If you ate an oyster a day, you wouldn't need to supplement with zinc!

Chromium – the secret of balancing blood sugar

The older you are, the less likely you are to be getting enough chromium[33] – an essential mineral that helps stabilise blood sugar levels and, hence, weight. The average daily intake is thought to be in the region of 28–35mcg, although an optimal intake, certainly for those with a weight and blood sugar problem, is around 200mcg. Chromium is found in wholefoods and is therefore higher in wholewheat flour, bread or pasta than refined products. (Flour has 98 per cent of its chromium removed in the refining process – another reason to stay away from overprocessed products.) Beans, nuts and seeds are other good sources, and asparagus and mushrooms are especially rich in it. In addition to the problem of low consumption due to eating refined and processed foods, it has been shown that typical Western diets high in refined food such as white bread, cakes, sweets and biscuits increase chromium losses because it is used up in processing sugar.

Chromium's role in insulin regulation was first proven in the 1970s.

We now know that the essential mineral increases insulin binding, increases the number of insulin receptors and also increases insulin effectiveness; all of which lead to improved glucose transport into muscle, fat and liver tissue, and therefore better glucose control.

Since chromium works with insulin to help stabilise your blood sugar level, appetite and weight, the more uneven your blood sugar level, the more chromium you use up. Hence a sugar and stimulant addict, eating refined foods, is most at risk of deficiency.

Two studies carried out at Bemidji State University in Minnesota have shown that chromium supplementation helps to build muscle and burn fat.[34] Because it helps to lower cholesterol as well as stabilise blood sugar levels, it is especially helpful for people at a high risk of developing diabetes.[35] And, in trials where chromium supplementation was taken by people who made no change to their diets, it had a small effect on weight loss compared with placebos.[36] The real benefit of chromium supplementation is that it reduces hunger, as well as fat and sugar cravings, and hence your appetite for the wrong foods. As a consequence, you lose more weight. This has been shown in both human and animal studies.[37] One study on people with 'atypical' depression (see page 111), supplementing 600mcg of chromium, found that half the volunteers reduced their food cravings and consequently lost weight, whereas those taking placebos gained weight.[38]

Whether or not you can achieve an optimal intake of chromium from diet alone is debatable. It is therefore wise to take supplements of this fatburning mineral as well as eating wholefoods. The best form of chromium is chromium polynicotinate, which means it's bound with vitamin B_3 (also called nicotinic acid). Most good multivitamins will contain 30mcg of chromium, but you can help balance your blood sugar and reduce sugar cravings more quickly by taking 200–400mcg a day for the first three months of the Holford Diet. Chromium supplements, usually in 200mcg amounts, are readily available in any health-food shop.

Slimming pills – the next generation

I'm hardly a fan of slimming pills. Few actually work, and those that do often act like stimulants: speeding up your metabolism and giving you short-term weight loss – and potential *long*-term problems. Over time, some may end up slowing down your metabolism, and may even promote weight gain. This category includes ephedra (now banned), guarana and other sources of caffeine. Others, such as conjugated linolenic acid (CLA for short) promised great results on animal studies, but failed to deliver significant weight loss in human trials.[39]

There are two, however, that I like and recommend: hydroxycitric acid (HCA for short) and 5-hydroxytryptophan, or 5-HTP.

HCA curbs your appetite

HCA is extracted from the dried rind of the tamarind fruit (*Garcinia cambogia*), which you may know from Indian and other Eastern cuisines. HCA is not a vitamin, but it will help you lose weight. Originally developed by the pharmaceutical giant Hoffman-LaRoche, it has been proved to slow down the production of fat and reduce appetite. It has been extensively tested and found to have no toxicity or safety concerns.

HCA works by inhibiting the enzyme that converts sugar into fat. The carbohydrate in a meal is first used to provide fuel and short-term energy stores as glycogen. Any excess is then converted to fat by the enzyme ATP-citrate lyase. HCA dampens down the activity of this enzyme. Evidence of HCA's fatburning properties has been accumulating since 1965.[40] For example, participants in one eight-week, double-blind trial reported an average weight loss of 5.03kg (11lb 2oz) per person, compared with 1.9kg (4lb 3oz) on a dummy pill.

HCA also reduces the synthesis of fat and cholesterol. Animal studies have confirmed this, and it may be that HCA has a role to play in helping those with high triglyceride (fat) or blood cholesterol levels. There is also evidence that HCA may enhance the burning of calories and increase energy levels. According to John Sterling, whose company BioCare was among the first to introduce HCA to the UK, 'People are reporting very positive results. HCA doesn't help everybody, but it is helping about 50 per cent of those who've tried it.'

A recent trial conducted by the University of Maastricht in the Netherlands confirms that HCA acts as a powerful appetite suppressant, reducing weight with no harmful effects. In the study – which was the best kind, a so-called double-blind, placebo-controlled, randomised, crossover trial – 12 men and women were given a tomato-juice drink three times a day for two weeks. They then had a two-week break. Following this, the group were divided up, unbeknown to them. Some participants drank tomato juice with a placebo, others drank one containing 300mg of HCA, three times a day for the next two weeks.

Only those taking the HCA-loaded drink ate less – a total of 15 to 30 per cent fewer calories. However, they didn't report that they tried to eat less, tried to restrict their diet or experienced any loss of enjoyment regarding their food. They just happened to eat less. They also lost more weight, averaging 450g (1lb) extra weight loss a week.[41] HCA is both effective and safe for promoting weight loss.[42]

I recommend taking HCA, especially during the first three months of the Holford Diet. You need 2,250mg a day of Garcinia Cambogia extract, containing at least 50% HCA. Most supplements (see Resources) provide 750mg per capsule, so take one capsule three times a day, ideally anywhere from immediately before, to 30 minutes before, a main meal.

5-HTP helps you 'think thin'

Have you ever thought about why you get hungry? You might think the obvious answer is because you haven't eaten. But that isn't always true, is it? And don't you often find yourself craving something sweet even though you just ate more than enough food?

The two most powerful controllers of your appetite are your blood sugar level and your brain's level of serotonin, the 'happy' neuro-transmitter. Serotonin is made from an amino acid, or building block of protein, called *tryptophan*. Many people have low levels of this vital brain chemical and feel depressed as a result. This is especially true of people on weight-loss diets, most of which are notoriously low in tryptophan.

But that isn't all. Serotonin controls appetite. The more you have, the less you eat – and the less you have, the more you eat (most people eat more when they are depressed, and low in serotonin).

If you are low in serotonin, one of the quickest ways to restore normal levels, and normal mood, is to supplement your diet with a special form of tryptophan called 5-hydroxytryptophan, or 5-HTP for short. It's found in meat, fish and beans, although in rather small amounts. But one, the African griffonia bean, contains significant amounts, and extracts of this are sold as 5-HTP supplements.

It's not just speculation that 5-HTP works: it's been proven to make you feel happier and want to eat less. Although it's been known for some time that giving 5-HTP to animals causes a reduction in appetite, followed by a loss in weight,[43] two recent studies, conducted by Dr C. Cangiano and colleagues at the Department of Clinical Medicine, University of Rome (La Sapienza) in Italy, show that 5-HTP does the same thing in overweight people.

In the first study, 20 obese volunteers took either 5-HTP (900mg) or a placebo for 12 weeks. During the first six weeks, volunteers could eat what they liked. During the second six weeks the volunteers were recommended a low-calorie diet. In both phases those taking 5-HTP consistently ate less, felt more satisfied and consequently lost weight.[44] What was particularly interesting was that they ate less carbohydrate.

The second study gave 25 overweight non-insulin-dependent diabetic volunteers either 5-HTP or a placebo for two weeks, with no dietary restriction. They could eat what they liked. In the words of the researchers, 'Patients receiving 5-HTP significantly decreased their daily energy intake, by reducing carbohydrate and fat intake, and reduced their body weight.'[45]

Why the reduced craving for carbohydrates? Imagine two breakfasts. One is an Atkins-style bacon and eggs, high in protein. The other is cornflakes with chopped banana and a muffin. Which will give your serotonin a boost, thereby satisfying you the more? If you think about it logically, you'd say the protein-rich, hence tryptophan-rich, breakfast. But you'd be wrong. It's the cornflakes, banana and muffin breakfast.

Why? Even though the bacon and eggs do contain tryptophan, it has a hard time getting from your blood into your brain – it just doesn't compete well with all the other amino acids in these high-protein foods. However, it does get into the bloodstream. So what drives it into your brain? The answer is insulin. Insulin, which is released by a high-carbohydrate breakfast, carries tryptophan into the brain, and gives you a mood boost. What this means is that when you are feeling tired, hungry and a little blue you crave something sweet, not a sausage. Sound familiar?

Top Tip

A low-GL carbohydrate-only snack raises the brain's level of serotonin, which makes you happier and reduces sugar and carbohydrate cravings. If you're particularly prone to such cravings replace one of your twice-daily carb-and-protein snacks with a low-GL carbohydrate-only snack such as strawberries.

One big secret of successful weight loss is to (a) ensure you have enough serotonin so that you have less desire to eat in excess; and (b) keep your blood sugar level, and your insulin release even, so that you don't have increased appetite due to blood sugar dips. Remember: too much insulin drives blood sugar into body fat, whereas too little means low serotonin levels and increased carbohydrate cravings. It's a careful balancing act and one that the Holford Diet takes into account.

Fatburning supplements put to the test

To test the effects of the diet, with or without supplements, we conducted a survey of 72 Holford dieters who had followed the diet for an average of 17 weeks.[46] Those who said they had followed the diet with reasonably high compliance reported an average weekly weight loss of 770g (1lb 11oz), compared to those who had followed the diet with low-compliance, who reported an average weekly weight loss of 400g (14oz).

Those with high dietary compliance who took a multivitamin and any two or more of chromium, *Garcinia cambogia* extract (containing HCA) and 5-HTP reported a higher average weight loss (900g/2lb per week) compared to those who didn't take supplements (590g/1¼lb per week). Those who only took a multivitamin also reported a slightly higher average weight loss compared to the non-supplemented group (625g/1lb 6oz/week). See the diagram below.

Of the 72 respondents, 27 reported having more energy, 20 said they had better skin and 28 described the diet as easy. There were many

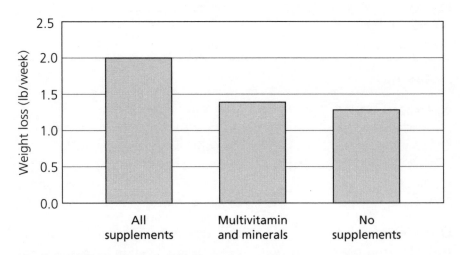

Effects of supplements on weight loss

other reported benefits including fewer cravings for sweets and stimulants, improved mood, less bloating and better sleep.

Many people have tried the Holford Diet with and without supplements. It works either way, but there's no question that these supplements really do make a difference.

Here's what I recommend to maximise weight loss.

Fatburning supplements – the basics

I recommend that you supplement your well-balanced diet with fatburning vitamins and minerals, to ensure your metabolism is working at peak efficiency. The ideal intake is different for every individual and can be worked out individually for you by a nutritional therapist (see page 432). However, the chart below gives a good approximation of the optimal supplement levels for an average person, given they're eating a healthy, balanced diet.

Vitamins	Optimum daily intake
Vitamin A	1,500mcg
Vitamin B$_1$ (thiamine)	25mg
Vitamin B$_2$ (riboflavin)	25mg
Vitamin B$_3$ (niacin)	50mg
Vitamin B$_5$ (pantothenate)	50mg
Vitamin B$_6$ (pyridoxine)	50mg
Vitamin B$_{12}$ (cobalamine)	10mcg
Folic acid	200mcg
Biotin	50mcg
Vitamin C	1,000mg
Vitamin D	15mcg
Vitamin E (d-alpha tocopherol)	100mg

Minerals	Optimum daily intake
Calcium	200mg
Magnesium	150mg
Iron	10mg
Zinc	10mg
Manganese	3mg
Chromium	30mcg

In summary, what this means is taking, on a daily basis:

Daily supplements

> 2 × multivitamin/mineral
> 1 × vitamin C 1,000mg

Most health-food shops can help you find supplements to meet these levels in the simplest and least expensive way, choosing from a variety of good brands. Decent, high-strength multivitamin/mineral supplements will tell you to take two a day – you just can't get these optimum levels in one tablet. Supplements should be taken with food, preferably with breakfast, or spread throughout the day, since it is during the day that we make most energy and hence need a good supply of these nutrients.

Fatburning supplements – pulling out the stops

During the first three months, if you want all the help you can get in stabilising your appetite and sugar cravings, I recommend the combination of HCA, 5-HTP and chromium. Some supplement companies provide these in combination (see Resources). These are the optimal daily levels:

	Optimum daily intake
Garcinia cambogia extract (contains HCA)	2,250mg
5-hydroxytryptophan (5-HTP)	100–200mg
Chromium	200–400mcg

Bear in mind that 5-HTP is much more effective at normalising the brain's serotonin levels if taken with some carbohydrate, such as a piece of fruit. This will also help prevent the minor abdominal discomfort that a small minority of people get when they take 5-HTP. My advice, therefore, is to supplement both your morning and afternoon snacks with 50mg of 5-HTP.

A word of caution: don't take 5-HTP if you are on serotonin-reuptake inhibitor drugs (SSRIs) such as Prozac, Xeroxat, Paroxetine or Lustral, to name just a few. These drugs block the reuptake of serotonin, whereas 5-HTP provides the brain with the raw material to make enough in the first place. (Logically, 5-HTP should be a more effective antidepressant with fewer side effects. It is – and if you want the proof, see my book *New Optimum Nutrition for the Mind*.) Theoretically, taking both could overload you with serotonin. Although I know of no case as such, I don't recommend taking both anti-depressant drugs and 5-HTP.

Also take 200mcg of chromium twice a day, with your midmorning and afternoon snack. Both these supplements tend to reduce sugar cravings and make you feel less hungry and more satiated.

HCA works best before meals. Most supplements supply 750mg per tablet or capsule. You need three times this amount to make a difference, so take one capsule up to 30 minutes before each meal.

All these supplements are easy to find in most health-food shops.

Summary

- Supplement with a high-strength multivitamin and mineral, usually taken in two daily doses, plus vitamin C every day.

- Supplement with additional chromium, HCA and 5-HTP, especially if you are prone to sugar cravings and have poor appetite control, for the first three months.

Part Four shows you how you do all this.

17

Step 5: Do 15 Minutes of Exercise a Day

The body is designed to be active. If you've ever truly enjoyed exercise – be it anything from a brisk walk in the park to trekking in the Himalayas – you'll know that wonderful feeling of being at ease and at one with your body. But, even if you've hated exercise, were 'bad at sports' as a child and wouldn't touch an activity holiday with a bargepole, you'll find that the kind of exercise I advocate is amazingly easy to get into, and enjoy.

Exercise is the final puzzle piece in the fatburning picture. Let's take a look at why, and how, it works.

Why exercise?

If you haven't led a very active life, or did once but have gradually become more sedentary, it's not surprising. Life in the West conspires against it. Cars, remote controls, food processors, takeaway deliveries, 'home entertainment centres', escalators, lifts . . . every year, there are more gadgets and mod cons that do away with the need to expend energy. Ultimately, all roads here lead straight to the sofa, and, if you give in, couch-potato syndrome awaits.

Once that happens, it's all too easy to pile on the pounds. There is no doubt that part of the reason for the massive increase in the number of overweight people is that we are becoming less active.[47] And not only does less activity mean fewer calories burned, but it also interferes with the body's appetite mechanisms, rate of metabolism and ability to keep blood glucose levels stable. In other words, some exercise is essential for the body's chemistry to stay 'in tune'.

Now, according to calorie theory, exercise is a poor method of losing weight. After all, running a mile burns up only 300 calories. That's equivalent to two slices of toast or a piece of apple pie. But this argument misses three key points.

1. The effects of exercise are cumulative. OK, so running a mile a day burns up only 300 calories. But if you do that three days a week for a year, that's 22,000 calories! Also, the number of calories you burn up depends on how fat or fit you are to start with. The fatter and less fit you are, the more benefit you'll derive from small bouts of exercise.

2. Moderate exercise decreases your appetite. A degree of physical activity is necessary for appetite mechanisms to work properly. Those who do not exercise have exaggerated appetites and hence the pounds gradually creep on.

3. Exercise boosts your metabolic rate. The most important reason why exercise is a key to weight loss is its effect on your metabolic rate. According to Professor William McArdle,[48] exercise physiologist at City University, New York, 'Most people can generate metabolic rates that are eight to 10 times above their resting value during sustained cycling, running or swimming. Complementing this increased metabolic rate is the observation that vigorous exercise will raise metabolic rate for up to 15 hours after exercise.'

The dynamic duo: diet and exercise

Combining diet and exercise is the best way to lose weight. Weight lost through restrictive dieting is often half fat and half lean tissue, such as muscle. Since muscle burns up more energy (calories) than fat, the less muscle you have, the slower your metabolism is. Combining the Holford Diet with a good exercise programme ensures you lose fat, not lean muscle. The best kind of exercises to help to burn fat efficiently are brisk walking, jogging, cycling, swimming, aerobic dance, stepping, cross-country skiing, circuit training or any aerobic exercise that is steady, continuous and of a certain intensity.

Such exercises also tone the body, reduce the risk of osteoporosis, increase muscle tissue and reduce one's body fat percentage (high ratios of body fat to lean tissue have been linked to heart disease, diabetes and some cancers). They will strengthen your heart and lungs, reduce your risk of heart disease, help control stress and improve circulation.

Exercise improves insulin sensitivity

But exercise does more than make you leaner. It also helps regulate body chemistry that's essential for fatburning. According to Vanessa Hebditch of the British Diabetic Association, 'Being overweight reduces insulin sensitivity so the risk of developing diabetes is higher. However, there is proof that exercise increases insulin sensitivity, thereby reducing risk.' Many studies have shown that exercise helps regulate blood sugar levels, increases the body's sensitivity to insulin, and decreases blood lipids (fats) while also helping to burn body fat.[49]

Exercise is especially important in middle age because we are less likely to be able to maintain an even blood sugar level as we age.[50] A study of 87,000 women aged between 34 and 59 showed that those taking vigorous exercise at least once a week reduced their risk of diabetes by a third, compared with those who didn't workout.[51] Unsurprisingly, our sensitivity to insulin decreases with age, along with our control of blood sugar. But physical activity in middle and old age improves insulin sensitivity, therefore helping to stabilise blood sugar levels and weight.[52] Athletes have vastly improved blood sugar control, enhanced insulin sensitivity and faster metabolic rates.[53]

And there's more. High-intensity exercise, such as aerobics, reduces insulin levels and raises glucagon levels. This means you improve your production of good prostaglandins, boost circulation (and thus the supply of oxygen and nutrients to cells) and increase your ability to burn fat.

Anaerobic exercise such as using weights doesn't burn fat in the same way, or to the same extent. If it is intense enough, though, it may release human growth hormone (controlled by good prostaglandins), which builds muscle and burns fat.

In short, exercise offers a huge array of benefits. If you haven't really got into it before, it opens up an undiscovered world of vitality, health and sheer enjoyment.

Top Tip

Go for a stroll after a meal, especially if you tend to get sleepy after meals. It helps to stabilise your blood sugar and insulin level.

How much exercise?

Exercise shouldn't mean a fanatical struggle for some mythical level of fitness. The important thing is merely to stay within the 'training heart rate zone' for your age. Appendix 5 shows you how to work this out (see page 413).

The most traditional formula for calculating your 'training heart rate zone' is to subtract your age from 220. This allows you to estimate your maximum heart rate. This is not the level at which you need to work, this is the predicted maximum your heart can perform at. Once you have calculated your maximum, it is one small step to calculating your training zone.

An overweight, out-of-condition person may reach their training-heart-rate zone by walking just a few hundred yards. A fitter, leaner person may have to walk briskly for at least five minutes to push their pulse up to their training zone. This is why you need to monitor your pulse while exercising to make sure you do not over- or underexercise, and achieve the best fatburning benefits. As you get fitter and leaner, you'll find that you will have to push harder – perhaps by walking faster or adding more hill walking to your programme – to reach your training zone.

According to surveys, the best benefits in terms of longevity come from expending more than 2,000 calories a week. Walking uses up approximately 300 calories an hour, so you'd need to walk for six hours a week. Jogging is twice as efficient, so you'd need to do only three hours a week. The more overweight you are, the more calories you burn up, so you may need to do only two hours.

If you are doing the right kind of exercise, all you need to do is 15 minutes a day. And this will be enough both for losing weight and trimming your figure. If you want to confine your exercising to the working week, you can do 21 minutes Monday to Friday and leave the weekend free. Alternatively, you may choose to 'double up' and exercise three times a week for 35 minutes. It doesn't sound that difficult, does it? And it isn't.

When to exercise

The best time to exercise is two hours after eating. If you exercise first thing in the morning, make sure you have breakfast straight after. Even better, if you aim to eat some fruit, perhaps an apple, with your breakfast, have half before you exercise, then the other half with breakfast.

Don't exercise late at night. Exercise promotes adrenal hormones, including cortisol. Cortisol should be lowest at night as too much can make it hard for you to sleep. Also, if possible, exercise in natural daylight, because you'll make vitamin D in your skin, which means stronger bones.

One great way to up your general level of exercise is simply to get more active generally. Use the stairs instead of the lift; walk or cycle instead of driving everywhere; run around with your kids, or take up a sport. There are many ways in a day to develop fitness, and soon this way of living will become a habit.

The fat way	The fit way
Take a lift	Use the stairs
Use a trolley when shopping	Use a hand basket
Drive to work	Walk or cycle some of the way
Drive to the shops	Walk to the shops
Spend the evening watching TV	Take up an active hobby
Get other people to bring you a drink when they get their own!	Get up and get your drink yourself and get theirs
Use powered tools for gardening or DIY work	Use manual tools when it's just as quick
Go upstairs as little as possible at home	Run upstairs as often as possible
Use automatic car washes	Wash the car yourself
Stick children in front of TV	Actively play with them
Discuss things sitting down	Go for a walk where possible

The more you exercise, the less you eat

Contrary to popular belief, moderate exercise actually decreases your appetite. According to new evidence on appetite research, both animals and humans consistently show a decreased appetite where there are small increases in physical activity. One study looked at an industrial population in West Bengal, India. Those doing sedentary work ate more and consequently weighed more than those doing light work. As the level of work increased from light to heavy, workers ate more, but not relative to their energy output. The result was that the heavier the work, the lighter the worker.

Job classification	Daily caloric intake (calories)	Body weight (kg/lb)
Sedentary	3,300	67kg (148lb)
Light work	2,600	53.5kg (118lb)
Medium work	2,800	51.7kg (114lb)
Heavy work	3,400	51.25kg (113lb)
Very heavy work	3,600	51.25kg (113lb)

Building muscle, burning fat

Having the right balance of hormones, especially insulin – the fat-storage hormone – helps the body to use protein and, if you're exercising, to turn the protein you eat into muscle. And muscle, in its turn, burns fat. Thus the exercise plan I've outlined above works brilliantly with the Holford Diet to turn you into a lean and healthy fatburner.

A word of warning for the scale-watchers, though: when you start a committed exercise programme, and lose fat and gain lean muscle, you will lose inches faster than pounds. In the first month you'll look trimmer and feel fitter but may lose less weight than you wished. This is because muscle is denser, and hence heavier than fat. In other words, 450g (1lb) of muscle takes up less space than 450g (1lb) of fat.

Remember, the enemy is not so much your weight, but having too high a body-fat percentage. So check this every month using the chart in Appendix 1 (page 375), rather than jumping on the scales only. The more lean muscle you gain, the more ability you'll have to burn fat – and that's what counts.

How do you fit the food around your exercise? Generally, as I've said above, it's good to eat a balanced meal one to two hours before training. Or you can have a light snack half an hour before. Drink plenty of water while you're exercising and eat either a balanced snack or a light meal within an hour of finishing a hard workout. Don't let yourself get so hungry that you eat the wrong food. Glucose drinks, energy bars and the like abound, but by now you'll realise that they're not the way to go for fatburning.

Now we're ready to look in depth at how you're going to put all the pieces together, in Part Four.

Summary

- Exercise at least 15 minutes a day, or 35 minutes three times a week.

- Choose aerobic types of exercise that raise your heart rate into the training zone.

- Choose exercise that helps you to build more muscle, which, in turn, burns fat.

PART FOUR

The Action Plan

18

In a Nutshell

The Holford Diet is not a gimmick. It has been tested over 20 years of clinical experience, and is backed by hundreds of scientific trials. It is the best way of helping you lose weight and gain health, easily and enjoyably, because it works with your body's natural design. All you have to do is get your blood sugar balance back to normal, to kick-start your body's own formidable fatburning ability. And in this section I'll show you how – every step of the way.

The key principles behind the Holford Diet are explained in Part Three. Make sure you understand these before you start.

If you're ready – here are the ground rules:

Food

Out

- **Avoid sugar** in its many disguises, refined foods and foods that contain fast-releasing carbohydrates with a high-GL score – that is, above 10 ⓖⓛ per serving.

- **Avoid foods high in saturated, hydrogenated, processed fats or damaged fats**, such as sausages, fried food and junk food.

- **Eliminate any foods you're allergic to**. You can do an avoidance/ reintroduction test, but in the long run it's better to have a proper quantitative IgG ELISA test. (After three months you can reintroduce the foods you tested positive for, ideally not eating them every day.)

In

- **Eat no more than 40 ⓖ a day**, choosing foods that contain low-GL carbohydrates, below 10 ⓖ per serving.

- **Eat low-GL carbohydrates with protein-rich foods**.

- **Eat whole, unadulterated food, high in soluble fibre** (beans, lentils, oats etc.).

- **Eat foods high in the essential fats** omega-3 and omega-6, with an emphasis on omega-3 fats from fatty coldwater fish, seeds and their oils.

Drink

Out

- **Limit or avoid alcohol**. Ideally, drink no more than three small glasses of wine, half-pints of beer or lager, or single measures of spirit a week.

- **Limit or avoid caffeinated drinks**. Ideally, drink no more than one regular coffee or two weak teas a day. Avoid all caffeinated fizzy drinks.

In

- **Drink the equivalent of eight glasses of water a day**, including non-caffeinated herbal teas or diluted juices.

Supplements

In

- **Supplement your diet with a high-strength multivitamin and mineral (twice daily), plus vitamin C, every day**.

- **Supplement your diet with additional chromium, HCA, 5-HTP or konjac extract** (glucomannan fibre) if you are prone to sugar cravings and have poor appetite control, for the first three months.

Exercise

In

● **Exercise at least 15 minutes a day**, or 35 minutes three times a week.

Each one of these makes a difference in its own right. Put them all together and amazing things can happen, because the whole is far greater than the sum of its parts. This is the most effective way to reduce body-fat percentage, lose excess weight and gain health without a rebound effect. Do all this for 30 days and you will switch your body's metabolism from storing fat to burning fat. You will be a fatburner.

Putting all this into practice is even simpler than it sounds. In essence, all you have to do is:

● **Eat any recommended breakfast, lunch or dinner, plus two of the snacks**.

● **Take the recommended supplement programme every day**.

● **Do fatburning exercise on a regular basis**.

There are two ways to do this. Either follow the four weeks of sample menus, together with recipes, in Part Five. Or, for the more independent among you, or any time you're eating out (including working lunches), you can devise your own regime using the chart on pages 386–401. Simply follow the golden rules, and you'll be following the Holford Diet.

Whichever way you choose, it's a good idea to stick to the Week 1 menu. This will give you a good idea about quantities, and how to prepare some of the fatburning foods that may be new to you.

Exercise is important for everybody. Combining the Holford Diet with a regular exercise programme (at least three times a week) will undoubtedly give you top results.

It's as simple as that!

One of the first things you'll feel is the satisfaction – you won't have that starved feeling some diets give you. According to Hilary Evans, the first ever Holford dieter:

❛ *I have never felt hungry on this diet.* ❜

She lost over 9.3kg (1st. 6lb).

Chances are you'll also feel more energised and alert within days of starting the Holford Diet. Beyond that, it just gets better.

Now let's look at what you need to do before you start.

19

Getting Ready

Getting ready for the diet is a bit like a warm-up before you exercise. You need a week to prepare: restock your fridge with fatburning foods, find the best alternative foods and drinks and your nearest suppliers, and get used to some of the new foods.

As I said in Part Three, if you're addicted to coffee, tea, chocolate, alcohol and/or cigarettes, you'll need to cut them all out of your life when you start the diet. I realise that cutting out cigarettes might take a bit more time, although you'll be surprised how a combination of resolve, modern techniques for quitting and getting into the fatburning way of life will help cut the cravings. This is also a great time to try out your exercise options (see Chapter 28) and fit them into your weekly routine.

Remove temptations

You'll also need to remove any edible temptations. Start by using up or throwing away any of the foods you'll need to avoid (these are outlined in the following chapters) from your fridge or larder. This is a great time to have people round for dinner! Restock your kitchen with the recommended foods and drinks. Do the same at work.

Some of the foods on this diet may be new to you, but all of them are readily available from your local health-food shop, supermarket or good greengrocer's. There's a shopping list for you, as well as guidance on how to prepare foods that may be new to you, in Chapter 24.

Setting your targets

Most people start diets hoping to lose in a month what they gained in a year. They vow never to eat chocolate again and to exercise every day. This approach usually ends in failure.

Remember, the purpose of the Holford Diet is to reprogramme your body to burn fat. Although it is specifically designed for you to lose weight, equally important is changing your body's chemistry so that you become more inclined to burn unwanted fat than to store it. This takes about 30 days. Once this is achieved, losing weight becomes much easier.

In the meantime, you don't want to start out like a rookie in diet boot camp. So here's my advice on easing into this new way of eating and exercising.

Be realistic

Be realistic, and take it one step at a time. Set yourself targets for changing your diet and taking exercise that you know you will reach. The weight will look after itself. It is far better to take one step towards permanently changing your lifestyle than to take four steps forward and four steps back because you were overambitious to start with.

After all, we often eat because we are under pressure or stressed. Boredom, frustration, anger or a lack of direction all lead to feelings that can be temporarily suppressed with food. Even making small dietary changes is, to begin with, stressful. It takes time to adjust. So don't add to your stress by expecting too much from yourself and then failing to meet your targets.

Be patient

It took years to get that fat. Does it really matter if you take months, rather than weeks, to lose it? Our impatience drives us towards the countless 'get-slim-quick' diets that have been shown, time and time again, not to produce long-term results.

It is very hard for the body to lose more than 900g (2lb) of actual fat in a week, although you can also lose a lot of excess fluid when you stop eating something you're allergic to. Anything more rapid is likely to be mainly the short-term loss of fluid caused when you eat too little carbohydrate for energy production, leaving the body to break down stores of glycogen. Glycogen is stored with water – hence the apparent loss of fat that's really loss of water.

Obviously, this won't be happening with the Holford Diet: good-quality, low-GL carbs are an important part of it, as is a sure and steady weight loss.

What results can I expect?

According to studies on the Holford Diet, the average weight loss achieved is 450–900g (1–2lb) a week over a 12-week period. That's 6.3–12.7kg (1–2st.) in less than three months. It is better not to lose weight faster than this. Weight loss of over 900g (2lb) a week will not be all fat loss.

Generally speaking, a good target during the first 30 days is to lose 2.7kg (6lb). This is easily achievable on the Holford Diet. But don't forget that your body-fat percentage is far more important than your weight, so don't rely on your scales as the only means for checking your progress. As you begin to make more lean muscle you won't lose so much weight, because lean muscle is heavier than the fat you burn off. But you will lose inches, since muscle is more compact than fat.

Making muscle is good news, not only because you'll look leaner. Muscle cells are more metabolically active and therefore have the capacity to burn off fat, whereas fat cells don't. So, as you make more lean muscle, your ability to burn fat increases. Therefore, with the Holford Diet, you'll be able to lose weight and inches consistently, month after month, as well as gaining health and vitality.

How do you measure your body-fat percentage? You can do this roughly on a week-by-week basis using the equation in Appendix 1. If you do have access to the equipment for measuring it, perhaps at your gym, aim to reduce it by 10 per cent each month until you reach the optimal level of not more than 15 per cent for a man and 22 per cent for a woman.

The chart in Appendix 1 shows your ideal weight range for your height. These figures are calculated from life insurance figures. If you're within your ideal range, I recommend that you don't aim to lose more than 1.8kg (4lb) a month until you reach your target. If you are above the ideal range, your target should be no more than 3.6kg (8lb) a month.

Week-by-week planning

When setting your target, it is good to have long-term and short-term objectives. Let's call your long-term objective your goal. What weight would you like to be, ideally? The following questions help to give you a realistic yardstick to go by. What do you weigh now? What, in your opinion, is your ideal weight? How does that compare with the chart in Appendix 1? When were you last that weight? What is the most you've ever lost on a diet?

When you've answered these questions, you'll have a good idea of your ultimate goal. Once you've set it, you can work out your target, week by week, and fill it in on the charts on pages 408–12. For example, if you want to lose 6.8kg (15lb), your target after one week would be to weigh 680g (1½lb) less and so on for ten weeks, when you achieve your goal.

Now you are ready to get fatburning! The next three chapters tell you what to eat for breakfast, lunch, dinner and snacks.

20

What to Eat for Breakfast

First of all, don't skip breakfast. It's the most important meal of your day. You may feel that the old adage 'Breakfast like a king ...' is being taken down and dusted off, but it's absolutely true, and here's why.

When you wake up, your blood sugar is low because you haven't eaten. So you need to eat. But many people in the grip of a firm resolve to lose weight make the fatal mistake of trying not to eat anything for as long as possible. Unless propped up with liquid stimulants (coffee or tea), nicotine, or instant sugar in the form of a piece of toast or a croissant, that resolve becomes weaker and weaker as your blood sugar level dips lower and lower, until the chances of making the right food choices become smaller and smaller. So you buckle under the strain and end up bingeing on high-GL foods. Sounds familiar?

That's why you must eat breakfast. The only question is what and how much. Nutritionists at Oxford Brookes University set out to test this by giving children either a low-GL breakfast or a high-GL breakfast, then measuring who ate the most as children helped themselves to a buffet lunch. Although both breakfasts were rated as equally satisfying by the children immediately after eating, by lunchtime those who'd had the high-GL breakfast were hungrier and ate more food.[1] Exactly the same thing has been shown in adults too.[2]

The message is clear. Eat a low-GL breakfast. It will satisfy you for longer so you'll eat less later.

There are two ways to do this. The simplest is to choose from any of the Holford Diet breakfasts listed on page 312. These are already calculated to give you no more than 10 Ⓖ, plus the right amount of protein and essential fats.

Or you can 'do it yourself'. The DIY Holford Diet breakfast is also very straightforward. The fundamental rules are shown in the diagram overleaf.

Breakfast

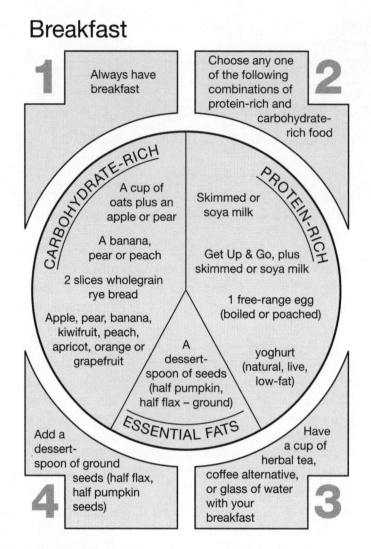

The Holford Diet: breakfast

There are five fundamental breakfasts that give you the correct balance of both carbohydrate and protein. These are:

Carbohydrates		Protein
Cereal/fruit	+	seeds/yoghurt/milk
Fruit	+	yoghurt/seeds
Fruit	+	Get Up & Go/milk
Bread/toast	+	egg
Bread/toast	+	fish (such as kippers)

The question is which and how much cereal, fruit, toast and so on? Let's kick off with the cereal-based breakfast, sweetened with fruit rather than sugar.

The best cereal-based breakfasts

A good cereal-based breakfast needs to include a low-GL cereal, a low-GL fruit as a sweetener and a source of protein and essential fats. The goal, remember, is no more than 10 🄶ᴸ.

In the chart below you'll see how much of the following six cereals you can have to total 5 🄶ᴸ. As you can see, the best 'value' in terms of your appetite are oat flakes, either cooked as in porridge or eaten raw, just as you would cornflakes. Basically, you could eat as much as you like, given that one very large bowl (75g) will fill anybody up.

Cereal	5 🄶ᴸ
Oat flakes	2 servings
All-Bran	1 serving
Unsweetened muesli	1 small serving
Alpen	half a serving
Raisin Bran	half a serving
Weetabix	1 biscuit

Below you can see how much of these six fruits you could eat to equal 5 🄶ᴸ.

Fruit	5 🄶ᴸ
Strawberries	1 large punnet
Pear	1
Grapefruit	1
Apple	1 small
Peach	1 small
Banana	less than half

So your best bet out of these would be to have porridge or raw oat flakes with as many strawberries as you could eat. Alternatively, you could have a bowl of All-Bran and a grapefruit, or a bowl of unsweetened muesli with a small grated apple. Or you can build up your own breakfast using the full GL Chart in Appendix 2 on page 383.

As far as protein is concerned, there's some in milk (or in soya milk, if you're allergic to dairy). Rice milk is high-GL and best avoided.

Yoghurt (unsweetened) is also high in protein. So, have a spoonful of yoghurt, some milk or some soya milk on your cereal if you'd like to.

Another source of protein, as well as countless vitamins, minerals, essential fats and fibre, is seeds. I recommend you have a tablespoon of ground seeds on your cereal as well. This really adds flavour and, by giving yourself the essential fats you need, you won't crave less desirable food sources of fat.

Top Tip

Smart animals – from parrots to people – eat seeds. Seeds are incredibly rich in essential fats, minerals, vitamin E, protein and fibre. You need a tablespoon a day for 100 per cent health. Here's the magic formula:

1. Take a glass jar that has a sealing lid and half-fill with flaxseeds (rich in omega-3), then fill the remaining half with a mixture of sesame, sunflower and pumpkin seeds (rich in omega-6).
2. Keep the jar sealed and in the fridge to minimise damage from light, heat and oxygen.
3. Put a handful of the seed mixture in a coffee/seed grinder, grind up and put a tablespoon on your cereal. Store the remainder in the fridge and use over the next several days.

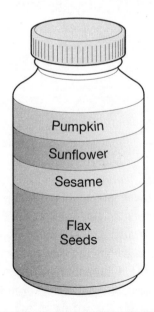

The best cereal-based breakfast is Fatburner Muesli, made by mixing porridge oat flakes, oat bran and ground seeds, fresh berries and yoghurt. See the recipe on page 313. A serving has a GL of 8 and is completely satisfying.

The best yoghurt-based breakfasts

If you are fond of yoghurt, you could dispense with the cereal altogether and have yoghurt, fruit and seeds. Let's take a look at how this adds up. In the chart below you'll see how much yoghurt you can eat for 5 ⓖ. (A small pot of yoghurt is 150g/5½oz.)

Yoghurt	5 ⓖ
Natural yoghurt	2 small pots (300mg)
Non-fat yoghurt	2 small pots
Low-fat yoghurt with fruit and sugar	less than 1 small pot (100g/3½oz)

So, provided you choose a yoghurt that doesn't have added sugar, you can eat two small pots, and sweeten it with any of the fruits you like from the fruit chart on page 240, plus a tablespoon of ground seeds.

Breakfasts based on Get Up & Go

Get Up & Go is a powder that you blend with a piece of fruit, choosing from any of the 5 ⓖ servings of fruit shown earlier and 350ml (12fl oz) skimmed milk (or sugar-free soya milk if you are allergic to dairy).

Get Up & Go is made from a special blend of quinoa, brown rice and soya flour, giving an excellent quality of protein. This is balanced with carbohydrate, mainly from whole apple powder, together with oat bran, rice bran and psyllium husks for added soluble fibre, plus sesame, sunflower and pumpkin seeds and some almond meal, cinnamon and natural vanilla for flavour. In addition, it has added vitamins and minerals, including 50mcg of chromium and 1,000mg of vitamin C, plus all the B vitamins.

When it's made up, it's guaranteed to fill you up until lunchtime, and yet is only 283 calories. The best fruits to add to Get Up & Go are strawberries, raspberries, a soft pear, blackcurrants (which you can buy in cans in apple juice) or banana. If you use banana, use only half a fruit. Get Up & Go provides about 5 ⓖ, so you're looking for no more than another 5 from the fruit you blend in with it. (See page 436 for Get Up & Go stockists.)

The best egg-based breakfasts

Although it is true that more than half the calories in an egg come from fat, the kind of fat depends on what feed the chicken has been given. Most eggs come from battery chickens. These chickens are unhealthy and their eggs are high in saturated fat, so eggs from battery chickens are not suitable.

However, there are egg producers that give their chickens feed rich in fatty acids, for example flaxseeds. These brands include Columbus, Intelligent Eating and Goldenlay. These are both free-range and rich in omega-3 fats, and much better for you than ordinary eggs. I recommend you have no more than six eggs a week on the Holford Diet – preferably omega-3 eggs, though free-range or organic eggs are OK. Have either two small eggs, or one large egg, at one meal. Poach, boil or scramble them, but don't fry them, because the high heat damages the essential fats.

What to eat with your eggs

As eggs are pure protein and fat, what carbohydrate can you have with them? If this is your entire breakfast you can use up your entire 10 🄶🄻 quota by having any of the following bread servings.

Bread and oatcakes	10 🄶🄻
Oatcakes	4
Pumpernickel-style rye bread	2 thin slices
Sourdough rye bread	2 thin slices
Rye wholemeal bread (yeasted)	1 slice
Wheat wholemeal bread (yeasted)	1 slice
White, high-fibre bread (yeasted)	less than 1 slice

As you can see, your best-'value' breads are oatcakes or Scandinavian-style pumpernickel (sonnenbrot- or volkenbrot-type) breads, or sourdough rye bread, made without yeast. Unlike the light, white, fluffy 'fake' breads we've been conditioned to eat (which are full of air, super-refined and nutritionally inferior), sourdough and the like are real breads – substantial, fibre-rich and delicious. You may find the change a bit of a shock at first, but you'll discover that they are very satisfying.

Real breads are better for the following reasons. First, is the way they're processed, which I discussed in Part Three. Second, they have far fewer additives, use coarsely ground flours and, in the case of sourdough, have no added yeast. All this keeps the GL score lower.

The lowdown on grains

Some grains are better than others because of the type of carbohydrate, or sugar, they contain. Wheat and corn are high in a fast-releasing sugar called amylopectin, whereas barley, rye and quinoa are higher in one called amylose, which is slower-releasing. Most rice, by the way, has a high GL score, because it contains a large proportion of amylopectin. Basmati rice, however, has more amylose and is therefore slower-releasing. Brown basmati is best.

Of the grains, oats are among the best. Whereas the GL of wheat varies depending on what's done to it, oats are the same whether you're eating whole oat flakes, rolled oats or oatmeal, as used in oatcakes – all have a low glycemic effect.[3]

Kippers, anyone?

Kippers (which are smoked herring) have gone out of fashion, but they make a fabulous fatburning breakfast – tasty and highly nutritious. Rich in protein and omega-3 fats, one kipper and any of the bread portions shown above will meet your needs for a fatburning breakfast.

Now let's move on to snacks, since that's the next thing you are going to eat.

21

What to Eat for Snacks

The Holford Diet is all about enjoying your food while losing weight and boosting health, and snacks give you even more scope for enjoyment. But what to eat? Those with sugar sensitivity are likely to reach for snacks that compensate for changes in blood sugar levels and hormonal responses. Most commercial snacks are incredibly high in sugar or fat. It won't surprise you that a Mars Bar is almost two-thirds sugar with the rest mainly fat; but even some so-called 'muesli' bars are deceptively unhealthy, made with refined sugar and masses of hydrogenated fat.

However, research shows clearly that 'grazing' (eating little and often) is healthier for you than 'gorging' (having one or two big meals in the day).[4] Grazing helps keep your blood sugar level even and this makes overeating far less likely, as you'll never experience any between-meal hunger pangs. For this reason I recommend you have a mid-morning and a mid-afternoon snack. The ideal snack is one that provides no more than 5 ⒼⓁ and also some protein.

The simplest snack food is fruit. Let's see what you'd need to eat to stay within 5 ⒼⓁ for your snack.

Fruit	5 ⒼⓁ
Berries	1 large punnet
Plums	4
Cherries	1 small punnet
Pear	1
Grapefruit	1
Orange	1
Apple	1 small (can fit into the palm of your hand)
Peach	1 small
Melon/watermelon	1 slice

Berries, plums and cherries are your best-'value' fruit snacks. Berries include strawberries, raspberries, blueberries, blackberries and any others that you can get your hands on in season. You can further slow down the GL score of these fruits by eating them with five almonds or two teaspoons of pumpkin seeds. Other than chestnuts, almonds are the best nut, because they have the most protein compared with calories. Pumpkin seeds are also high in protein and in omega-3 fats. Flaxseeds are the highest for omega-3 but are too small to make good snacks, and need to be ground up because they have a hard outer coating.

Another snack option would be some kind of bread with a protein-based spread. Cottage cheese, hummus and peanut butter are good examples. Deliciously rich-tasting hummus is low in GL and tastes great with oatcakes, on rye bread or with a raw carrot (see recipe on page 329). (A large carrot is still less than 5 ⓖ). If you like peanut butter, buy the kind with no added sugar. A slice of any of the bread servings below with either hummus or peanut butter gives you the right kind of low-GL carbohydrate with some protein to keep your blood sugar level even.

Oatcakes, and oats in general, are excellent as far as weight and blood sugar are concerned. Oats contain beta-glucans, a type of fibre that helps to slow down the release of glucose into the blood, lessen insulin response and also lower cholesterol and heart disease risk. Of all the grains, it's the best for losing weight, and for controlling your blood sugar.[5]

Watch out when buying oatcakes, though. Many contain sugar. The best are Nairns – not only are these oatcakes sugar-free but they also make organic types and they use palm fruit oil, which contains unsaturated fat, as opposed to palm oil, which is higher in saturated fat.

Bread and oatcakes	**5 ⓖ**
Oatcakes	2 biscuits
Pumpernickel-style rye bread	1 thin slice
Sourdough rye bread	1 thin slice
Rye wholemeal bread (yeasted)	half a slice
Wheat wholemeal bread (yeasted)	half a slice
White, high fibre bread (yeasted)	less than half a slice

So, here is a selection of 5 ⓖ snacks to choose from:

- A piece of fruit, plus five almonds or two teaspoons of pumpkin seeds.

- A thin slice of rye bread or two oatcakes and half a small tub of cottage cheese (150g/5½oz).

- A thin slice of rye bread/two oatcakes and half a small tub of hummus (150g/5½oz).

- A thin slice of rye bread/two oatcakes and peanut butter.

- Crudités (a carrot, pepper, cucumber or celery) and hummus.

- Crudités and cottage cheese.

- A small yoghurt (150g/5½oz), no sugar, plus berries.

- Cottage cheese plus berries.

As you can see, you won't be bored between meals, as there's masses of scope for mixing and matching. But these are only to give you an idea of what to expect. You'll find an array of snack recipes in Chapter 27, including Flageolet Bean Dip or Smoked Salmon Pâté with oatcakes and crudités, and Quinoa Tabouleh.

22

What to Eat for Lunch and Dinner

Main meals are really something to look forward to on the Holford Diet, as you'll see from the recipes and menus in Part Five. But how do you put it all together? The easiest way to get the correct nutritional balance is to imagine all the different foods on a plate. I showed you this method in Part One (page 89), and you'll find it described again below.

Half the plate will consist of very low-GL vegetables. These include peas, broccoli, carrots, runner beans, courgettes and kale, among many others. These vegetables, listed on pages 247–8, will account for no more than 4 ⓖ, and I'm going to show you how to prepare them in minutes. If you haven't been all that interested in veg up to now, you'll be amazed by how fresh and zingy they can taste when they're cooked in these ways.

The other half of your plate is divided into two, one for protein-based food such as meat, fish or tofu, and the other for more 'starchy' vegetables, pasta or rice, which account for 6 to 7 ⓖ. So, a quarter of what's on your plate is protein-rich, a quarter is carbohydrate-rich and half is made up of very low-GL vegetables. You'll soon get the hang of it. It's dead simple.

More fish, less meat

Let's kick off with the protein serving on your plate. Remember from Part Three that the overall amount of protein – by which I mean the protein contained in the various foods, not protein-rich foods – at each meal will be 20g (¾oz). The protein-rich food on your plate will provide

15g (½oz) of this, and the table below tells you how much you need to eat of each of these to get that 15g (½oz). (The one serving of carbohydrate-rich starchy vegetables and two servings of very low-GL vegetables will provide the remaining 5g/⅙oz.)

In the table below I've listed a lot of fish options and fewer meat options. Avoid red meat during the weight loss phase of the diet. White meat tends to be much lower in fat, and fish is much higher in the essential omega-3 fats, so, becoming a 'fishichicketarian' is a great way to lose weight and gain health. Does this mean you can never eat red meat again? Certainly not. Once you've attained your target weight you can have lean red meat once a week.

How big is a protein serving?

Food	Weight	Serving
Tofu and tempeh	160g	¾ packet
Soya mince	100g	3 tbsp
Chicken (no skin)	50g	1 very small breast
Turkey (no skin)	50g	½ small breast
Red meat (beef, pork, etc.)	50g	1 small serving
Quorn	120g	⅓ pack
Salmon and trout	55g	1 very small fillet
Tuna (canned in brine)	50g	¼ can
Sardines (canned in brine)	75g	⅔ can
Cod	65g	1 very small fillet
Clams	60g	¼ can
Prawns	85g	6 large prawns
Mackerel	85g	1 medium fillet
Oysters	–	15
Yoghurt (natural, low fat)	285g	½ large tub
Cottage cheese	120g	½ medium tub
Hummus	200g	1 small tub
Skimmed milk	440ml	about ¾ pint
Soya milk	415ml	about ¾ pint
Eggs (boiled)	–	2 small or 1 large
Quinoa	125g	large serving bowl
Baked beans	310g	¾ can
Kidney beans	175g	⅓ can
Black-eye beans	175g	⅓ can
Lentils	165g	⅓ can

Starchy vegetables

As we saw on the plate on page 89, carbohydrate-rich 'starchy vegetable' servings should be roughly the same size or weight as protein servings. But this depends on how each food weighs up. For example, if you are eating chicken with rice, the serving size of rice is somewhat larger than the piece of chicken for each to be roughly the same weight, because chicken is dense and heavy and rice is relatively light.

Remember, starchy vegetables will account for a maximum 7 🕒 of your meal (out of a total of 10 🕒). Let's take a look at what quantity of different starchy vegetables you can eat to keep within that limit, leaving 3 🕒 for the very low-GL veg that occupy half the plate. (All figures in brackets are cooked weights.)

Starchy vegetables	7 🕒
Pumpkin/squash	big serving (185g)
Carrot	one large (160g)
Swede	big serving (150g)
Quinoa	big serving (130g)
Beetroot	big serving (110g)
Cornmeal	a serving (115g)
Pearl barley	a small serving (95g)
Wholemeal pasta	half a serving (85g)
White pasta	third of a serving (65g)
Brown rice	a small serving (70g)
White rice	a third of a serving (45g)
Couscous	a third of a serving (45g)
Broad beans	a serving (30g)
Corn on the cob	half a cob (60g)
Boiled potato	three small potatoes (75g)
Baked potato	half (60g)
French fries	tiny portion (45g)
Sweet potato	half (60g)

As you can see, there are some obvious winners. Wholemeal pasta – for example spaghetti – and brown rice are much better than white pasta and white rice. (As we saw earlier, brown basmati rice has the lowest GL score of all the different types of rice.) Swede, carrot and squash are much better than potato. Boiled potato is better than baked potato, which is in turn better than French fries.

Some of these foods may be new to you. If so, you'll be bowled over by, say, the nutty flavour of quinoa and the smooth, rich texture of the squashes. If you love pasta, switching to the wholemeal variety is painless. These wholegrain versions cook the same, but you can eat more of them than the refined variety and stay slim.

Top Tip

Try a new food every week. For example, have you ever eaten barley or quinoa? Barley can be cooked like rice and is very tasty in soups and casseroles. Quinoa – actually a seed rather than a grain – takes only 13 minutes to cook and is packed with extra protein, iron and vitamins.

Beans and lentils

It's telling that beans and lentils are no longer widely eaten in many of the world's fattest nations. These are the best foods for both balancing your blood sugar and giving you the right mix of protein and carbohydrate. It's this rare double whammy that keeps their GL score low. (Another reason why lentils and soya – also a bean – are so low is that they contain a substance that prevents the digestion of amylose, therefore slowing down its release further.) Soya also keeps your arteries healthy by lowering the 'bad' LDL cholesterol. A serving a day, either as soya milk or tofu, can lower your LDL cholesterol by over 10 per cent.

If a meal contains beans and lentils you can be quite generous with the portion size, because you are getting both the protein and the carbohydrate from the same food.

However, when you are eating these foods as your source of protein, combine with only *half* the serving size of a carbohydrate-rich food, instead of an equal serving. This is, of course, because you're already getting a significant amount of carbohydrate in the beans.

This is how much you can eat, assuming you are not eating another starchy vegetable, to stay within 7 **ᴳᴸ**. (Most regular cans of beans provide around 225–245g/8–8½oz of beans.)

Beans and lentils	**7 ⓰**
Soya beans	2 cans
Pinto/borlotti beans	¾ can
Green/brown lentils	¾ can
Baked beans	½ can
Butter beans	½ can
Split peas	½ can
Kidney beans	½ can
Chickpeas	½ can

If you're not vegetarian, you may be relatively unfamiliar with beans and lentils. You may have encountered dhal, baked beans, hummus or cassoulet, but never actually thrown a packet or can of lentils or beans into your shopping basket. These are great foods, immensely satisfying in flavour and texture, and they feature in all of the world's great cuisines – as well as kitchen classics such as beans on toast. You'll be making mouthwatering dishes with them, from hummus and Flageolet Bean Dip to Lentil and Lemon Soup, Tabouleh and a fiery chilli, to name just a few.

Top Tip

Eat your food slowly. Chew each mouthful 20 times, as this will further 'slow-release' the carbohydrate in your food.

Unlimited vegetables

Now it's time to move on to the other half of your plate. This is made up of what I call the 'unlimited vegetables'. Of course, there are limits, but these are vegetables for which a serving is less than 2 ⓰. A serving of peas, for instance, is a cup (approximately115g/4oz).

Unlimited vegetables

Asparagus	Cabbage	Endive
Aubergine	Cauliflower	Fennel
Beansprouts	Celery	Garlic
Broccoli	Courgette	Kale
Brussels sprouts	Cucumber	Lettuce

Mangetouts	Radish	Spring onions
Mushrooms	Rocket	Tenderstem broccoli
Onions	Runner beans	Tomato
Peas	Spinach	Watercress
Peppers		

If the word cabbage makes you think of watery soup, and runner beans have always been something you pushed around on your plate, be prepared: I have some seriously delicious recipes for lots of different vegetables. You'll end up eager to find new ways of eating vegetables – and, what's more, you'll be looking amazing, thanks to the vitamins, minerals and other phytonutrients they're brimming with.

So, to recap: I want you to eat two servings of unlimited vegetables, one serving of 'starchy' vegetables and one serving of protein-based food. Together, they'll help you feel full at the end of every meal.

Vegetarians

If you're a strict vegetarian, you'll need to eat more tofu, beans, lentils, soya produce and Quorn than usual to achieve the target for protein intake. A serving size of tofu for a main meal is 160g (5¾oz), which is roughly three-quarters of a packet. Part Five contains a number of recipes and ways to use tofu – the vegetarian fatburner's best friend – along with recipes using a variety of beans and lentils. And many of the recipes containing chicken or fish can be adapted by replacing them with tofu, and I make a point of mentioning this. (For more detailed general advice for vegetarians, see Chapter 26.)

Fats and oils

This diet is not low-fat; you'll be able to eat enough to keep you satisfied. As far as fats and oils go, what's important is which fats you use, and how you use them.

Creams

If you want to make a savoury dish creamier, try adding a teaspoon of tahini (sesame spread) or a tablespoon of coconut milk or coconut cream.

Salad dressings

When using seed oils for salad dressings, pick either flaxseed oil or a blend of oils that gives at least one part of omega-3 fats to one part of omega-6 fats. These seed oils need to be cold-pressed and stored in a lightproof container.

A good seed-oil blend is Udo's Choice (see page 436 of Resources). Also good is walnut oil. You can lightly drizzle these oils onto vegetables instead of adding butter.

Cooking oils

For steam-frying (see below) and sautéing, use a small amount of butter, coconut butter or olive oil. Coconut butter adds a great flavour to steam-fries.

Cooking methods

All carbohydrate foods release their carbohydrate somewhat faster once cooked. The longer you cook something and the higher the temperature, the faster-releasing the food becomes. It is therefore best to eat food as close to raw as possible.

This doesn't mean endless salads. You can steam, poach, steam-fry and boil food without cooking it to death. Next best is baking and grilling. Worst is frying, particularly deep-frying.

Steaming

The best way you can cook green, leafy, less starchy vegetables is by steaming, as it preserves a lot of their vitamins and minimises any raising of GL. The method can be used with any food and is very successful with fish – but perhaps not ideal with starchy vegetables, which require longer cooking, or with red meat. Many different kinds of steamers are available, or you can improvise with a colander, pan and lid. Steam less-starchy vegetables until they are crisp-tender (*al dente*), so that they are still bright and fresh.

Poaching

Poaching is useful for making delicious water-based sauces while you cook. For example, you could cook fish in a vegetable broth flavoured with ginger, garlic, lemongrass, spices and wine (the alcohol boils off).

Steam-frying

I use steam-frying frequently in the Holford Diet because it adds loads of taste without compromising on health. The great advantage of this style of cooking is that the lower temperature of steaming doesn't destroy nutrients to anything like the extent that frying does and you use only a small amount of oil, if that. As with other cooking methods, aim to keep veg *al dente*.

To steam-fry, use a shallow pan or a deep frying pan with a thick base and a lid that seals well. You can steam-fry without oil by first adding two tablespoons of liquid to the pan – this can be water, vegetable stock, soy sauce or a little watered-down sauce that you'll use for the dish. Once it boils, immediately add some vegetables, 'sauté' rapidly for a minute or two, turn up the heat, add a tablespoon or two more of the liquid and clamp the lid on tightly. After a minute, add the remaining ingredients. Turn the heat down after a couple of minutes and steam in this way until cooked.

Alternatively, add a teaspoon to a tablespoon of olive oil, butter or coconut oil to the pan, warm it, add the ingredients and sauté. After a couple of minutes, add two tablespoons of liquid as above and clamp the lid on. Steam the ingredients until done.

Boiling

When you boil foods, this raises the GL more than steaming but less than baking. Changes can be kept to a minimum by using as little water as possible, keeping the lid on, and cooking the food as whole as possible. Also, eat all vegetables *al dente* – a little crisp, not soft.

Waterless cooking

For waterless cooking you will need specially designed pans in which you can 'boil' foods by steaming them in their own juice, or 'fry' foods with no oil. Both methods are excellent, for preserving both nutrients and flavour.

Baking

This method is useful, especially if the food is large and has a thick skin (such as a whole or half pumpkin). Avoid coating food with oil, because the oil will oxidise during cooking, which creates free radicals (highly reactive, harmful molecules). You can roast a potato without adding oil. The higher the temperature and the longer you cook something, the higher the GL becomes.

Grilling

For foods that contain fat, grilling is less damaging than frying, but browning or burning a food does create free radicals. Try to avoid barbecued food, or at least ensure that what you eat is not charred.

Frying

Keep frying to a minimum, and avoid deep-frying altogether. When you do fry, use butter, coconut oil (saturated fat) or olive oil (monounsaturated) rather than other vegetable oils (polyunsaturated oils), as these are much more prone to oxidation.

Microwaving

Although admittedly fast, microwaving is a problematic cooking method. As food cooks in its own water, it seems better than most cooking methods for preserving the water-soluble vitamins B and C. A Spanish study, however, found that microwaved broccoli lost vast amounts of major antioxidants (nutrients working to rid the body of free radicals) compared with steaming.

Moreover, the temperatures reached in fat particles are very high, so avoid microwaving oily fish: it will destroy the essential fats it contains. And remember that microwave ovens do give off electromagnetic radiation, which can be detected even from six feet away.

If you must microwave, it is better to use lower voltage/heat settings for longer. Cover dishes to encourage steaming, although you do need to leave some room for steam to escape.

Top Tips

● Buy foods as fresh and unprocessed as possible and eat them soon afterwards.

continued

- Eat more raw food. Be adventurous. Try raw beetroot and carrot tops in salad.
- Cook foods as whole as possible, slicing or blending before serving.
- Use as little water as possible, preferably steaming, poaching or steam-frying.
- Fry foods as infrequently as possible.
- Favour slow-cook methods that introduce less heat.
- Don't overcook, burn or brown food.

What to limit and avoid

The trick with any diet is to fill yourself up with the good stuff so there's little room left for less desirable foods. Some of the goodies, however, such as oily fish, still need to be limited because, although they contain valuable fats, too much of any fat is bad for you.

Foods to limit

The chart below shows you which foods to limit. Some of these are included in the recipes in specific amounts because they contain important nutrients. Some are high in fat, whereas others are high in sugar, so do not eat more than the recommended amounts.

Dried fruit	choose fresh fruit instead or soaked dried fruit
Coconut	can be used in small amounts to flavour dishes
Seeds	limit to four teaspoons a day maximum, or one heaped tablespoon
Nuts	same as seeds (don't have both, and seeds are better)
Salad dressings	stick to the measures given in Part Five
Avocados	twice a week, maximum
Vegetable oil and butter	use sparingly, as in the recipes
Tahini (sesame spread)	use a small amount instead of butter
Fatty fish such as herring, mackerel, tuna, kippers	three times a week, maximum
Chicken (no skin), game	twice a week, maximum
Milk and yoghurts	stick to skimmed milk and low-fat yoghurt
Eggs	six a week, maximum

Foods to avoid

These foods are high in fat and/or fast-releasing sugar, or are devoid of nutrients, so they're best strictly avoided. Once you have attained your target weight they may be eaten on a rare occasion.

High-fat meats including beef, pork, lamb, sausages and processed meats

Lard, dripping, suet and gravy

Deep-fried foods

Cream and shop-bought ice cream

High-fat spreads and mayonnaises

All cheeses except cottage cheese, low-fat quark or fromage frais, and half-fat
   Cheddar cheese

Rich sauces made with cream, cheese or eggs

Sugar, sugar-laden sweets and foods with added sugar

Pastries, cakes and biscuits

White bread

Snack foods such as crisps

23

Drinks, Desserts and Sweets

So far, we've looked only at food. But what about drinks – including alcohol? You'll have a broad choice of hot drinks and juices, and will be able to have a few convivial glasses of wine a week. And there are plenty of mouthwatering desserts in Part Five to choose from, as well as sweets that won't overshoot your GL allowance by a mile, and are available at your local health-food shop.

As you now know by heart, the food you eat will have 40 ⑮ a day. On top of this, the GL allowance for drinks, desserts and sweets is 5 ⑮. Your daily 5 ⑮ could be a glass of juice or wine, a fatburner dessert or even some chocolate – just not all four in the same day.

As before, if you're drinking a lot of coffee or tea, getting through a fair bit of chocolate, drinking alcohol fairly frequently – or doing all three – you will need to stop all of them for at least two weeks to a month when you start the Holford Diet. Thus, any withdrawal symptoms will be short-lived: the nutrients and supplements you're taking in will be getting to grips with the bottoming out of your blood sugar. You could feel a bit rough for several days, but this will dissipate fast.

Gradually, you should see any cravings for super-sweetness or alcohol begin to disappear. By the time you're ready to reintroduce the odd piece of chocolate, cup of tea or glass of Sancerre, the switchover to fatburning will have begun and you'll be able to handle the occasional treat without encouraging any imbalance in blood sugar.

Cold drinks

The best drink for fatburning is water – I suggest you drink the equivalent of 2 litres (3½ pints), or approximately eight glasses, a day. If that seems an enormous amount, be aware that you can factor in any herbal teas, coffee substitutes and juices you drink. Leaving a bottle on your desk at work makes it easier to remember to keep it topped up. When you're thoroughly hydrated, you'll feel much better in every way. This is a habit that will become second nature – like the rest of the Holford Diet.

Fruit juices, whether concentrated or fresh, have a relatively high GL because the fibre has been removed. The best is cherry juice (made with a concentrate called CherryActive) and apple juice, although even this should be drunk diluted – half juice, half water, or, even better, two-thirds water, one-third juice.

Here's how much you can drink for 5 ⓖⓛ.

Drink	5 ⓖⓛ
Tomato juice	1 pint
Carrot juice	small glass
CherryActive	30ml, diluted with 250ml water
Grapefruit juice, unsweetened	small glass
Apple juice, unsweetened	small glass, diluted 50:50 with water
Orange juice, unsweetened	small glass, diluted 50:50 with water; or juice of one orange
Pineapple juice	half a small glass, diluted 50:50 with water
Cranberry juice drink	half a small glass, diluted 50:50 with water
Grape juice	an inch's worth of liquid!

Stay away from all fizzy, sweetened, caffeinated drinks and sugar-sweetened cordials. You can use cordials sweetened with apple juice concentrate, which contains more slow-releasing fructose, rather than grape juice concentrate, which has a much higher GL score.

A good rule of thumb is to have no more than one glass of juice a day, diluting it as you need to in order to have no more than 5 ⓖⓛ a day. So have, say, either a glass of carrot juice, or a diluted apple juice.

Top Tip

Drink slowly. Sip rather than gulp your drinks. This helps to slow-release the sugars in fruit juice, as does diluting them.

Alcohol

The effect of alcohol is similar to that of sugar in that the liver can process it into fat. To help regain your blood sugar balance, ideally I recommend avoiding all alcohol during the first two weeks of starting the Holford Diet.

Pure alcohol has no GL as such but that doesn't mean you can have as much as you like. I recommend that you limit your alcohol intake, in any event, to no more than 1 unit of alcohol. That means half a pint of beer or a glass of wine.

However, you also need to stick to the 5 ⓖ-a-day rule for all drinks or desserts. So, assuming you've had no GL drinks (for example, just water, teas, etc.) or desserts, you've got up to 5 ⓖ for drinks. As you'll see from the chart below, from a GL point of view the best is neat spirits, then white wine, red wine and finally beer. Beer has the highest carbohydrate content, double that of red wine and eight times that of white wine.

So, if you are a beer drinker, the ideal is half a pint *every other day*, or choose a low-carb beer or lager. However, the odd glass of, ideally, dry white wine or red wine, or perhaps a single spirit with a little juice, keeps you within your limits. If you choose dry white wine you've still got 4 ⓖ for a dessert or perhaps a small glass of diluted apple juice.

	ⓖ	Units	Daily max
Beer/lager (300ml/½ pint)	10	1	150ml/ (¼ pint)
Red wine (115ml/3½fl oz) small glass	2	1	1
White wine	1	1	1
Spirits (30ml)	0	1	1
Spirits + orange juice (125ml/4fl oz juice)	6	1	1 small
Vodka + coke (125ml/4fl oz coke)	8	1	1 small

● Assumption that alc. carbs = 100 GI
● Max of 5 ⓖ a day (if no other drinks/desserts) or 1 unit, whichever is greater

---

Top Tip

Have you ever tried a Virgin Mary (tomato juice, Worcester sauce and a touch of Tobasco, ice and lemon)? It's a delicious low-GL non-alcoholic drink that you can ask for in any bar, that fills you up but is only 2GLs.

Hot drinks

Refer to page 160 for a full discussion of coffee, tea and all their permutations. By now you'll know that, whether you're addicted to endless cuppas or are a real espresso fiend, you'll need to abstain completely for two weeks to a month on the diet. Luckily, there are many wonderful, non-addictive alternatives around – really delicious and inventive herbal teas as well as excellent coffee substitutes – so it should be positively enjoyable to do so. After all, when you're fizzing with energy from diet alone, stimulants lose their sparkle pretty fast.

That said, when the time comes, you can reintroduce weak tea. Drinking it from time to time shouldn't be a problem. Coffee has several addictive substances in it, however, and should be reserved as the occasional treat.

Top Tip

If you're addicted to coffee try a Teeccino with some frothed milk and a touch of cinnamon. If you're addicted to tea try rooibos (red bush) tea with milk.

Sugar and sweets

Sugar is perhaps a greater addiction than many people realise, and kicking the habit could prove a little tough (see page 158). But your taste buds will become acclimatised. Fruit will help when you crave something sweet (see the list on page 392 for the low-GL fruits). Also, get used to diluting fruit juices with water, as outlined above. Once you're sugar-free, the odd sweet food is no big deal.

Many 'sugar-free' foods use grape juice concentrate as a sweetener. They might as well use glucose. Some use apple juice concentrate and, as it's high in fructose, it is much better for you. Some health-conscious drinks contain blue agave cactus nectar, which is better still.

The best sugar-free alternative is xylitol (see page 433 of Resources). It is a natural sweetener found in many fruits and vegetables, but has a much lower GL score: a seventh that of sugar and half that of fructose. Plums, for example, are naturally high in xylitol and hence taste sweet but have a very low GL score. So, if you are addicted to having three teaspoons of sugar in your tea, cutting down to one teaspoon of xylitol will cut your GL load by 14.

Sugar	**5 ⓖⓛ**
Xylitol	10 teaspoons
Blue agave cactus nectar	10 teaspoons

Fructose	5 teaspoons
Lactose	2 teaspoons
Sucrose	1 heaped teaspoon
Honey	1 teaspoon
Glucose	1 teaspoon
Malt	1 teaspoon

Chocolate

As we've seen, chocolate is full of sugar and cocoa, which contains stimulating substances including caffeine, theobromine and theophylline. Higher-quality dark chocolate tends to have less sugar, but obviously more of the stimulants. Some chocolates even use some of the 'healthier' sugars described above. But the fact is that, whichever way you cut it, chocolate is addictive and contributes to blood sugar problems and hence weight gain. When you're two weeks to a month into the diet, you may well find you've lost any cravings for it. But, if you still fancy some here and there, limit it to once a week.

So, how much equals 5 ⒼⓁ?

Sweets	5 ⒼⓁ
Fruitus oat and fruit bar	1 bar
Rebar fruit and vegetable bar	½ bar
Muesli bar	less than ½ bar (12g/½oz)
Regular chocolate bar, milk or plain	less than ¼ bar
Mars Bar	⅕ bar

One way of quitting the chocolate or sweets habit is to find good alternatives, which luckily abound in health-food shops. One of my favourites are Panda Liquorice bars, which are sweetened with molasses.

But you can't munch on these all the time, either; they'll simply keep your sweet tooth going. And be aware, too, that many so-called healthy bars are packed with sugar, hydrogenated fat and other not-so-healthy ingredients – so always check labels.

Desserts

It's the same story with desserts. If you eat a lot of desserts, or if you are insulin resistant, you will probably crave something sweet at the end of each meal. It is very important to break this habit because, if you don't, it will keep your blood sugar level seesawing. It takes only three days in most cases to stop the craving. So, after your initial stimulant- and sugar-free period, limit desserts to one a week, perhaps at the weekend.

You'll find wonderful recipes for fatburner desserts in Part Five, including Chocolate Ice Cream, and Kiwi and Coconut Pudding. These don't exceed 5 ⒼⓁ and aren't loaded with saturated fats. Don't have desserts when you are eating out (see Chapter 25), because almost all restaurant desserts are heavily loaded with sugar and saturated fat.

You can have a 5 ⒼⓁ dessert with your meal and leave out one of your snacks, but having the snack is better because this way you will be grazing rather than gorging. This helps to keep your blood sugar level even, which, as we've seen, prevents weight gain.

So, in summary, once you've started the diet, you can be drinking unlimited hot drinks such as Teeccino, rooibos tea or herbal teas a day, and one glass of diluted juice a day. After you've gone through two weeks to a month with no coffee, tea, sweets or alcohol, you can have some alcohol instead of juice on that day: a small glass of wine, a small beer or a shot of spirits up to a maximum of three times a week; or six pieces of chocolate, or a fatburner dessert, once a week. And don't forget your 2 litres (3½ pints) of water a day.

But, whichever option you choose, the goal for your drinks, sweets and desserts is to keep within 5 ⒼⓁ a day. Enjoy!

24

Shopping

Everything you need for the Holford Diet is easily available in the supermarket, greengrocer's and, for a few speciality items, your local health-food shop.

Some of the ingredients may be new to you, so this chapter will tell you where to get them and give you some guidance on what to do with them. Below you'll find a shopping list containing all you need to get stocked up and ready for fatburning.

This list includes anything that lasts for a week or more. Fresh fruits and vegetables form a large part of what you eat and need to be stocked up on a regular basis, but you may want to check the recipes and menus in Part Five first to see what you'll need. When buying fresh fish, ideally eat it on the day you buy it, otherwise freeze it to use another day that week. As for supplies from the health-food shop, these are becoming far cheaper than they once were, as demand is growing. And some items once available exclusively from such stores, such as wholemeal pasta, are now widely available from supermarkets. So scout around for products and prices that suit you.

Your shopping list

From the supermarket

Foods for the fridge

Apples, bananas, pears, oranges, raspberries (fresh or frozen), gooseberries or cooking apples, rhubarb, blackcurrants

Mushrooms, celery, spring onions, avocado, parsley, carrots, beansprouts, potatoes and sweet potatoes, peppers, courgettes, aubergine, onions, garlic, cucumber, lettuce, lemons, frozen peas

Fresh root ginger

Skimmed milk

Very low-fat, live natural yoghurt (with no additives)

Cottage cheese, low-fat quark or fromage frais, half-fat Cheddar cheese, such as
  Shape

Very low-fat mayonnaise

Free-range eggs, ideally omega-3-rich

Tofu – plain, smoked and marinated pieces

Tahini

Cod, haddock, mackerel, herring, salmon (go for wild salmon if possible)

Store-cupboard staples

Rolled oats and oat flakes

Wheatgerm

100 per cent rye, pumpernickel-style rye bread

Oatcakes (the best are Nairns sugar-free variety)

Brown rice

Soba noodles

Bulgur (cracked wheat)

Couscous

Millet

Wholemeal spaghetti and other wholemeal pasta

Wholemeal flour

Chickpeas, various dried beans, lentils

Cooked chestnuts

Raw (unroasted/unsalted) mixed nuts, cashew nuts, almonds, walnuts

Sunflower, sesame, pumpkin seeds and flaxseeds

Flat leaf parsley and basil plants

Raisins, dried apricots

Canned pineapple chunks (unsweetened, in juice)

Tinned tomatoes, tomato purée

Tuna fish in brine

Anchovies in olive oil (drain on kitchen paper before use)

Sardines in tomato sauce

Olive oil (cold-pressed, extra-virgin)

Cider vinegar

Balsamic vinegar

Dried herbs and spices (turmeric, cumin, paprika, cayenne pepper,
  coriander)

Honey
Vanilla essence
Herbal teas

From the health-food shop

Foods for the fridge

Alfalfa seeds or sprouts
Seed oil blends such as Udo's Choice or Omega 3:6:9 (Higher Nature)

Store-cupboard staples

Instant vegetable stocks (Vecon, Hugli, Morga, Marigold and the like)
Tamari (an alternative to soy sauce)
Yeast extract – low-salt (Natex)
Wholemeal lasagne and macaroni, and wholemeal or buckwheat spaghetti
Millet
Quinoa
Pear and apple spread (a sugar-free alternative to jam)
Sugar-free jam (Whole Earth or Meridian)
Get Up & Go (Biocare)
Dandelion coffee (Symingtons)
Barleycup, Caro or Teeccino

How to use the more unusual foods

In Part Five, you'll be discovering how to cook with all these foods. For now, here's a little background on some that may be new to you.

Quinoa is actually a seed rather than a grain, and looks much like millet. It was once eaten by the Inca and was reputed to be the source of their empire's strength – and it is still eaten widely in the Andes. The flavour is slightly nutty and something like rice, and it's an excellent source of protein, as well as slow-releasing carbohydrate.

You cook quinoa like rice, adding up to three times as much water as quinoa and cooking it for about 13 minutes. It's best eaten as an accompaniment to, for example, a steam-fry or casserole. You could also add it to a soup to thicken it up or eat it cold as part of a salad, much like couscous, and it makes a tasty pilaf cooked with onions, brown rice and peas. (Rinse thoroughly before use.)

Tofu is, in terms of protein quality, second only to quinoa – and is also an excellent source of both protein and slow-releasing carbohydrate. Both tofu and quinoa, when eaten with carbohydrate-rich foods, slow down the release of their sugars.

Tofu is made from the soya bean and is something like a bland cheese. It comes in different textures: soft (good for desserts or making things 'creamy') or hard (better for steam-fries and main meals). While rather flavourless itself, it rapidly absorbs the flavour of any sauce. So if you are cooking a Chinese steam-fry flavoured with soya sauce, garlic and ginger, the tofu will readily soak up these flavours and taste delicious. With plain tofu, you need to drain off the liquid first.

You can also buy tofu ready flavoured – smoked, marinated or braised (but avoid fried tofu). These varieties, which are firmer than plain tofu and already delectable-tasting, make an excellent substitute for meat or chicken in steam-fries, stews and casseroles. You can also add flavour to tofu by marinating it for 20 minutes before you cook with it. You can even make a tofu steak (see alternative suggestion for Tuna Steak with Black-Eyed Bean Salsa), or include it in sandwiches. I recommend suppliers who guarantee soya that has not been genetically modified, such as Cauldron Foods.

Lentils and beans are excellent and inexpensive foods that are very much underused in traditional British cooking. Both lentils and beans need to be boiled in plenty of water. Lentils, depending on the type, take between 15 and 25 minutes. Beans need to be soaked overnight then boiled, usually for up to two hours. You can buy pre-soaked, cooked beans and green/brown lentils in cans that you can simply drain and add to recipes.

If you've never cooked with beans, you'll soon become an enthusiast. Their taste and texture are very satisfying, and, as they're such a large part of cuisine around the world – from India, Mexico and South America to the Far East – the range of dishes you can make from them is huge. Hummus and other dips, chilli, casseroles, lentil roast and soups are only part of the story, as you'll see in Part Five.

Salad ingredients are now part of virtually everyone's diet but they can be used much more imaginatively than most people think. With a few exceptions, most vegetables can be eaten raw. Raw, uncooked and grated beetroot, cabbage, broccoli, courgettes and carrot tops can all be used along with peppers, tomatoes, grated carrots, baby sweetcorn and a variety of green leafy vegetables such as watercress, rocket, lettuce, chicory, red cabbage and spinach. You can also add marinated tofu pieces, almonds and, less frequently, avocados, to increase the protein content. There are plenty of salad and salad-dressing recipes to choose from in Part Five.

Tahini is a spread made from sesame seeds and their oil. As it's high in essential fats, it's a lot better for you and more flavourful than butter. I use tahini on bread and toast instead of butter, and often add some to savoury dishes at the end for a creamier texture and added flavour. Use in moderation, as instructed in the recipes, and store in the fridge.

Seeds contain vitamins, minerals, protein, fibre and essential fats. They are therefore a superfood, yet many people shy away from them because of fat phobia or simply ignorance about how to use them. Flaxseeds (linseeds) and pumpkin seeds are the best for the essential omega-3 fats, whereas sesame and sunflower seeds are the best for omega-6 fats. A combination of all four, stored in a glass jar in the fridge to minimise oxidation, then ground in a coffee grinder, makes a great addition to any cereal. A tablespoon gives you a good daily intake of essential fats plus lots of other key nutrients, including bone-building calcium, magnesium and zinc. They're best uncooked or thrown in at the last moment of cooking, such as in a steam-fry, since heating them lowers the quality of their essential fats.

Seed-oil blends need to be cold-pressed and preferably organic, stored in a lightproof container and kept refrigerated. The best blends of oils are those that provide omega-3 and omega-6 fats, usually by combining flaxseed oil, pumpkin seed oil, sesame oils, sunflower oil or borage oil. Two such oils are Udo's Choice, available from good health-food shops and internet suppliers (see Resources) and Omega 3:6:9 (from Higher Nature – see Resources). Seed-oil blends can't be cooked, so they're for adding to soups at the end of cooking, or to cereals, vegetables and salad dressings.

25

Eating Out

You don't need to stay in every night, slaving over a hot stove (or a salad bowl) on the Holford Diet. But when it comes to eating out you will need to be choosy. As I've said, I travel the world on lecture tours and I always find excellent restaurants as I go, simply by choosing Chinese, Japanese, Malaysian or Thai establishments.

The reason? These countries have the leanest, healthiest people, and much of that is down to the way they eat. And, because the Chinese, for instance, have emigrated to so many countries around the world, it's usually possible to find a Chinese restaurant at least, whether in the US, Canada, Australia, Continental Europe, South America – or the Far East! But this doesn't mean you can't eat French, Italian, Mexican, Indian or other foods. You just need to know what to order.

The trick, as ever, is to fill yourself up with the good stuff. That means having a starter and a main course, or just a main course, but not a dessert. It also means avoiding any breads, prawn crackers or the like. In fact, it's best to ask the waiter to take it away, thus removing the temptation. Instead, ask them to bring some olives, or a dish of hot pickles. Order water and say you won't be drinking anything else.

When you are choosing items from the menu, watch out for the hidden sugar and high-GL carbohydrates in sauces, pickles and dips. For example, all Thai restaurants do very tasty fishcakes and spring rolls. The fishcakes are better than the spring rolls because they have more protein. Both come with a sweet sauce, and you'll need to leave this on the side.

Where possible, choose food that hasn't been deep-fried. So go for boiled noodles rather than fried, or boiled rice rather than fried rice. Share a portion between two or even three people. Remember: you want about the same weight of carbohydrate food as protein-rich food, such as a steamed or poached fish.

Japanese restaurants are great, especially if you like fish. All offer wonderful fish dishes, from teriyaki salmon to sashimi. (Sushi isn't as good because it includes a lot of sweet white rice.) This can be very satisfying without filling you up with fast-releasing carbohydrates or saturated fat.

Always order some vegetable dishes, whether it's a salad or a side order of green beans or broccoli. Make sure you eat your greens and, if you haven't had enough, order some more.

By the time you get to the end of your main course you should be full. This is the time to make your exit, asking for the bill and letting your perhaps dejected waiter know that the food was so good and so filling that you don't want coffee or dessert!

Most of all, remember who is in charge of what goes into your mouth. Think of the menu as only a small selection of what's on offer, opening up the possibility of ordering 'off menu'. For instance, if you like the sound of the fish, but not the cream sauce, ask for it without, or swap to another method of cooking. Ask what's in various dishes and have a look around at what other people are eating.

Indian food uses a lot of vegetables, beans and lentils, but there's also a lot of hidden sugar and fat in some of the sauces. You have to choose very carefully indeed in an Indian restaurant, so I'd recommend going to them only as an occasional treat. The same applies to cheaper Italian restaurants that specialise in pizza and pasta. These dishes are based on high-GL carbohydrates and the pasta can come with fatty, cheese or creamy sauces, so they're best avoided. But authentic Italian and French restaurants will have plenty of excellent main dishes, such as grilled chicken, plus good salads and vegetables, so be on the lookout for these.

Here are some typical items from Chinese, Thai, Japanese, Malaysian or Indian restaurant menus to choose, or avoid.

Choose

Sashimi (Japanese raw fish dish)
Fish/chicken teriyaki
Tom yum soup
Thai fish/chicken/prawn tikkas, curries (but avoid the creamier ones listed under 'Avoid' below)
Fish/chicken satay (peanut-based sauce)
Indian bhunas or baltis – ask for less oil
Steamed fish and other non-fried fish dishes

Tofu-based dish

Omelettes

Noodles with vegetables, such as chop suey (share a portion)

Vegetable dishes such as chana masal or dhal (Indian) or stir-fried beansprouts, bamboo shoots, water chestnuts or mushrooms (Chinese)

Avoid

Fried fish/meat

Sweet-and-sour dishes

Creamy curries such as kormas and masalas

Rice (unless brown, then share a portion)

Potato dishes

Bread such as naans and chapattis

Prawn crackers

The fallback in any restaurant is to choose something simple, without sauces containing unknown ingredients. So you can't go wrong with grilled fish or chicken and vegetables or salad.

Restaurants are a good proving ground for your new relationship with food. Now that you understand so much more about why you feel the way you do and what food has to do with it, make good food your friend. Become the master of your own weight and health by becoming the master of your diet.

The best way to do this is to get your hands dirty preparing your own meals. Experiment. Make mistakes. Try new foods. Get involved with creating a way of eating that really works for you.

Choose to follow this diet because it makes sense and you want to change. I guarantee the results will be worth it. I want you to make this *your* diet, and simply use what's in this book as a springboard. That means finding the balance between eating out and eating in, breaking your addictions and having the odd treat. Be moderate in everything, including moderation.

26

Fatburning for Vegetarians

Being vegetarian is generally healthier than being a carnivore, but you have to know what you are doing. The key is making sure you get enough protein, vitamin B_{12} and iron (see Chapter 16), and don't live off dairy and wheat, which are the most common allergy-provoking foods.

The Holford Diet's emphasis on vegetables and plant-based protein makes it very easy for vegetarians and vegans to follow. There are a number of delicious dishes listed in Chapter 34 that are suitable for anyone avoiding meat and fish, from Mushroom Pilaf and Quinoa Tabouleh to Thai-Style Vegetable Broth and Borlotti Bean Bolognese. The diet has also been designed to be as versatile as possible, so that you can simply substitute tofu or pulses such as chickpeas or kidney beans for the meat or fish in any unsuitable recipes.

To make this easier for you, in Part Five I have given recommendations for suitable replacements alongside recipes in the meat and fish sections, where appropriate. This is a good opportunity to try a wider range of recipes using some of the most useful vegetarian and vegan-friendly ingredients that are on offer. We've already had a look at some of these in Chapter 22, but let's delve a little deeper here and see how they can be used as dietary staples.

Soya stars

Plain, marinated and smoked tofu (see page 263) are the protein stars of the vegetarian Holford Diet. You can now buy imaginative flavours of marinated tofu, such as sesame and ginger, or almond and hazelnut. Silken tofu is a very soft type that is useful for blending to thicken sauces, dips or smoothies. Tempeh is made of fermented soya beans, and has a much nuttier taste and firmer texture than tofu. Rather like Marmite, it is not for everyone, but I love it. There are a number of recipes in the vegetarian section of the main meals in Chapter 34 that make use of soya products; for example, Japanese Noodles and Chilli.

Finger on the pulse

I've already discussed beans and lentils in Chapter 22, and as a vegetarian you're very likely highly familiar with legumes and pulses such as chickpeas and kidney beans. But we'll be cooking with many others, such as the delicious green-hued flageolet (Flageolet Bean Dip has a very delicate flavour and is a delicious and unusual alternative to hummus) and black-eyed beans (which add a great texture to salsas, and can be added to Gazpacho). If you have previously dismissed lentils as mushy and bland, try Puy lentils cooked with a little vegetable stock. These brown, shiny lentils hold their shape and texture when cooked, and are rightly considered a delicacy in France.

With the grain

You've seen how amazing quinoa is already. Containing all the essential amino acids for our protein requirements, it's a nutritionally perfect food as well as being versatile, working as both carbohydrate and protein in a meal. You can use quinoa in all kinds of dishes, such as salads (Quinoa Tabouleh), main dishes (Roasted Vegetables with Mediterranean Quinoa), and even desserts (Coconut Quinoa Pudding).

But good grains and seeds don't stop there. You can experiment with couscous, bulgur wheat and millet, which are excellent served with all sorts of casseroles. And the range of available yeast-free pumpernickel and other low-GL breads, as well as delicious flaked grains, increases yearly.

Not from the cow

If you are vegan, you can substitute soya milk or rice milk for dairy milk. Rice milk has a much higher GL and is therefore not so good. There are other milks now available in health-food shops, from oat milk to quinoa milk. These have a lower GL.

27

Supplements

Good nutrition is achieved by eating the right foods, *and* by supplementing. There is no question that the levels of many nutrients required to help your body function at its best are above those easily achieved by diet alone. Such optimal levels of nutrients can also help you to reprogramme your body to burn fat. If you want to know more about the vitamins and minerals that help you to burn fat, refer back to Chapter 16.

If you have never taken supplements before, you may find they have many beneficial side effects. In a survey at the Institute for Optimum Nutrition (ION), 79 per cent of people, after six months on a supplement programme, reported improved energy, whereas 61 per cent felt physically fitter, and had fewer colds.

The basics

The starting point for any supplement programme is a good, all-round multivitamin and mineral supplement (usually taken twice a day) plus 1,000mg of vitamin C. Do check that the multivitamin/mineral you've chosen meets the amounts shown on page 203. You'll also probably need to supplement your diet with chromium (200mcg) separately – check the label on your multi.

So an ideal supplement programme looks like this:

	Breakfast	Lunch	Dinner
High-strength multivitamin and mineral	(as directed)		
Vitamin C 1,000mg	1		
Chromium 200mcg	1		

Note that, if you're having Get Up & Go for breakfast, you won't need to supplement it with vitamin C that day, as it already includes 1,000mg.

If you are struggling with your appetite or sugar cravings, I recommend you add hydroxycitric acid (HCA) and 5-HTP:

	Breakfast	Lunch	Dinner
HCA (250mg)	1	1	1
5-HTP (50mg)	1	1	1

HCA helps encourage fatburning and is good for everyone. Take up to 30 minutes before each meal.

5-HTP is especially good for those with sugar cravings and a tendency to mild depression. If you crave something sweet when your mood is low, try 5-HTP. It is best absorbed either on an empty stomach or with a piece of fruit. Try with your mid-morning and mid-afternoon snack.

For details on suppliers and brands of supplements I recommend, see page 435 in Resources.

Fibre supplements

Generally speaking, fibre is not something you add to food. It's in food anyway, unless a food manufacturer has processed it out. The Holford Diet is a high-fibre diet. However, there is one special kind of fibre that can help you to lose weight by slowing down the release of carbohydrates. It is called glucomannan and comes from the Japanese konjac plant (see Chapter 13, page 154, for more details).

Three grams of glucomannan a day has been proved to assist weight loss. Konjac fibre, which is 60 per cent glucomannan, comes in 500mg capsules. It's recommended that you take nine of these capsules a day. Take three, with a large glass of water, three times a day just before meals. As it swells to a hundred times its volume by absorbing water, it is very important to drink a large glass of water whenever you take konjac extract or glucomannan. Suppliers are given on page 436.

The when and how of supplements

Vitamin and mineral supplements are best taken with food and, if they are involved in energy regulation, during the day (B vitamins, for example, can disturb sleep so should not be taken at night). They should also be taken *every* day. Although most people notice the effects of taking them after 30 days, it is best to stick to a supplement programme for three months to really see the difference.

There are no dangers with taking any of these supplements on a long-term basis. However, once you've achieved your desired weight, you may wish to stop taking HCA, 5-HTP and additional chromium. These are included specifically to help stabilise your blood sugar levels. Most decent multivitamin and mineral supplements will provide around 30mcg of chromium, which is enough when you're on the maintenance phase of the Holford Diet.

28

Exercise

Although the main thrust of the Holford Diet is food, we've also seen how exercise helps you to keep your blood sugar level even and to burn fat. But it's important to do the right kind, and this is a combination of aerobic exercise and resistance or toning exercise.

To be a fatburner, the minimum you need to exercise is 15 minutes a day, or 35 minutes three times a week. The exercise programme you choose needs to include both aerobics, which burns fat directly, and toning exercises, which build muscle that burns fat. If you are significantly underlean (see page 221), you may need to do more to build up enough lean muscle to keep you thin.

Earlier I suggested that you start to experiment with some of the exercises in this chapter right before you start the diet, to get used to including it in your week. Take that time to find an exercise routine that suits you. You may wish to join a gym, get a workout video and find a friend to do it with so you can keep each other motivated. Set yourself a specific time to exercise during the day. You may wish to double the time you exercise, and do it every other day, which will let you have more days off.

If you've never really exercised, or are very overweight or unfit, it's best to go to your local gym and get advice from a fitness instructor before you start. It's important, too, to let your doctor know what you're doing so that he or she can advise, if necessary.

Aerobic exercise

Your aerobic exercise has to be intense enough to raise your pulse rate into the training zone (see Appendix 5, page 413), but not so intense that you exceed your capacity to produce muscular energy using the oxygen you breathe. Sprinting, for example, is too intense – it demands more oxygen than is available, so the muscles switch to making energy anaerobically. This results in a build-up of toxic by-products.

You may never have done aerobics, but don't view it as a hard slog before you've begun. It can be hugely fun. Think of swimming, a volleyball game with friends or colleagues, or a long ramble through stunning countryside.

Here are just some of your choices:

Walking	Aerobics
Rambling	Dance classes
Jogging	Cycling
Swimming	Team sports
Circuit training	DVD workouts

But whichever you choose, you need to follow the same golden rules with each:

1. Warm up first. This is especially important if you are unfit and overweight. Warming up is necessary to prepare the body for an increased level of activity. The body needs time to transport the oxygen you breathe into your muscles. Gradually increasing a walk from a slow to medium pace gives the body the time that is needed. Or, when swimming, starting with breaststroke before you move on to front crawl may be a good way to slowly increase the intensity.

If you start too quickly, inevitably you will start to feel uncomfortable and will need to slow down in order to continue. This can be discouraging if you are new to exercise. Take two to three minutes to warm up. Think of it as a gradual increase rather than stop–start. It's like driving a car – you need to pull away in first gear and work your way up through the gears, slowly building up to a level you can maintain. If you tried to pull away in top gear when driving a car, it would struggle and stall. In the same way, you will feel very uncomfortable very quickly if you do not warm up.

Remember: you warm up to work out, you don't work out to warm up.

2. Exercise at a level that keeps you in your training zone for at least 15 minutes. If you are swimming, for example, don't stop every couple of lengths. It is better to swim more slowly and keep going than to stop frequently and catch your breath. If you are attracted to team sports such as tennis, badminton, squash or football, the trick is to keep moving. Short bursts of activity won't do you much good for developing aerobic fitness, which is what burns fat.

The purpose of training in your training zone is to develop your aerobic fitness. This will in turn increase your body's ability to use fat as a fuel. As you get fitter the body increases the cells where it produces energy. These cells (mitochondria) increase in size and number with activity that is continuous in nature and of a moderate intensity. They can turn you into an incredibly efficient fatburning machine. It is no surprise that distance runners and cyclists have the highest levels of these cells. Your goal is to build up to a level that allows you to keep exercising continuously for up to 35 minutes.

How will you know if you are exercising within your training zone? Well, it will be a faster pace than your normal walking speed but not so fast that you can't continue to talk to someone else at the same time.

If you are new to exercise, it is best to start by increasing how many times you exercise and how long you exercise for, before you increase the intensity of the exercise. Think: 'more active, more often'.

3. Set yourself a realistic goal and gradually increase it. Here's an example. If you like jogging round your local park, you might find that one circuit takes you ten minutes. In your second week, can you get that time down to nine minutes? Or you could increase the distance and/or how often you do it. In the beginning, make it easy to reach your goal. Then week by week, reach for higher goals. When you achieve them you'll know you're really fatburning – you'll be seeing, and feeling, the results.

Find some time in your schedule when you can do some exercise, and make a date with yourself. As a benchmark, see how long you can exercise in your training zone. Let's say five minutes. Now that you know what you can manage, make sure you do five minutes of exercise more frequently. Your goal is to build up to three to five times a week. Alternatively, you may want to increase the time. Again, with five minutes as your starting point, try to add just one minute each time you exercise. Too often people try to add too much at the beginning, become uncomfortable, do not achieve their goal and become discouraged.

Here's an example. If you plan to do more exercise, you may want to start with 10 minutes, three times a week. You could aim to add one minute each time you exercise, thereby gradually increasing the total duration. This would mean that in the first week you would complete three sessions: one of ten minutes, one of 11 minutes and one of 12 minutes. Within four weeks you will have doubled the time you initially exercised for, but the increase will have been so gradual that you'll hardly have noticed it.

	Monday	Wednesday	Friday	Total minutes
Week1	10	11	12	33
Week 2	13	14	15	42
Week 3	16	17	18	51
Week 4	19	20	21	60

Within two weeks you will have reached the recommended 15-minute minimum and you can then focus on increasing the frequency.

Alternatively, you may want to increase the frequency first. This would require you to plan 15 minutes of exercise into your day. In the first week you might manage to fit in two 15-minute sessions. The following week you should aim to find time to add another session. This should continue gradually, and soon you'll find that you are exercising for 15 minutes every day.

Once you have achieved this, you should try to find time elsewhere in your schedule so that you could carry out two 15-minute sessions in a single day. Perhaps you could look at alternatives to driving or taking public transport to work: if you cycle, or get off your bus a few stops earlier, you could gain 15 minutes of exercise when travelling in and another when travelling home.

Your goals need to be achievable and manageable. You are better off planning and attaining small goals that build your success rather than aiming too high initially. Remember that just becoming more active is an achievement. Finding time to be more active and planning exercise may be your initial goal.

4. Vary the exercise so that you don't get bored. Variety can add a dimension to your exercise routine. In the same way that you don't plan to eat the same meals every day, you can vary the types of exercise that you do. This will also allow you to work different muscles and develop your general fitness.

Try to find activities that you enjoy. If you don't enjoy one form of exercise, try something else. Finding the right environment can be very important.

Exercise won't always be fun. At times you may find it uncomfortable, time-consuming or solitary. However, ask any one who exercises on a regular basis and they will tell you that although they don't always enjoy the sessions they do enjoy the results.

5. Exercise with a friend, at a gym, or in classes for extra motivation. When you start to plan your exercise programme consider several options.

Who do you want to exercise with? Some people prefer to exercise in groups or with other like-minded people. However, others prefer to exercise alone and use the time to think. You may want both. Time passes more quickly when you are with someone else.

Where do you want to exercise? The gym can be a really good place to get support. The fitness instructors want to help and they enjoy developing new exercise programmes for people. However, you may prefer to do exercise classes. If you're not sure which would be most effective, ask for advice. Remember that you want something that is aerobic in nature rather than a 'legs, bum and tums' class, which is better for toning.

Plan to reward yourself with something other than food for completing certain targets. These rewards can be symbolic or practical: a new piece of training gear, a massage or a new book – anything that will motivate you to achieve your goal.

6. Drink plenty of water before, during and after exercising. The body is two-thirds water and you lose significant amounts of it through sweat and breathing. Drink a glass of water for every half hour of exercise.

7. Cool down when you finish and stretch the muscles you've been exercising. If you have been exercising for 15 minutes take two to three minutes to cool down before starting your stretches. The cool down is the opposite of the warm up. Again, if you think of your body as a car, you would not change from fifth gear to first in one go. So make sure you slow down gradually.

Stretching will promote recovery as well as relaxing your muscles, but it is often neglected. It is essential that you stretch the muscles you have worked to reduce the risk of injury. Depending on which muscles you've been working, stretch them immediately after exercising. It is best to hold a stretch and count to 20, rather than stretching, then releasing, then stretching again.

8. Keep it up. The real benefits of exercise are seen after weeks or months, not days. Make exercise a part of your daily routine.

It can be quite an achievement to plan and complete exercise on a daily basis. Remember that every exercise session you complete takes you closer to your goal, whereas every session missed keeps you further away. Try not to focus only on the physical changes to your body, as this does not recognise your accomplishment in being a regular exerciser (with all the planning and organisation this entails).

Don't think of it as taking up exercise, but as giving up being inactive.

The psychological benefits of exercise are just as well established as the physical benefits. You won't just enjoy a healthier, more efficient body but you will also sleep more soundly, have more energy for other tasks and think more clearly.

Toning exercises

By toning specific muscle groups you can lose inches as well as pounds. As we've seen, the more muscle you build, the greater your ability to burn fat: muscle uses up more calories. Some workouts include both aerobic and toning exercises. Alternatively, you could do a mainly aerobic exercise one day and a mainly toning exercise another.

The trick for toning exercises is to get some good advice. Your local gym is probably the best place for that. If you prefer to exercise as part of a group, ask your gym for an exercise programme. Classes focusing on toning exercises (such as 'legs, bums and tums') are very popular and you will often have a variety to choose from. Many celebrities swear by yoga – if you can't attend a class you could try one of the yoga DVDs on sale. There are different types of yoga and you need to find a style and level of class that suits you.

Ask your gym instructor to include compound exercises in your workout. These exercises use the large muscle groups and help keep the total number of exercises to a minimum.

Typical exercises used in circuit classes can be completed at home. Traditional press-ups and their modifications can be performed in the living room as well as many of the other bodyweight movements.

Here is an example of a set of exercises that could be performed one after another in circuit fashion, to give you the toning effects you want. (For detailed descriptions of the exercises please visit www.theholforddiet.com.)

Example circuit workout			
Exercise	Circuit 1	Circuit 2	Circuit 3
Squats	10	12	15
Press-ups	10	12	15
Sit-ups	10	12	15
Upright rows	10	12	15
Back extensions	10	12	15
Triceps dips	10	12	15
Lunges	10	12	15
Side leg lifts	10	12	15
Lateral raises	10	12	15
Biceps curls	10	12	15

You do not have to start by doing all of the exercises at once or all three circuits the first time; you can build up to completing this over a period of time.

Psychocalisthenics

One of my favourite exercise routines is Psychocalisthenics®. You can learn it in five hours, by DVD or, ideally on a course, and do it in about 15 minutes wherever you are.

Psychocalisthenics is a precise sequence of 23 exercises that leave you feeling fantastic. I've been doing it for over 20 years and I've yet to find anything that keeps me trimmer and makes me feel better – which isn't bad for 15 minutes a day! Each exercise is driven by the breath and, somehow, my body feels lighter, freer and thoroughly oxygenated after this simple routine, which anyone can do.

Psychocalisthenics is the brainchild of Oscar Ichazo. Ichazo founded the Arica School in the 1960s as a school of knowledge for the understanding of the complete person. A practitioner of martial arts and yoga since 1939, Ichazo developed Psychocalisthenics to be a daily routine that can be done in less than 20 minutes. At first glance it looks like a powerful kind of aerobic yoga. 'In the same way that we have an everyday need for food and nourishment we have to promote the circulation of our vital energy as an everyday business,' says Ichazo.

Whereas most exercise routines simply treat the body as a physical machine that needs to be worked to stay fit, Psychocalisthenics is designed to generate both physical fitness and vital energy by bringing mind and body into balance. The key lies in the precise breathing pattern that accompanies each physical exercise. Energy generation happens when you have stable blood sugar, plus a good supply of oxygen. According to Jane Alexander of the *Daily Mail*, 'Psychocalisthenics is exercise, pared to perfection. I wasn't sweating buckets as I would after an aerobics class. But I had exercised far more muscles. I was clear-headed and bright rather than wiped out.'

The best way to learn Psychocalisthenics is to do a short course. For details see www.patrickholford.com/psychocalisthenics. You can also teach yourself from a DVD, but it is best to learn it 'live'.

My ideal weekly fatburning exercise regime is to do Psycho-calisthenics every other day, three or four times a week; walk, run, swim or cycle three times a week; and do one Ashtanga yoga class a week that involves 'resistance' training, building muscle more than stamina. Enjoy experimenting and finding your favourite routine – once you've done this, it'll be easier to stick to it.

For exercise enthusiasts

If you are already an exercise enthusiast and are clocking up a significant amount of time each day doing exercise you'll find that the 40 ⓖⓛ rule for the food you eat might not fill you up. The same also applies if you are very tall, while the reverse applies if you are very short. The chart opposite helps adjust the total number of GLs you eat, based on your height and your average level of exercise.

Average exercise per day (mins)

	0	15	30	45	60	90	120
5 ft	35	35	40	45	45	50	55
5 ft 3	40	40	40	45	50	55	60
5 ft 6	40	40	40	45	50	55	60
5 ft 9	40	40	45	50	55	60	65
6 ft	45	45	50	55	60	65	70
6 ft 3	50	50	55	60	65	70	75
6 ft 6	55	55	60	65	70	75	80

29

Monitoring Your Results

Once you've got going on the Holford Diet, you will feel and see the results. You may not be able to measure your new energy levels – but you can certainly monitor the pounds you're dropping and the inches you're losing. And here's how.

Weigh and measure yourself at the start of this diet and at the end of every week. Always weigh yourself in the morning, before breakfast, without clothes. Keep monitoring your progress week after week. If you have a bad week, notice what effect that is having on your progress, and get back on course. If you reach a 'plateau', don't worry. This can happen. You can encourage weight loss by following the diet more precisely. Soon, you'll find what you need to do to lose weight, and, once you've reached your ultimate goal, what you need to do to stay there.

There's a Holford Diet Progress Report for each of the first four weeks in Appendix 4. Fill out the report for week one, setting your long-term goal weight and your weekly target weight (see page 229 for how to figure these out). You'll need an accurate pair of scales and a tape measure. Since scales do vary, it's best to weigh yourself on the same ones each week. For the measurements, always take your waist measurement and the widest part your thighs or your hips. For your thigh measurement, take the average of your left and right thighs.

Waist–hip ratio and total inch loss

I recommend that you also work out your waist–hip ratio. This is your waist measurement divided by your hip measurement. The reason is that it's one of the most important measures in relation to your health. Abdominal weight gain is associated with insulin resistance and the risk of diabetes; much more so than with hip and thigh weight gain. The average ratio in Britain is 0.90 for men and 0.79 for women. Once you're above 0.95 for men or 0.85 for women, you do have an increased risk of obesity-related diseases. Broadly speaking, if your waist is greater than 102cm (40in) (men) or 86cm (34in) (women), you need to lose weight. (Obviously, this does depend a bit on your height.)

Your total inch loss is the sum of all the inches you have lost from measurements of your bust or chest, waist, hips and thighs. (If you've lost 2.5cm/1in from each, your total loss is 10cm/4in.)

Progress, week by week

At the end of each week, ask yourself honestly how well you've stuck to the diet and exercise programme. There's a space on the Progress Report to rate yourself out of 100 per cent. This will help you to stay on course. If, at the end of the week, you feel your targets are too hard or too easy, you can adjust the rate of progress you're aiming for.

You'll also find a spare Holford Diet Progress Report that you can copy for subsequent weeks.

With a little help from your friends...

Let your friends and your family know what you are doing. Show them this book. Maybe they'll want to join in too! Doing the diet with a friend is great, because you can then give each other support. Encourage your family to support you by being tolerant with the new foods you'll be preparing, and not tempting you with forbidden foods. When you're invited to dinner, let your hosts know about the diet. And when you throw your own dinner party, use the recipes in Part Five. There are plenty that are elegant enough for a formal meal, and they're all delicious.

You may also find it extremely helpful to carry out this diet with the help of a nutrition consultant, who can help you to get started and will work out a personalised vitamin programme for you. He or she can also keep you on track and provide you with moral support and tips on how to deal with any problems you may have. (See the section on nutrition consultations in Resources, page 432.)

Breaking the rules

Very few people stick to diets 100 per cent, 100 per cent of the time. No doubt there will be the odd occasion when you break the rules. This is not a disaster. In fact, it can be a good idea to give yourself two meals a month when you can eat what you like. This will help you to deal with special occasions and celebrations. So enjoy yourself.

Remember, though, that the more you break the rules, the slower your progress will be. And if you are really addicted, say to double espressos or binge drinking after work, be careful. You can't consume any of these substances in excess and keep your weight down or health up. They have a nasty habit of creeping back into your life and are best avoided if you really feel you can't control your consumption of them.

If you do indulge at a friend's wedding, or find yourself unable to resist pizza and *gelato* on your Italian holiday, the most important thing to do is to get back on track the next day. In one experiment, two groups of slimmers were given an identical milkshake to drink. One group was told it was high in calories, the other that it was low. Each group was then given an unlimited amount of ice cream. Which group, do you think, ate more?

The answer was the group that had been told the milkshake was high in calories. This shows a very common pitfall among dieters – the 'If I've broken my diet I might as well go the whole hog' syndrome. Don't do it. If you blow it one day, get back on track the next.

The first 30 days

If you have more weight to lose and feel good on this diet, keep going for up to 90 days. An excellent target weight loss for an obese person is to decrease body fat percentage by 10 per cent each month or to lose 8.5kg (18lb 12oz) in 90 days. The balance of protein, carbohydrate and fat in the Holford Diet (25 per cent protein, 50 per cent carbohydrate, 25 per cent fat) helps to reprogramme your body to burn fat. This reprogramming is especially important for those of you with a degree of insulin resistance who show signs of sugar sensitivity (see the questionnaire on page 61), and sometimes it takes longer than 30 days.

If you've achieved your goal you can ease up by eating 50 🄶🄻 a day. Chapter 32 is all about how to maintain your weight and health. But first let's look at what to do if this diet simply isn't working for you.

30

What if it's Not Working?

Say you're on Week 4 of the diet, and you've really stuck with it. Congratulations! You've sorted out your coffee addiction, you're feeling much more energetic, and you can definitely see the gloss back in your hair with all the omega-3s you're getting. You love the recipes and your new running regime. There's just one problem: you haven't shed a pound.

I can understand how frustrating this must feel. It's at this point that I have to say that no single diet works for everyone, for the simple reason that there are many different causes of overweight or obesity.

But I also have to say that, in truth, I haven't yet had a case of a person failing to lose weight after they looked at all the possible reasons below, and discovered the one that's holding them back.

So let's look at them.

You're not losing weight, but you are losing inches. This is OK for now. What it means is that you are making lean muscle, which is heavier, but has the capacity to burn more fat. Keep going. The weight loss will follow.

You are still insulin-resistant. Have you quit alcohol, sugar and/or caffeine? If not, and you're not losing weight, you'll have to bite the bullet and give them up.

You're not exercising. Exercise really does help kick-start your metabolism. If your weight isn't shifting, then up your levels of activity.

You're not taking the supplements. Supplements do make a difference and, in addition to the basic multivitamin and vitamin C, the combination of chromium, HCA and 5-HTP definitely gives you the edge in appetite control. They are well worth taking.

You have a hidden allergy. Don't underestimate this factor. Many people fail to lose weight until they have their food allergies and intolerances checked. Your weight can really get stuck until you remove an offending food. Have a food intolerance test (see Resources, page 435) and avoid your food allergies.

You are oestrogen-dominant. Hormonal imbalances, especially of the thyroid, can stop you losing weight. You need to get this checked by your doctor. You should also be tested for an underactive thyroid (see below).

Hormone imbalances and weight gain

It is not at all uncommon for weight gain to be precipitated by hormonal changes. In fact, according to the MyNutrition Survey ION conducted on almost 30,000 people, those with hormonal issues were twice as likely to have problems losing weight. For some women, the pounds pile on during pregnancy, only to stay on after the birth. For others, going on or coming off the pill or HRT can trigger weight gain.

A common time for weight gain for many women is in the premenopausal years (usually from 40 onwards) and even more so at the menopause, when menstruation ceases. Even more common than weight gain is a change in weight distribution, which we'll look at now.

Apples and pears

Are you an apple, or a pear? Excess weight on the hips and thighs, resulting in a pear-shaped body, is associated with excess oestrogen, the feminising hormone. Too much upper-body and waist gain is associated with excess androgens, the masculinising hormone.

These hormonal differences are partly genetic and partly a consequence of how we live. Some people have more active adrenal glands, a factor encouraged by a stressful and competitive lifestyle. This leads to the release of more adrenal hormones, such as cortisol and adrenalin, as well as androgens, which all help to build protein and muscle.

Hence these 'adrenal types' tend to be more muscular and have more weight in the top half of their bodies. For such people it is very important not to live off adrenal stimulants (see Chapter 12) and to keep fat intake down. Too much fat, coupled with prolonged stress and a lack of exercise, leads to obesity. In fact, too much of the adrenal hormone cortisol can also lead to too much oestrogen (produced in the adrenal glands and fatty tissue, as well as the ovaries) which can lead to lower-body weight gain, too.

The two key female hormones are oestrogen and progesterone. They're produced mainly in the ovaries and need to be in balance with each other. An increasingly common problem is that a woman produces too much oestrogen in relation to progesterone. The problem usually stems from a progesterone deficiency, rather than actual excess oestrogen.

Progesterone is produced by the ovaries only once the egg has been released, at ovulation. If a woman doesn't ovulate (which is increasingly common as a woman approaches the menopause), then no progesterone is produced. After the menopause progesterone output falls to almost nothing, while oestrogen levels sink very gradually. Oestrogen is the 'feminising' hormone: it helps to lay down fat as storage, especially on the hips and thighs, creating a more curvaceous shape. This is why so many women gain weight in these places after the age of 35.

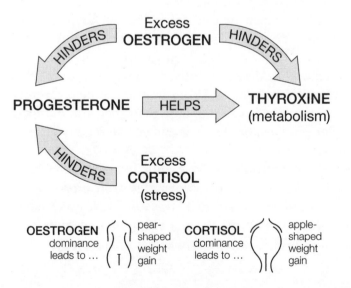

Hormones and their effects on weight distribution Too much oestrogen (or not enough progesterone) competes with the thyroid hormone thyroxine, resulting in a slow metabolism and weight gain, especially on the hips and thighs. Too much cortisol, the stress hormone, also affects thyroid function, slowing down the body's metabolism which leads to weight gain, especially around the middle.

Full details on this subject are given in my book *Balancing Hormones Naturally*, co-authored with Kate Neil (Piatkus).

Men, too, can suffer from oestrogen dominance. This is most likely to occur when their level of the male hormone, testosterone, is low, as this counteracts the feminising effects of oestrogen. A diet high in meat, dairy and pesticide-sprayed foods can make a contribution to developing oestrogen dominance.

If you suspect you have a hormonal imbalance and that this is contributing to your excess weight, the best thing to do is to see a nutritional therapist who can work with your doctor to have the necessary tests done and organise appropriate treatment if necessary.

Thyroid problems

The thyroid gland, found in the area at the base of the throat, controls your rate of metabolism by releasing a hormone called *thyroxine*, which stimulates cells to speed up energy production. Although they make up a relatively small percentage, some people with persistent weight problems do have underactive thyroids, which produce insufficient thyroxine. Excess oestrogen can also interfere with thyroid function.

Some people have an underactive thyroid because their immune system is attacking their thyroid tissue. This is known as autoimmune thyroid disease. You can have this checked by having an 'antithyroid antibody test'. One in every ten people who test positive has undiagnosed coeliac disease (gluten sensitivity). It seems that you can become allergic to a food, and your immune system can then attack a part of you, thinking it's the food, perhaps because the food and you share similar proteins. So the next thing to do is get yourself tested for hidden food allergies.

If you've done everything I've mentioned in this chapter and it still isn't working, I recommend that you get professional advice from a qualified nutritional therapist. They can investigate your particular problem or perhaps give the necessary support and guidance you need. There are details on how to find one near to you on page 432.

31

Controlling Emotional and Obsessive Eating

Eating is very nearly the first thing most of us do in life. Within minutes of being born, a baby receives sustenance from its mother. But suckling provides far more than food, as Harry Harlow's monkeys showed us.

In this famous experiment from the 1950s, infant monkeys were presented with the choice of two surrogate mothers: constructed dummies complete with teats. One provided nourishment, the other no milk but the tactile experience of fur. The baby monkeys chose the tactile sensation rather than food – comfort, over nourishment.

Eating is emotive

For baby humans, the tactile sense and security of the breast is soon associated with food. Eating is an emotive business. And, later in life, eating can become associated with pleasing, rebelling, imitating, rewarding – even punishment. For example, the girl who eats sparingly, like her mum, because she also wants to be thin; the boy who eats certain foods because they 'make him big and strong' and develops aversions to other foods; the rebellion against 'eat it up or you won't get any pudding'; the reward of sweets if you do something good, or the comfort of sweets when you're hurt. By adolescence, a multitude of psychological factors govern when, how, what and how much we eat.

Does any of this ring bells? Do you reach for chocolate when you're upset? Do you gain or lose weight when you are in love? Do you reward yourself with food? Do you always finish what's in front of you? Are you a fussier eater when you feel unhappy? Do you eat more when you are out with the lads?

'Five hundred people were asked what they fear most in the world and 190 answered that their greatest fear is "getting fat",' wrote Kim Chernin in *The Obsession*, a book about hunger. The fear of fat, and the love and hate of food, is a real social problem of epidemic proportions. With this fear, there has been a rapid rise in maladaptive eating behaviour, compulsive eating, crash dieting, bulimia (weight control by vomiting) and anorexia nervosa.

Conflicting images

At least 95 per cent of the sufferers of eating disorders are women, and there is little doubt that social pressures play a significant role. Torn between the advertising images of the sexual 'perfect' woman and the perpetual sensory bombardment with tantalising foods; between the image of the thin and sensuous woman, designed to attract her man, and the caring, providing, 'earth mother' image associated with fat, twenty-first-century women feel they must be all things to all people. And twenty-first-century men are also meant to bring home the bacon, yet look like Brad Pitt. But who has the time, the money or the inclination to live in gyms with today's work pressures?

There's a simple set of exercises to get a handle on emotional eating so you have more choice about how to eat, rather than being a victim of your immediate desires or emotions. The exercises are divided into three steps called 'the three As':

Awareness
Acceptance
Action

Step 1: Awareness

Become aware of why you eat – when, how, what you eat, your beliefs, facts and fantasies about eating, being fat, being thin. To get the most benefit from these exercises answer each question accurately and write down your answer on a separate sheet of paper.

1. What do you weigh?

2. What is the heaviest you have ever been?

3. What is the lightest?

4. What is your ideal weight?

5. How long have you been overweight?

6. What personality characteristics do you associate with being fat?

7. What personality characteristics do you associate with being thin?

8. What do you fear most about being overweight (think about this in relation to health, sex, relationships, work and so on)?

9. What do you like most about being overweight?

10. Imagine you're at a party and you are your ideal weight. What feelings would you experience? How would this change the way you relate to the people around you?

11. Now imagine you become very overweight. How do you feel now, and how does this change the way you relate to others?

12. If you were your ideal weight, how do you think your life would change (think of your feelings, relationships, sex, career, clothes, sports)?

When?

At this stage do not reason 'why', just observe your own behaviour in relation to eating – the hows, whens, whats. Now make a comprehensive list of all the circumstances that precipitate eating for you, other than hunger, for example:

> I eat when I'm bored
> I eat when I get home from work
> I eat when …
> I eat when …

What?

The next exercise will take a little longer.

Keep a food diary for one week, listing the circumstances, feelings before and feelings after each meal or snack, as well as detailed listings of what, and how much you ate.

This can be done as follows:

Day 1 (time)	Food/drink	Circumstances	Feelings before	Feelings after
Example: Monday 9.00 am	Cup of coffee	Need to wake up	Tired	Bit more energy

Be precise in your answers. This will help you become aware of the situations in which you eat, as well as showing you what you eat. You may find that there are some foods or snacks you feel guilty about, that you would rather not commit to paper. You may make excuses to yourself: 'I don't usually eat …' or 'It would have been rude to refuse.' Again, observe your own reactions as if you were watching your behaviour and thoughts, without judgement, on a TV screen.

How?

The next series of questions will help you examine how you eat. Answer these as precisely as possible.

1. What eating and mealtime rules did your parents teach you (such as, 'Always eat everything on your plate')?
2. Do you:
   a) eat your food very fast?
   b) eat your food at a normal rate?
   c) savour each mouthful and chew it well?
3. How fussy are you? What foods will you not eat and for what reasons?
4. When you shop for food do you:
   a) go for the best quality even if it's a little expensive?
   b) go for the best value in terms of money?
5. Do you enjoy cooking and preparing food?
6. Do you usually work, read or watch TV when you eat?
7. Do you have set mealtimes?
8. How much of what you eat is from snacks and nibbles?
9. Do you usually eat beyond the point of feeling full?
10. Do you prefer to eat with other people or by yourself?

Now go back over all the questions and make any additions or changes until you are sure that you have a comprehensive picture of all aspects of your eating behaviour (if there are aspects of your eating behaviour that are not covered by the questions, write these down too). Review your eating behaviour by reading your answers back to yourself as if you were reading an impartial commentary on someone else.

Step 2: Acceptance

All eating behaviour, however destructive or counterproductive, has a purpose. We may overeat to help us deal with anger or boredom, or as a rest after a hard day. Sometimes we overeat because we *want* to be fat. For some people being fat is a mark of authority. Suzie Orbach, in *Fat is a Feminist Issue*, cites a number of clients for whom fat was a rebellion against the sexy, dependent, ineffective model imposed on women. By being fat one could be stating, 'I'm a real person with ambitions and independence.' Fat means many different things for many different people. For all, overeating has a purpose, is a means for compensation. The first step to acceptance is to understand this.

Only by seeing your eating behaviour as it is – and understanding that, in the past and the present, this behaviour has been an attempt to compensate, find pleasure or security – is it possible to eat (and on occasions overeat) without guilt or remorse. However, to accept our habits is not to give in, to surrender to food. It's a step nearer to being in control of your eating behaviour.

Acceptance is the opposite of resistance. To resist any desire or want means that desire will persist. Nothing really is solved. If you continually crave chocolate you can resist for only so long. You may overeat 'good' food with the hope that your craving for chocolate will go away. You may believe that eating chocolate is bad, that you're bad, and as you give in to this irresistible urge you may have feelings of guilt and self-disgust at your unhealthy tastes and lack of willpower. With these feelings can come more desire to eat, to compensate for these feelings. It is better to accept your initial desires and to understand them.

As an exercise in acceptance, go to your favourite food shops and buy all the foods you like most, whether 'good' or 'bad'. Stock up your fridge and larder with all the foods you could possibly want. For one week eat what you want, how you want it. If what you really want is the dessert, start with this.

Step 3: Action

We are all programmed to survive. We have a built-in mechanism that makes us hungry when we are deprived of nutrition. Any baby will cry if it wants food. If the food doesn't satisfy the baby's nutritional needs it will still feel hungry. We are no different.

For many of us hunger is rarely the motive for eating. We have learned that eating suppresses feelings, that certain foods are addictive, that it is sociable to eat and encourage others to eat. We have learned how to eat against our instincts. Only by unlearning these habits is it possible to discover or uncover our inbuilt desire to eat nutritious food in the right quantities.

From the questions on the previous pages you will have a list of when you eat and what you eat, as well as the feelings associated with eating. These are some of the commonest 'whens' from clients at my clinics:

- I eat when I'm bored.

- I eat when I'm happy.

- I eat when I'm frustrated/angry/upset.

- I eat when I'm sexually frustrated.

- I eat when I'm tired.

- I continually nibble after work from 6.00 pm onwards.

- I eat when I'm under pressure at work.

According to the psychologist Oscar Ichazo, these are examples of using eating to compensate for feelings we cannot handle. For instance, boredom may result from having more energy than we know how to deal with. Drinking or overeating is one way to dissipate that energy, leaving us psychologically in balance. It's as if we had a steam boiler full of energy, and when the pressure builds up we experience negative feelings like frustration or boredom. To compensate, we must let off steam by opening safety valves, one of which is gluttony, which includes overeating. Others include panic, phobia, overexertion, cruelty and toximania (such as getting drunk).

Ichazo calls these 'doors of compensation' because we develop the habit of losing energy through one 'door' or another. I've discussed these more fully in my book *Beat Stress and Fatigue*, Piatkus). If, for example, gluttony is one of your favourite doors (using food to excess), or toximania, then the goal is to find a better way to deal with the situation you are compensating for.

Breaking the habits

The object of the next exercise is to break each part of your overeating habits initially for a period of one week. Only then are you in a position to decide whether curbing overeating is the most effective way to deal with the particular situation. With objective awareness and acceptance of our eating behaviour and the following exercise, habitual eating becomes easier to stop.

Exercise: breaking the habits

Pick a 'when' such as, 'I eat when I'm frustrated.'

Question 1. Is there any way you can deal with the situation directly? For example, how can you most effectively express the anger/frustration to achieve the results you want? Depression is often anger without enthusiasm!

Question 2. Is there any way you can deal with the situation indirectly? For example, go for a run, call a friend, do some housework energetically, beat the hell out of a rug, or rip the weeds out of your garden instead.

Set your target. Now set yourself this target for the next week:

'I eat as much as I want, when I want, and I do not eat when … [I'm frustrated].'

Write this down on a card and keep it in a prominent place. When you have completed your first target, reward yourself by doing something you really enjoy. You are now in a position to choose whether eating is the best way of dealing with this 'when' situation. You are in control.

Now move on to your next 'when'. Ask yourself Questions 1 and 2 each time this situation arises. Set your target for the next week and write this down on a card and keep it in a prominent place. Do this for each 'when' until you've completed your list.

Remember: *you* are not your eating behaviour. Your eating behaviour consists of habits you have consciously or unconsciously learned as a result of experiences in the past. Some of these habits are still useful and some of them are not. By stopping each eating habit for a week you are in a position to choose how, when and what you eat. You are in control.

These simple exercises will help you get a handle on emotional and obsessive eating, helping you to follow my diet to its successful conclusion.

32

Maintenance

As I said at the start, the Holford Diet is all about optimum health, and weight loss is just one facet of this. It's a diet for life, and that's why 90 per cent of the principles covered in this book are consistent with ongoing good health and weight maintenance. However, there are some aspects of the diet that you don't need to keep up forever.

Once you have lost most of the weight you wanted to lose, are feeling full of energy and vitality, and have lost any cravings for stimulants and sugary foods (check your score on the Are You Insulin-Resistant? questionnaire on page 61), you don't need to keep eating quite so much protein every day. You can reduce the amount from 25 per cent of your daily calories to between 15 and 20 per cent. The chart below shows you what this means in practice.

Protein servings on the maintenance diet

Food	Weight	Serving
Tofu	85g	½ packet
Soya mince	72g	2 tbsp
Chicken (no skin)	35g	¾ very small breast
Turkey (no skin)	35g	¼ small breast
Quorn	85g	¼ pack
Salmon	40g	¾ very small fillet
Tuna (canned in brine)	35g	⅕ can
Sardines (canned in brine)	55g	½ can
Cod	45g	¾ very small fillet
Clams	45g	⅕ can
Prawns	60g	4 large prawns
Mackerel	60g	¾ medium fillet

Oysters	–	11
Yoghurt (natural, low-fat)	205g	¼ large tub
Cottage cheese	85g	¼ medium tub
Hummus	140g	¾ small tub
Skimmed milk	300ml	c. ½ pint
Soya milk	300ml	c. ½ pint
Eggs (boiled)	–	1½
Quinoa	90g	5 heaped tbsp
Baked beans	225g	½ can
Kidney beans	125g	¼ can
Black-eyed beans	125g	¼ can
Lentils	120g	¼ can

But, although you eat less protein-rich food, you'll eat more carbohydrate-rich food. Go by the chart on page 89, but this time aim to eat between half to two-thirds of the protein portions given, and one and a half to twice the carbohydrate portion. This means upping your daily GL score for what you *eat* from 40 to 55 points, which will include unchanged GLs of 10 for two snacks, and 5 for drinks, sweets and desserts. So each meal will have 15 🄶🄻.

As a result, you'll have to alter some of the recipes a bit to up the proportion of carbohydrate-rich foods. The chart below gives you some guidelines on common combinations.

Protein-rich food	Carbohydrate-rich food (cooked weights)
¾ small breast/3 slices chicken	1 medium serving brown rice (150g)
¾ small fillet salmon	1 serving wholewheat pasta (175g)
¼ medium pot cottage cheese	6 small (new) boiled potatoes (150g)
¼ can beans	6 oatcakes

Everyone is different, so you'll have to experiment with ratios of carbohydrate and protein until you find what suits you best. Your best guide is your body and your instincts. Eat what works for you.

Supplements for life

Although it's a great idea to keep supplementing your daily diet with a good high-strength multivitamin and mineral twice a day, plus 1,000mg of vitamin C, you don't need to keep taking additional chromium (provided there's 40mcg or more in your multi), or HCA or fibre supplements forever. So you can safely stop these, too, when you've achieved your final weight. Chromium is particularly helpful at keeping your blood sugar level stable, so if you ever find yourself craving stimulants or sweet things – perhaps when you're under a lot of stress – you may find it helpful to take additional chromium for a few weeks.

Stimulants – don't drift back

One of the most important, yet most difficult, times to stay on track is when you're stressed. This is when the old familiar stimulants (tea, coffee, chocolate, cigarettes, sugar) remind you of their existence. If you've really been addicted to one or more of these, don't let them creep back, even when you've achieved your final goal. The daily use of any stimulant is a bad sign. The odd cup of weak tea or coffee when you eat out or on holiday, or the odd chocolate dessert, is no big deal, though.

100 per cent health

Losing weight and gaining all that energy is just the beginning. Why not go all the way, and start to incorporate into your diet and lifestyle all the advice given in my books *The Optimum Nutrition Bible* and *Optimum Nutrition for the Mind*? Each encourages you to go deeper in both your understanding and application of optimum nutrition, to help you achieve higher and higher levels of health in all aspects of mind and body. And you can produce even more delectable gourmet dishes with *The Optimum Nutrition Cookbook*, *The Low-GL Diet Cookbook* and *Food GLorious Food* (see Recommended Reading).

PART FIVE

Food, Menu Plans and Recipes

33

Menus

You may have followed diets with insipid low-fat recipes, or, in the case of high-protein regimes, super-rich and filling ones. The Holford Diet is all about freshness, flavour, zing – and satisfaction. And there's no end to the variety of meals you can make that fit within the Holford Diet principles.

Ciara S is typical of the many successful Holford dieters who contact us to say how much they enjoyed our recipes:

> *I am becoming more and more adept at making the yummy recipes in the book! Seriously, I cannot understand why everyone hasn't adopted this way of eating! Healthy, interesting and, most importantly, utterly delicious!*

So now is the time to get to grips with all the new ingredients in your fridge and larder. I'll start with a menu plan for the first four weeks, which I recommend you follow for at least the first week so that you get a clear idea of the quantity and balance of foods on this diet. Once you're familiar with them and with the basic rules, you can use these recipes and your imagination to create a feast of fatburning gastronomic delights.

Should you wish to do it your own way and work out your menus yourself, that's fine too. You can swap meals around from one day to another. However, do bear in mind that each day of menus is well balanced. The menus are also balanced for fat, giving you two measures of the essential fats (explained on page 172) each day.

If you make up your own daily menus, make sure you are not getting too much or too little essential fat. Don't pick, for example, the highest-fat recipe and have that every day. Oily fish, for example, occurs in the menus no more than three times a week. So, as you work out each day's menu, ensure you have enough variation. Also, be sure to ring the changes with your snacks. Try a ripe pear with pumpkin seeds; a couple of oatcakes with a dollop of hummus; cottage cheese with berries; or a handful of delicious Spiced Chickpea Chews (page 372). The various snack ideas are featured in Week 1 so substitute the ones you like for the standard snack of fruit and nuts or seeds, given in Weeks 2 to 4.

Bear in mind that puddings are a treat I recommend having just once a week, starting in Week 3.

If you're a vegan or vegetarian, you've got recipes that are suitable as they are, and others in which you can substitute tofu, tempeh or other protein sources for the fish or chicken given. Chapter 26 also has useful information and suggestions for the rich array of options this diet offers you.

Please note the portion sizes you should consume for the following, as either snacks or components of a meal:

- Nuts or seeds – 50g

- Berries – ½ cup unless stated otherwise

- Steamed vegetables (taken from the 'unlimited' table on pages 247–8) – half a dinner-plateful, unless stated otherwise

Week one

Note: all weights for pasta and rice are cooked weights (half this amount to give the dried weight you need to cook).

Day 1

Breakfast	Scots Porridge with berries *or* one chopped apple *or* pear and milk
Lunch	Apple and Tuna Salad with three oatcakes
Dinner	Steam-Fried Vegetables served with 70g (2½oz) brown basmati rice
Snacks	Pear with pumpkin seeds/two oatcakes with hummus
Drinks	Unlimited water, herbal teas and coffee alternatives, plus one glass of diluted juice

Day 2

Breakfast Fatburner Muesli
Lunch Fatburner Sandwich with Green Salad
Dinner Chicken Tandoori with 70g (2½oz) brown basmati rice
and steamed vegetables
Snacks Apple with sunflower seeds/cottage cheese with berries
Drinks Unlimited water, herbal teas and coffee alternatives, plus
one glass of diluted juice

Day 3

Breakfast Fruit Yoghurt/Yoghurt Shake
Lunch Beany Vegetable Soup with two oatcakes
Dinner Pasta with Pumpkin Seed Pesto
Snacks A punnet of strawberries/one thin slice of rye bread with
peanut butter
Drinks Unlimited water, herbal teas and coffee alternatives, plus
one glass of diluted juice

Day 4

Breakfast Scots Porridge with berries *or* one chopped apple *or* pear,
and milk and yoghurt
Lunch Quinoa Tabouleh
Dinner Tuna Steak with Black-Eyed Bean Salsa and Rocket and
Watercress Salad
Snacks An apple and five almonds/two oatcakes and peanut butter
Drinks Unlimited water, herbal teas and coffee alternatives, plus
one glass of diluted juice

Day 5

Breakfast Fatburner Muesli
Lunch Fatburner Baked Potato with Coleslaw
Dinner Chicken Chermoula with Oriental Green Beans
Snacks A small yoghurt with blueberries/crudités (one carrot,
two celery sticks and five broccoli florets) and hummus
Drinks Unlimited water, herbal teas and coffee alternatives, plus
one glass of diluted juice

Day 6

Breakfast Fruit Yoghurt/Yoghurt Shake
Lunch Walnut and Three-Bean Salad with Green Salad
Dinner Chestnut and Mushroom Pilaf with steamed spinach and broccoli
Snacks Pear with pumpkin seeds/two oatcakes with hummus
Drinks Unlimited water, herbal teas and coffee alternatives, plus one glass of diluted juice

Day 7

Breakfast Scrambled Egg with one thin slice of rye toast
Lunch Stuffed Peppers with Green Salad
Dinner Thai Baked Cod with 70g (2½oz) brown basmati rice and Crunchy Thai Salad
Snacks Apple with sunflower seeds/cottage cheese with berries
Drinks Unlimited water, herbal teas and coffee alternatives, plus one glass of diluted juice

Week two

By now you'll be getting a taste for the fatburner recipes. Note the ones you like, and remember that you can exchange lunches or dinner from one day with another day. However, keep your choices varied, as some meals are less balanced than others. By Weeks 3 and 4 you can add one dessert per week, and continue to introduce new and delicious recipes.

Day 1

Breakfast Scots Porridge
Lunch Fatburner Sandwich with Green Salad
Dinner Ratatouille Sausage Bake with three steamed baby new potatoes and a quarter of a plateful of broccoli
Snacks Two pieces of fruit with nuts/seeds
Drinks Unlimited water, herbal teas and coffee alternatives, plus one glass of diluted juice

Day 2

Breakfast Fatburner Muesli
Lunch   Thai-Style Vegetable Broth, Crunchy Thai Salad
Dinner   Trout with Puy Lentils and Roasted Tomatoes on the Vine
Snacks   Two pieces of fruit with nuts/seeds
Drinks   Unlimited water, herbal teas and coffee alternatives, plus one glass of diluted juice

Day 3

Breakfast Fruit Yoghurt/Yoghurt Shake
Lunch   Smoked Salmon Pâté on two thin slices of toasted rye bread
Dinner   Thai Green Curry with a quarter of a plateful of steamed mangetouts
Snacks   Two pieces of fruit with nuts/seeds
Drinks   Unlimited water, herbal teas and coffee alternatives, plus one glass of diluted juice

Day 4

Breakfast Scots Porridge
Lunch   Flageolet Bean Dip with crudités (one carrot, two celery sticks and five broccoli florets) and three oatcakes
Dinner   Roasted Vegetables with Mediterranean Quinoa
Snacks   Two pieces of fruit with nuts/seeds
Drinks   Unlimited water, herbal teas and coffee alternatives, plus one glass of diluted juice

Day 5

Breakfast Fatburner Muesli
Lunch   Fatburner Baked Potato with Green Salad
Dinner   Dhal (Lentil Curry) with 70g (2½oz) brown basmati rice and steamed broccoli
Snacks   Two pieces of fruit with nuts/seeds
Drinks   Unlimited water, herbal teas and coffee alternatives, plus one glass of diluted juice

Day 6

Breakfast Fruit Yoghurt/Yoghurt Shake
Lunch Chestnut and Butterbean Soup with two oatcakes
Dinner Spiced Turkey Meatballs with 85g (3oz) of wholegrain spaghetti and one courgette sliced lengthways and grilled
Snacks Two pieces of fruit with nuts/seeds
Drinks Unlimited water, herbal teas and coffee alternatives, plus one glass of diluted juice

Day 7

Breakfast Boiled Egg with one thin slice of rye toast
Lunch Gazpacho, Baba Ganoush and one thin slice of rye bread
Dinner Chicken Dumplings with Chilli Dipping Sauce, with 85g (3oz) soba (buckwheat) noodles and steam-fried pak choi
Snacks Two pieces of fruit with nuts/seeds
Drinks Unlimited water, herbal teas and coffee alternatives, plus one glass of diluted juice

Week three

Day 1

Breakfast Scots Porridge
Lunch Green Bean, Olive and Roasted Pepper Salad in one wholemeal pitta bread
Dinner Borlotti Bean Bolognese with two steamed courgettes
Snacks Two pieces of fruit with nuts/seeds
Drinks Unlimited water, herbal teas and coffee alternatives, plus one glass of diluted juice

Day 2

Breakfast Fatburner Muesli
Lunch Hummus with crudités (one carrot, two celery sticks and five broccoli florets) and four oatcakes
Dinner Fajitas with Mediterranean Tomato and Courgette Salad
Snacks Two pieces of fruit with nuts/seeds
Drinks Unlimited water, herbal teas and coffee alternatives, plus one glass of diluted juice

Day 3

Breakfast Fruit Yoghurt/Yoghurt Shake
Lunch Beany Vegetable Soup with two oatcakes *or* one toasted pitta bread
Dinner Garlic and Lemon Roast Chicken with two small boiled new potatoes and steamed broccoli
Chocolate Coconut Cookies
Snacks Two pieces of fruit with nuts/seeds
Drinks Unlimited water, herbal teas and coffee alternatives, plus one glass of diluted juice

Day 4

Breakfast Scots Porridge
Lunch Blueberry and Cottage Cheese Salad with three oatcakes
Dinner Chickpea Curry with 70g (2½oz) brown basmati rice *or* 50g (1¾oz) couscous, and steamed runner beans
Snacks Two pieces of fruit with nuts/seeds
Drinks Unlimited water, herbal teas and coffee alternatives, plus one glass of diluted juice

Day 5

Breakfast Fatburner Muesli
Lunch Fatburner Baked Potato with Mediterranean Tomato and Courgette Salad
Dinner Stuffed Peppers with Tomato and Red Onion Salad
Snacks Two pieces of fruit with nuts/seeds
Drinks Unlimited water, herbal teas and coffee alternatives, plus one glass of diluted juice

Day 6

Breakfast	Fruit Yoghurt/Yoghurt Shake
Lunch	Walnut and Three-Bean Salad with Coleslaw
Dinner	Sticky Mustard Salmon Fillets with 100g (3½oz) quinoa and steam-fried leeks and peppers
Snacks	Two pieces of fruit with nuts/seeds
Drinks	Unlimited water, herbal teas and coffee alternatives, plus one glass of diluted juice

Day 7

Breakfast	Scrambled Egg with one thin slice of rye toast
Lunch	Lentil and Lemon Soup with three oatcakes
Dinner	Indian Spiced Chicken with 70g (2½oz) brown basmati rice and steam-fried veg
Snacks	Two pieces of fruit with nuts/seeds
Drinks	Unlimited water, herbal teas and coffee alternatives, plus one glass of diluted juice

Week four

Day 1

Breakfast	Scots Porridge
Lunch	Fatburner Sandwich with Tomato and Red Onion Salad
Dinner	Grilled Goat's Cheese on Portabella Mushrooms with mixed salad leaves (such as spinach, rocket and watercress) and dressing
Snacks	Two pieces of fruit with nuts/seeds
Drinks	Unlimited water, herbal teas and coffee alternatives, plus one glass of diluted juice

Day 2

Breakfast	Fatburner Muesli
Lunch	Spicy Pumpkin and Tofu Soup
Dinner	Chicken with Roasted Courgettes and Red Onion
Snacks	Two pieces of fruit with nuts/seeds
Drinks	Unlimited water, herbal teas and coffee alternatives, plus one glass of diluted juice

Day 3

Breakfast Fruit Yoghurt/Yoghurt Shake
Lunch Sardines on Toast with Celeriac Rémoulade
Dinner Nick's Beefburgers with Mexican Bean Dip and as much lettuce as you can squeeze into a toasted wholemeal pitta bread
Individual Berry Cheesecake
Snacks Two pieces of fruit with nuts/seeds
Drinks Unlimited water, herbal teas and coffee alternatives, plus one glass of diluted juice

Day 4

Breakfast Scots Porridge
Lunch Chestnut and Butterbean Soup with a Green Salad on the side
Dinner Tarragon and Lemon Roast Chicken Breast with 70g (2½oz) brown basmati rice and Mediterranean Tomato and Courgette Salad (or steamed vegetables)
Snacks Two pieces of fruit with nuts/seeds
Drinks Unlimited water, herbal teas and coffee alternatives, plus one glass of diluted juice

Day 5

Breakfast Fatburner Muesli
Lunch Fatburner Baked Sweet Potato with Rocket and Watercress Salad
Dinner Grilled Burgers with one wholemeal pitta bread and mixed salad leaves (such as spinach, rocket and watercress) with either French Dressing or Tahini Dressing
Snacks Two pieces of fruit with nuts/seeds
Drinks Unlimited water, herbal teas and coffee alternatives, plus one glass of diluted juice

Day 6

Breakfast Fruit Yoghurt/Yoghurt Shake
Lunch Mexican Bean Dip and crudités (one carrot, two celery sticks and five broccoli florets)
Dinner Trout with Puy Lentils and Roasted Tomatoes on the Vine with steamed courgettes
Snacks Two pieces of fruit with nuts/seeds
Drinks Unlimited water, herbal teas and coffee alternatives, plus one glass of diluted juice

Day 7

Breakfast Boiled Egg with one thin slice of rye toast
Lunch Quinoa Tabouleh with Tomato and Red Onion Salad
Dinner Chestnut and Mushroom Pilaf with mixed salad leaves (such as spinach, rocket and watercress) and either French or Tahini Dressing
Snacks Two pieces of fruit with nuts/seeds
Drinks Unlimited water, herbal teas and coffee alternatives, plus one glass of diluted juice

34

Recipes

In the end, all diets stand or fall by their recipes. Huge amounts of research, care and thought may have gone into the principles behind them, but, if the food itself is tasteless or monotonous, the diet will fail.

The Holford Diet passes this test with flying colours. I promise you wonderful flavours, intriguing textures, fantastic freshness and great variety. I've borrowed from the best in world cuisine to create dishes bursting with health and flavour. Hundreds of thousands of people have found these recipes seriously delicious, so, if you're ready, let's get going on them.

Almost all the recipes are sugar-free, using the natural sweetness present in food, or they use xylitol, a natural plant sugar that has all the taste of sugar but a third of the calories, and does not disrupt your blood sugar, giving it a very low GL. Another added bonus is the fact that it protects your teeth from cavities.

The recipes are also high in fibre, so you don't need to add any. The foods used are naturally high in key vitamins and minerals. I recommend you buy the freshest ingredients, organic if possible, since these tend to contain more nutrients as well as being chemical-free.

As this diet is mainly based on fresh vegetables, fruits, beans, lentils and wholegrains, with some fish and chicken, you will find it very economical, too. You may, however, need to vary the fruits and vegetables depending on what's in season.

To follow the diet, all you need to do is select a breakfast, lunch and dinner for each day, based on the menus in the previous chapter. Not all the recipes have exactly the same balance of nutrients, so if you don't want to follow the menu plans it's best to vary your choices.

Note that, unless otherwise stated, all lunches and main meals, except for things like sandwiches, give quantities for two people. If there's only one of you, halve the portion sizes or make enough for two meals and pop one in the fridge. (Note also that I often suggest you season a dish with Solo, a special kind of salt; for more on this product, see Resources, page 433.)

Bon appétit!

Add to your repertoire

There are even more of our delicious low-GL recipes in *The Holford Low-GL Diet Cookbook*, by Patrick Holford and Fiona McDonald Joyce (Piatkus). Once you have achieved your weight and move on to 'maintenance' there are yet more delicious GL-friendly recipes in *Food GLorious Food*, by Patrick Holford and Fiona McDonald Joyce (Piatkus).

Note: Cup measurements are used for some of the quantities to make it quicker and easier for you to measure them. One cup measures 250ml (8fl oz); ½ cup is 125ml/4fl oz.

Breakfasts

Yes, it's true: breakfast *is* the most important meal of the day. It's all down, literally, to your body's sugar level, which is at its lowest ebb first thing in the morning. If you go to work very early, take your breakfast to work and have it during the first break you take. All breakfast recipes are for one person. (For the size of a serving of various kinds of fruits, see page 392.) Remember: breakfast can have a maximum 10 🔴.

GL scores

Recipe	Page number	🔴
Get Up & Go with berries	313	10
Fatburner Muesli	313	7
Scots Porridge	314	8
Fruit Yoghurt or Yoghurt Shake	314	10
Scrambled Egg on rye toast	315	9
Boiled Egg with rye toast	315	10

Get Up & Go is a powdered breakfast drink, which is blended with skimmed milk or soya milk and banana or berries. Nutritionally speaking, it is the ultimate breakfast: each serving gives you more fibre than a bowl of porridge, more protein than an egg, more iron than a cooked breakfast and more vitamins and minerals than a whole packet of cornflakes. In fact, every serving of Get Up & Go gives you at least 100 per cent of every vitamin and mineral and a lot more of some key nutrients. For example, you get 1,000mg of vitamin C – the equivalent of more than 20 oranges.

Get Up & Go is made from the best-quality wholefoods, ground into a powder. It contains no sucrose, no additives, no animal products, no yeast, wheat or milk, and it tastes delicious. Each serving, with 300ml (½ pint) of skimmed milk or soya milk and some fruit, provides fewer than 300 calories and, when mixed up, only 10 ⓖ, making it ideal as part of the Holford Diet. It is nutritionally superior to any other breakfast choice and is totally suitable for adults and children alike. It is fine to have this for breakfast every day, if you choose.

Make it up with berries or a soft pear. If you use a banana, have a small, less ripe banana or use half a larger banana. It is widely available in health food shops.

Get Up & Go

Serves 1
1 serving Get Up & Go powder
300ml (½ pint) skimmed milk or low-fat soya milk
1 small banana, or ½ larger banana, or 1 pear or 2 heaped tbsp berries

Blend milk, fruit and Get Up & Go powder.

Fatburner Muesli

This delicious muesli tastes best when the oats, bran and seeds are soaked overnight in enough water to cover them and the mixture is topped with berries and yoghurt when serving.

Serves 1
½ cup soft porridge oat flakes
½ cup oat bran
1 tbsp ground mixed seeds (see page 236 for the seed mix recipe)
as many berries as you want (strawberries, raspberries, blueberries)
2 tbsp plain, natural yoghurt

Scots Porridge

On a cold winter's day nothing could be more warming than porridge. Oats contain special factors that are known to promote a healthy heart and arteries, and are full of fibre and complex carbohydrates.

> Serves 1
> 300ml (½ pint) skimmed or soya milk
> 55g (2oz) porridge oats
> 2 tsp ground flaxseeds and pumpkin seeds
> 1 tsp honey

1 Put 300ml (½ pint) water and half the milk in a pan and sprinkle in the oats.
2 Bring to the boil and simmer for 3–5 minutes, stirring all the time.
3 Serve with the remaining milk, seeds and honey.

Fruit Yoghurt or Yoghurt Shake

Low-fat, live, natural yoghurt is a first-class food, unlike its commercial counterpart, in which most bacteria have been destroyed so that the yoghurt will have a longer shelf life. Live yoghurt is packed with friendly bacteria that have a spring-cleaning effect on your digestive system, as well as being a good source of protein. Use any fruit in season.

> Serves 1
> 280g (10oz) very low-fat live yoghurt
> 1 tsp honey
> 1 serving fruit, such as banana, apple, pear, berries, kiwi
> 2 tsp ground flaxseeds and pumpkin seeds

Combine all the ingredients. If you prefer, make a shake by processing the mix in a blender.

Scrambled Egg

Although eggs are rather high in fat, as part of a balanced diet they are a good source of protein and add variety. Limit to six a week.

Serves 1
1 large free-range egg
dash of skimmed or soya milk
1 tbsp chopped fresh parsley
small knob of butter
thin slice of rye toast, to serve

1 Beat the egg with the milk and parsley.
2 Melt the butter in a small pan over medium heat.
3 Pour in the egg mixture. Cook slowly, stirring constantly.
4 Serve with rye toast.

Boiled Egg

This simple breakfast makes a wholesome start to the day.

Serves 1
1 large free-range egg
very lightly buttered wholegrain rye toast, to serve

1 Add the egg to a pan of boiling water and cook for 3–4 minutes for soft-boiled.
2 Serve with the rye toast.

Salads, soups, dips and light meals

As you saw in the menus, you can include salads on the side with many of the main dishes. They add vitamins, crunch and flavour to mealtimes and are all fast and easy to prepare.

A number of the soups in this section can take the place of main dishes. There's a wide and delicious selection. To save time you may want to make enough soup for two or three days and store some portions in the fridge, or make it in even larger batches and freeze some. If you're in a real hurry, you could choose a serving of one of the better-quality soups now available commercially, such as Covent Garden fresh soups. Remember to include a serving of protein if you choose a vegetable soup, and to avoid the creamy ones.

Most of these recipes would make great packed lunches for work, too (just invest in an insulated flask for the soups), and I have included some dips and dressings to liven up salads and vegetable accompaniments.

Remember, salads and soups will make up a variable number of GLs within your ultimate meal allowance of 10 ⓖ.

GL scores

Recipe	Page number	ⓖ
French Dressing	317	0
Tahini Dressing	317	1
Rocket and Watercress Salad	318	3
Green Salad	318	3
Mediterranean Tomato and Courgette Salad	318	3
Crunchy Thai Salad	319	4
Tomato and Red Onion Salad	320	4
Coleslaw	320	3
Celeriac Rémoulade	320	2
Apple and Tuna Salad	321	4
Oriental Green Beans	321	2
Walnut and Three-Bean Salad	322	3
Green Bean, Olive and Roasted Pepper Salad	322	3
Quinoa Tabouleh	323	8
Blueberry and Cottage Cheese Salad	324	9
Rice, Tuna and Petits Pois Salad	324	7
Cottage Cheese, Radish and Watermelon Salad	325	10
Beany Vegetable Soup	325	8
Spicy Pumpkin and Tofu Soup	326	6
Chestnut and Butterbean Soup	326	4
Lentil and Lemon Soup	327	2
Thai-Style Vegetable Broth	328	2
Gazpacho	328	8
Mexican Bean Dip	329	4
Hummus	329	5
Flageolet Bean Dip	330	3
Baba Ganoush	330	3
Pumpkin Seed Pesto	331	0
Smoked Salmon Pâté	331	5

Recipe	Page number	Ⓖ
Smoked Trout Pâté	332	2
Hot-smoked Fish with Avocado	332	2
Curry Roasted Celeriac	333	5
Sardines on Toast	333	12
Sweet Potato Mash	334	7
Garlicky Butternut Squash and Aubergine	334	5
Smoked Salmon and Asparagus Omelette	335	1
Fish in an Oriental-style Broth	335	4

Salads

French Dressing

Use as little dressing as possible on salads; any unused dressing can be stored in the fridge for up to five days.

3 tbsp olive oil
2 tbsp Udo's Choice Oil, Omega 3:6:9 oil or olive oil
2 tbsp cider or balsamic vinegar
1 tsp French mustard
1 garlic clove, crushed

Put all the ingredients in a screw-top jar and shake vigorously.

Tahini Dressing

Use as little dressing as possible on salads; any unused dressing can be stored in the fridge for up to five days.

2 tbsp home-made French Dressing
1 tbsp tahini
or
½ tsp honey
1 tsp mustard
2 tbsp Udo's Choice Oil, Omega 3:6:9 oil or olive oil
1 tbsp tahini
juice of ½ lemon

Put all the ingredients in a screw-top jar and shake vigorously.

Rocket and Watercress Salad

Watercress is rich in iron and vitamin A and is delicious in salads.

Serves 2
2 good handfuls of rocket
a good handful watercress, torn
1 gem lettuce, torn into pieces
1 tbsp cress
1 tbsp French or Tahini Dressing, to serve

Combine all the ingredients and toss with the dressing.

Green Salad

This simple green salad is a good accompaniment to any meal. It's subtly different because of the aniseed flavour from the fennel and has plenty of crunch.

Serves 2
⅓ cos or other lettuce, torn into bite-sized pieces
¼ fennel bulb, finely sliced, or 2 tbsp fresh peas, uncooked
¼ cucumber, finely sliced
1 celery stick, finely sliced
1 tbsp French or Tahini Dressing, to serve

Combine all the ingredients and toss with the dressing.

Mediterranean Tomato and Courgette Salad

Raw courgette has a subtle flavour that makes an interesting change from cucumber.

Serves 2
3 tomatoes, thinly sliced
1 small courgette, very thinly sliced widthways (a mandoline is easiest for this)
6 large, fresh basil leaves, roughly torn
2 tsp olive oil

2 tsp balsamic vinegar
2 tsp pine nuts (lightly toasted in a dry pan, if time)
Solo sea salt and ground black pepper

Toss all the ingredients together.

Crunchy Thai Salad

This is a variation on one of the most popular street food dishes in Thailand, where it is freshly made to order with a pestle and mortar. It originally comes from the north-east of the country. Now you can save the airfare and make it in your own kitchen! (If you are not keen on hot food, leave out the chilli, although if you are careful to remove the inner pith and seeds you will find it provides flavour without excessive heat.)

Serves 2
¼ medium white cabbage, finely shredded
115g (4oz) mangetout and sugar snap peas, parboiled for 2 minutes and sliced
½ medium tomato, finely chopped
1 small, mild, red chilli, deseeded and very finely chopped
juice of 1 lime
½ tsp mirin (Japanese rice wine, available from supermarkets)
2 tbsp tamari or soy sauce
1½ tsp sesame oil
1cm (½in) piece root ginger, finely chopped
2 tbsp sesame seeds (toast in a dry pan over medium heat, shaking from time to time until golden)

Combine all the ingredients in a large bowl and toss well.

Tomato and Red Onion Salad

This classic salad is full of flavour and goodness.

Serves 2
1 beefsteak tomato, diced
½ red onion, finely sliced into rings
2 tsp extra-virgin olive oil
juice of ½ lemon
2 tsp balsamic vinegar
ground black pepper
small handful fresh basil leaves, torn

Toss all the ingredients together.

Coleslaw

Cabbage is packed with vitamins and minerals. So are carrots, which are high in vitamin A, and onions.

Serves 2
200g (7oz) red or white cabbage, finely shredded
85g (3oz) carrots, grated
½ small onion, finely chopped
1 tbsp low-fat mayonnaise
1 tbsp very low-fat live yoghurt

Mix all the ingredients well in a large bowl.

Celeriac Rémoulade

If you haven't eaten celeriac before, it's a revelation.

Serves 2
½ celeriac, peeled and thinly grated
½ tsp smooth mustard
2 tsp chopped fresh parsley
2 tbsp live natural yoghurt
Solo sea salt

Put all the ingredients in a bowl, stir well and serve.

Apple and Tuna Salad

Tuna is a fairly good source of essential fatty acids – which keep our hormones and brain in shape – as well as other vital nutrients and protein. Combining it with apple is a bit unusual, but highly successful in the flavour stakes.

Serves 2
175g (6oz) tuna in brine, drained
1 apple, chopped
1 celery stick, sliced
1 little gem lettuce, torn into bite-sized pieces
1 tbsp low-fat mayonnaise
85g (3oz) live natural yoghurt
2 tsp lemon juice
Solo sea salt and ground black pepper

Drain the tuna and mix well with the remaining ingredients.

Oriental Green Beans

Tender green beans go well with this dressing. This recipe works brilliantly with tofu steam-fries.

Serves 2
250g (9oz) young green beans, halved crossways
1 garlic clove, crushed
1 tbsp tamari or soy sauce
1 tsp sesame oil
1 tsp sesame seeds (toast in a dry pan over medium heat, shaking from time to time until golden)

1 Steam the beans gently for 3 minutes, or until tender.
2 Put the remaining ingredients in a bowl and stir together, then toss with the beans and serve warm.

Walnut and Three-Bean Salad

No foods are better than beans for satisfying your appetite and giving stamina. It helps if they're served in a delicious, crunchy salad such as this one.

Serves 2
400g (14oz) can mixed beans, such as haricot beans, chickpeas and
    flageolet beans
handful walnuts, roughly chopped
½ apple, cubed
2 tsp chopped fresh flat-leaf parsley or chives
1 tbsp olive oil
1 tbsp walnut oil (or olive oil)
juice of ½ lemon
1 celery stick, finely chopped
Solo sea salt and ground black pepper
mixed salad leaves, such as spinach, rocket and watercress, to serve

Combine all the ingredients and serve with mixed salad leaves.

Green Bean, Olive and Roasted Pepper Salad

A Spanish-style salad that goes well stuffed in a pitta pocket. As an alternative, why not add some black-eyed beans (5 **GL** per half-cup)?

Serves 2
2 medium free-range eggs
200g (7oz) French beans, trimmed
1 tsp red wine vinegar
1 tbsp olive oil
1 small red onion, finely chopped
2 roasted red peppers, finely chopped
handful black olives, stoned and halved
Solo sea salt and ground black pepper

1 Add the eggs to a pan of boiling water and cook for 8 minutes. Drain and put them into a bowl of cold water to cool. Peel and slice.
2 Steam the beans until *al dente*, then refresh under cold running water to keep the deep green colour. Dry on kitchen paper and put into a bowl.

3 Whisk the vinegar into the oil and season, then add to the beans and toss to mix.
4 Put the beans in a serving dish, stir in the onion, red peppers and olives, then gently place the egg over the top.

Quinoa Tabouleh

Using quinoa instead of bulgur wheat in this Middle Eastern dish provides first-class protein. You could double up the quantities and keep some in the fridge to take to work.

Serves 2
140g (5oz) quinoa
vegetable bouillon made up into a liquid (2 parts liquid to 1 part quinoa)
¼ medium-sized cucumber, sliced lengthways into quarters, then finely sliced horizontally
2 good handfuls cherry tomatoes, chopped to the same size as the cucumber
4 spring onions, finely sliced
good handful fresh mint, finely chopped
good handful fresh flat-leaf parsley, finely chopped
1–2 tbsp olive oil
1 tbsp lemon juice
2 tsp balsamic vinegar or to taste
Solo sea salt and ground black pepper

1 Bring the quinoa to the boil in a pan with the bouillon, then cover, reduce the heat and simmer for approximately 10–15 minutes, or until the liquid is absorbed and the grains are fluffy. Put the quinoa in a bowl and leave to cool.
2 When at room temperature, mix in the chopped vegetables and herbs, then add the oil, lemon juice and vinegar. Season. Taste to check the flavour and adjust accordingly.
3 Place in the fridge for at least an hour to allow the flavours to develop.

Blueberry and Cottage Cheese Salad

Blueberries are one of the best sources of bioflavonoids, which are powerful antioxidants. Here they contrast beautifully in colour and taste with apple and kiwi.

Serves 2
1 apple, thinly sliced
1 kiwi fruit, peeled and thinly sliced
2 tsp lemon juice
250g (9oz) cottage cheese
2 handfuls blueberries
4 fresh mint leaves, finely chopped

1 Arrange the apple and kiwi fruit on individual dishes.
2 Sprinkle with lemon juice and top with cottage cheese, blueberries and mint.

Rice, Tuna and Petits Pois Salad

This is unbelievably tasty – much more interesting than standard tuna mayo. Peas are delicious raw, and of course retain more vitamins this way.

Serves 2
115g (4oz) brown basmati rice
115g (4oz) tuna in brine, drained
1 tsp sesame oil
2 tsp tamari or soy sauce
2 tsp lemon juice
1 tbsp raw petits pois
1 carrot, finely sliced lengthways
1 spring onion, finely sliced
ground black pepper

1 Cook the rice according to the pack instructions and allow to cool.
2 Combine with all the other ingredients, tossing thoroughly to mix the flavours.

Cottage Cheese, Radish and Watermelon Salad

A refreshing, summertime salad. Don't remove the watermelon seeds, as they're packed full of nutrients.

Serves 2
⅓ cucumber, thinly sliced
¼ watermelon, sliced into thin triangles
6 radishes, trimmed and thinly sliced
250g (9oz) cottage cheese
2 tsp lemon juice
4 fresh mint leaves, finely chopped
ground black pepper

1 Lay the cucumber, watermelon and radish slices on a large platter and spoon the cottage cheese over the top.
2 Drizzle with the lemon juice, scatter with mint, and season.

Soups

Beany Vegetable Soup

This one-pot winter warmer is crammed full of fibre and is just the thing to take in a vacuum flask to work.

Serves 6
2 onions, chopped
3 celery sticks, finely chopped
3 leeks, sliced
450g (1lb) mixed root vegetables, such as carrot, swede and parsnip, peeled and chopped into bite-sized chunks
850ml (1½ pints) vegetable stock
2 × 400g (14oz) cans mixed pulses, drained and rinsed
2 tbsp roughly chopped fresh flat-leaf parsley
Solo sea salt and ground black pepper

1 Put the onion, celery, leeks, root vegetables, stock and seasoning in a large pan and stir. Cover and bring to the boil. Reduce the heat and simmer for 20 minutes.
2 Stir in the mixed pulses, then cover and simmer for 5–10 minutes, or until the vegetables and beans are tender.
3 Add the parsley, then check the seasoning before serving.

Spicy Pumpkin and Tofu Soup*

A wonderfully warming soup that is a completely balanced meal, with hidden protein power from the tofu.

Serves 4
1 tbsp olive oil
1 large onion, finely chopped
2 garlic cloves, crushed
2 large butternut squash, deseeded, peeled and diced
1½ tsp cumin
1 tsp ground coriander
¼ tsp chilli powder
½ tsp ground nutmeg
1 tsp fresh thyme, chopped
3 vegetable stock cubes dissolved in 1 litre (1¾ pints) hot water
1 packet Cauldron Organic Tofu, drained
salt and ground black pepper
parsley and chives, freshly chopped

1 Heat the olive oil in a large pan. Add the chopped onion and garlic, and gently cook over a low heat until the onion has softened.
2 Add the diced squash, cumin, coriander, chilli powder, nutmeg, thyme and stock. Bring to the boil, reduce the heat and simmer for 15 minutes, then allow to cool slightly.
3 Whiz the tofu in a food processor or blender and set aside.
4 Blend the soup and return to the pan. Whisk in the tofu using a balloon whisk, a tablespoon at a time, and gently reheat. Season to taste then add the fresh herbs and serve.

* Recipe courtesy of Cauldron Foods.

Chestnut and Butterbean Soup

Chestnuts have the lowest fat content of all nuts and a pleasantly sweet flavour that goes well with the smooth texture of the butter beans.

Serves 4
200g (7oz) cooked and peeled chestnuts (use vacuum-packed or canned to save time)
400g (14oz) can butter beans, drained and rinsed
1 onion, chopped

1 carrot, chopped
2 sprigs of thyme
1.2 litres (2 pints) vegetable bouillon or stock
ground black pepper

1 Place all the ingredients in a large pan and bring to the boil. Cover and simmer very gently for 35 minutes.
2 Purée the soup until smooth.

Lentil and Lemon Soup

The spices and lemony sharpness make this lentil soup anything but boring. It's a satisfying winter warmer.

Serves 4
1 tbsp olive oil
250g (9oz) onions, chopped
4 garlic cloves, coarsely chopped
250g (9oz) red lentils, rinsed
1.2 litres (2 pints) chicken or vegetable stock
1 tsp ground cumin
1 tsp ground coriander
juice of ½ lemon
Solo sea salt and ground black pepper

1 Heat the oil in a pan and add the onions and garlic. Cook over a low heat, stirring frequently, for 10 minutes, or until soft.
2 Add the lentils and cook for a further 2 minutes. Add the stock and bring to the boil, then reduce the heat to a simmer for 30–45 minutes, or until the lentils are almost soft.
3 In a non-stick frying pan, dry-fry the spices over a high heat for 1–2 minutes, or until they release their aroma, then add to the soup. Bring the soup back to the boil and add the lemon juice, then simmer for 5 minutes. Season lightly.

Thai-style Vegetable Broth

This soup is packed with flavour and phytonutrients.

Serves 4
4 thin slices fresh root ginger, cut into thin matchsticks
2 garlic cloves, cut into thin matchsticks
600ml (1 pint) vegetable bouillon powder
1 head pak choi, finely shredded
2 shiitake mushrooms, sliced
1 carrot, cut in half lengthways, then thinly sliced into half-moons
5 spring onions, sliced thinly at an angle
55g (2oz) firm tofu, cut into 1cm (½in) cubes
1 tbsp tamari or soy sauce

1 Put the ginger and garlic in a pan with the stock. Bring to the boil, cover and simmer for 3 minutes.
2 Add the vegetables and tofu, bring back to the boil and season with the tamari or soy sauce. Reduce the heat and simmer for 3 minutes.

Gazpacho

For a taste of Andalusia, serve this raw cold soup at alfresco meals, or keep for a perfect instant snack. It stores well in the fridge for up to a week. Add black-eyed beans to make it a main meal – and an ice cube or two on really sultry days.

Serves 6
3 peppers (red, yellow and orange are the sweetest), chopped
1 cucumber, chopped
1 red onion, chopped
3 celery sticks, chopped
400g (14oz) can chopped tomatoes
425ml (¾ pint) tomato juice
2 garlic cloves, crushed
½ jar of Peppadew sweet baby peppers, drained and chopped
Solo sea salt and ground black pepper

1 Put half the fresh vegetables in a food processor with the tomatoes, tomato juice and garlic, and process until smooth.
2 Add the remaining vegetables and the Peppadew peppers, and season with black pepper.

Dips

Mexican Bean Dip

This spicy red-bean dip is a tasty accompaniment to raw vegetables, but goes best of all with Nick's Beefburgers (see page 358) with lettuce in a pitta bread.

> Serves 2
> ¼ onion, finely chopped
> 2 garlic cloves, crushed
> ½ tbsp olive oil
> ¼ tsp chilli powder
> 140g (5oz) canned kidney beans, rinsed and drained
> 1 tsp lemon juice
> 85g (3oz) cottage cheese
> 1 tbsp yogurt
> Solo sea salt and ground black pepper

1 Sauté the onion and garlic gently in the oil for about 2 minutes, then add the chilli powder and cook for a further 3 minutes. Cool.
2 Blend all the ingredients to make a fairly smooth, creamy dip.

Hummus

Chickpeas have a unique taste, which combines well with tahini, a paste of ground sesame seeds, in this popular spread.

> Serves 2
> 400g (14oz) can chickpeas, drained and rinsed
> 2 garlic cloves, crushed
> 2 tbsp olive oil
> juice of ½ lemon
> 2 tsp tahini
> Solo sea salt
> a pinch of cayenne pepper, plus extra to garnish

1 Put all the ingredients in a food processor or blender and purée until smooth and creamy, adding a dash of water if necessary. Check the flavour and adjust according to preference.
2 Garnish with a little cayenne pepper.

Flageolet Bean Dip

This unusual and tasty alternative to hummus is delicious on oatcakes or with crudités.

> Serves 4
> 400g (14oz) can flageolet beans, rinsed and drained
> 5 spring onions
> 1 garlic clove, crushed
> handful flat-leaf parsley, finely chopped
> 2 tbsp lemon juice
> 1 tbsp olive oil
> about 1 tbsp water, if required
> Solo sea salt and ground black pepper

Put the beans, spring onions, garlic, parsley, lemon juice and oil into a food processor or blender, and blend until smooth. Add the water if necessary, then add the seasoning slowly, according to taste.

Baba Ganoush

I love this Lebanese aubergine dip on oatcakes or pumpernickel bread. Again, it's a great addition to a party, or can form part of a meze platter for an informal dinner, with Hummus and Quinoa Tabouleh (see pages 329 and 323). Just add green and tomato salads. Use live natural yoghurt as a healthier alternative to the traditional Greek yoghurt.

> Serves 2
> 2 garlic cloves, crushed
> 1 tbsp olive oil
> ½ aubergine, cubed
> juice of ½ lemon
> 25g (1oz) sesame seeds
> 25g (1oz) fresh coriander
> 115g (4oz) live natural yoghurt
> Solo sea salt and ground black pepper

1 Lightly sauté the garlic in the oil for 2 minutes, then add the aubergine. Add 1 tbsp or so of water to the pan, put on the lid and steam-fry the mixture for 8 minutes or so, until soft.
2 Put into a food processor or blender and add the remaining ingredients, then whiz until fairly smooth.

Light meals

Pumpkin Seed Pesto

This keeps in the fridge for 2–3 days and can be stirred through soup or pasta, or added to bean salads.

Serves 4
55g (2oz) raw pumpkin seeds
55g (2oz) flat-leaf parsley leaves
55g (2oz) basil leaves
2 garlic cloves, crushed
1 tsp Solo sea salt
2 tsp lemon juice
55g (2oz) grated Parmesan cheese
90ml (6 tbsp) pumpkin seed oil (roasted if possible) or 6 tbsp pumpkin seed butter instead of the separate seeds and oil (available from Totally Nourish – see Resources)

1 Put the pumpkin seeds in a blender or food processor with the herbs, garlic, Solo sea salt, lemon juice and Parmesan cheese. Whiz until the mixture is blended but retains some texture.
2 Add the pumpkin seed oil and mix until the pesto is an even consistency.

Smoked Salmon Pâté

The cannellini beans provide good long-term energy and are a healthier alternative to the cream used in most fish pâtés.

Serves 2
200g (7oz) smoked salmon trimmings
200g (7oz) canned cannellini beans, drained and rinsed
juice of ½ lemon
a drizzle of water or olive oil, if needed
1 tbsp chopped fresh parsley
1 tbsp chopped fresh dill
Solo sea salt and ground black pepper

Whiz all the ingredients in a food processor or blender until the mixture is smooth, adding a little oil or water to loosen the mixture if necessary. Chill before serving.

Smoked Trout Pâté

This reduced-fat pâté uses cream cheese instead of cream.

> Serves 2
> 2 smoked trout fillets, skinned, boned and flaked
> 200g (7oz) low-fat cream cheese
> juice of ½ lemon
> ground black pepper
> 1 tsp horseradish (optional)
> hot pitta bread triangles or rye bread, and salad, to serve

Whiz all the ingredients in a food processor or mash well with a fork. Serve with hot pitta bread triangles (5 ⊕ per half-slice) and salad, or with rye bread (5 ⊕ per slice).

Hot-smoked Fish with Avocado

The avocado provides healthy monounsaturated fat, and the fish gives plenty of omega-3 oils – just don't eat this more than once a week, to keep within your fat limit.

> Serves 2
> 2 fillets hot-smoked salmon or trout
> 5cm (2in) piece of cucumber, cut into bite-sized chunks
> ½ ripe medium-sized avocado
> juice of 1 lemon
> 1–2 tsp chopped fresh dill or chives
> 1–2 tsp chopped fresh flat-leaf parsley
> Solo sea salt and ground black pepper

1 Skin the fish and remove any bones, then flake into chunks. Place in a salad bowl with the cucumber.
2 Halve the avocado and cut one side into bite-sized pieces. (Leave the stone in the leftover half and drizzle this with lemon juice to prevent discoloration, then cover and put in the fridge for future use.) Add the avocado to the bowl with the lemon and herbs.
3 Season with pepper and Solo salt and gently mix together.

Curry Roasted Celeriac

An unusual accompaniment to meat or fish.

Serves 2
2 tbsp olive oil
¼ tbsp mild or medium curry powder
½ celeriac, peeled and chopped into 2.5cm (1in) chunks
2 garlic cloves, unpeeled
Solo sea salt and ground black pepper

1 Preheat the oven to 180°C/350°F/gas mark 4. Mix the oil and curry powder. Toss the celeriac and garlic in the mixture and season.
2 Put on a roasting tray and roast for 40–50 minutes, shaking the tray halfway through to recoat the pieces.

Sardines on Toast

This may take you back to your childhood. Sardines are endowed with lashings of omega-3 fats, and make a fast, delicious meal served this way. Just add a big green salad.

Serves 2
3 slices rye bread, cut in two
2 tbsp olive oil
2 tomatoes, sliced
175g (6oz) can sardines in brine, drained
ground black pepper

1 Toast the bread and drizzle with olive oil.
2 Put the tomato slices and sardines on the toast and season with black pepper.

Sweet Potato Mash

A delicious and lower-GL version of mashed potatoes. Serve with meat, fish or tofu and vegetables.

> Serves 2
> 1 medium sweet potato (unpeeled)
> Solo sea salt
> white pepper

1 Slice the sweet potato into thin circles, then steam for around 12 minutes, or until soft. Put into a bowl.
2 Season with Solo sea salt and pepper and mash with a fork.

Garlicky Butternut Squash and Aubergine

A wonderfully satisfying dish that goes well with anything from chicken to a simple Rocket and Watercress Salad (see page 318) with a good drizzle of Pumpkin Seed Pesto (see page 331) for protein.

> Serves 2
> ½ butternut squash, peeled and diced into 2.5cm (1in) pieces
> ½ medium aubergine, diced into pieces the same size as the squash
> 6 garlic cloves, unpeeled
> 1 tbsp olive oil
> 1 tsp cumin
> Solo sea salt and ground black pepper

1 Preheat the oven to 180°C/350°F/gas mark 4. Put the squash, aubergine and garlic into a bowl with the oil, cumin and seasoning, mixing until all the vegetables are covered.
2 Tip into a roasting tin and roast for 40–45 minutes, or until the vegetables soften and start to brown.
3 Do eat the roasted garlic if you like the taste, squeezing out the softened flesh with a fork, otherwise simply discard and enjoy the flavour that will have permeated the remaining vegetables.

Smoked Salmon and Asparagus Omelette

A sophisticated light supper – or even for breakfast in bed!

Serves 2
6 asparagus spears
4 free-range eggs
2 tsp olive oil
55g (2oz) smoked salmon, sliced finely
2 slices lemon
2 sprigs flat-leaf parsley
Solo sea salt and ground black pepper

1 Steam the asparagus until just cooked, then drain and set aside.
2 Beat the eggs with the seasoning.
3 Heat a medium frying pan and add the oil, allowing it to heat up and coat the whole pan. Pour the egg into the pan and gently move it around until the underside cooks through and colours slightly. Reduce the heat, loosen the base with a spatula and flip over to cook the other side for a minute or so until just firm, then cut in half and tip each half onto a separate plate.
4 Lay the salmon on one half of each slice and place 3 asparagus spears on top, then fold the other half over to create a triangle. Top with a slice of lemon and sprig of flat-leaf parsley and serve immediately.

Fish in an Oriental-style Broth

This dish is perfect for a special dinner.

Serves 2
150ml (¼ pint) vegetable bouillon
2 tbsp mirin (Japanese rice wine, available from supermarkets)
2 tbsp tamari or soy sauce
1 small chunk of root ginger, sliced
2 garlic cloves, crushed
2 lemon slices
2 small fish fillets (haddock, plaice or cod)
55g (2oz) broccoli, broken into very small florets
55g (2oz) carrots, peeled and coarsely grated
55g (2oz) pak choi, finely shredded
4 spring onions, thinly sliced
½ tsp sesame oil

1 Put the stock, mirin, tamari, ginger, garlic and lemon in a wok and bring to the boil.
2 Measure the thickness of the fish fillets at their thickest points, then reduce the heat under the wok and slide the fish in. Poach for 10 minutes for every 2.5cm (1in) of thickness, or until the flesh turns opaque and flakes easily.
3 Lift the fish out of the broth and remove the skin, then divide the fish between two soup bowls, cover and keep warm.
4 Bring the broth back to the boil and add the vegetables at 30-second intervals, cooking for a total of 2–3 minutes or until they are tender but very *al dente*. Remove the vegetables and add to the bowls.
5 Boil the broth for a further 30 seconds, then remove the ginger and lemon slices and stir in the oil. Ladle over the fish and vegetables, and serve immediately.

Main meals

From poached salmon to fajitas, there are enough delicious options here to keep you going through a year's worth of lunches, dinners and dinner parties. Vegetarian options are included for many, and meat eaters' options are also included for some of the vegetarian dishes. Generally speaking, the recipes are designed for easy adaptation, as far as protein is concerned. If the menu suggests a meal you prefer not to have, simply choose an alternative.

Recipes given are for two people unless otherwise stated. Some of these dishes can be prepared in advance and frozen.

GL scores

Recipe	Page number	ⒼⓁ
Steam-fried Vegetables with …	338	6–8
Fatburner Sandwiches	339	11–12
Fatburner Baked Potato or Sweet Potato	339	10–12
Tuna Steak with Black-eyed Bean Salsa	340	10
Sticky Mustard Salmon Fillets	340	1
Trout with Puy Lentils and Roasted Tomatoes on the Vine	341	11
Thai Baked Cod	342	1
Cod Roasted with Lemon and Garlic	342	0
Spicy Mackerel with Couscous	343	14
Grilled Herring	344	0

Fast and easy

Steam-fried Vegetables with ...

This is a healthier, lower-fat version of stir-frying. Versatility is the name of the game here. You can make this steam-fry with sauces ranging from Chinese to Mexican; throw in cauliflower and sugar snaps one night, carrots and mushrooms the next; use tempeh on Monday and chicken on Sunday – in short, anything goes. This is the perfect fallback recipe, using whatever's in the fridge and store cupboard for a truly tasty meal.

Vegetables

Use spring onions and garlic, then choose from carrots, broccoli, courgettes, cauliflower, sugar snap peas, runner beans, water chestnuts, mushrooms, beansprouts, peppers, bamboo shoots and so on, ensuring there's enough to fill half your plate. Cut the vegetables thinly to equal sizes so that they will cook in the same amount of time.

Seasonings

Thai: fresh coriander, green curry paste and a dash of coconut milk
Chinese: tamari or soy sauce, ginger and garlic
Japanese: ginger, tamari or soy sauce, teriyaki or yakitori sauce (try Kikkoman's, available in supermarkets)
Mexican: fajita or enchilada dry seasoning, or tomato salsa
Mediterranean: ½ jar tomato passata with chopped basil and flat-leaf parsley, and a few chopped black olives, if you like
Indian: chopped tomatoes with coriander, cumin and chilli powder to taste

Protein-rich foods

310g (11oz) tofu, or tempeh, cubed
or 115g (4oz) chicken, off the bone and cubed
or 140g (5oz) filleted fish, cubed

1 Put the spring onion and garlic in a large pan or wok and add the chosen seasoning. Cover and steam-fry over medium heat for 1 minute. Add the protein-rich food and stir-fry until cooked.
2 Add your choice of vegetables, stir-fry briefly, then add 1 tbsp water and clamp on the lid. Steam until the vegetables are cooked but still crunchy.

Fatburner Sandwiches

To make this low-GL sandwich, top two slices of rye bread or fill a wholemeal pitta pocket with any one of the following combinations.

Serves 1

115g (4oz) cottage cheese, with cucumber slices and chopped chives

or 140g (5oz) hummus and lettuce

or 1 small, roasted chicken breast (skin removed) and 1 sliced tomato

or 1 small smoked trout or salmon fillet with a smear of low-fat cream cheese or Pumpkin Seed Pesto (see page 331) and watercress

or 55g (2oz) canned salmon or tuna in brine, with cucumber and cress

or egg 'mayonnaise' (made with 2 small hard-boiled eggs, 1 tbsp cottage cheese, a chopped spring onion, salt and black pepper)

Fatburner Baked Potato or Sweet Potato

A baked potato can be a great base for a satisfying lunch. It's also available at many town and city sandwich shops in case you've forgotten to bring anything to work with you. All you need to remember is to choose a small potato so you don't overdo the carbs. Do eat the skins, as they're full of fibre. When making your own, cook them for as short a time as possible (around 50–60 minutes, at 220°C/425°F/gas mark 7), until done but still firm inside. Have them with any of the fillings below and a large salad or Coleslaw (see page 320). A sweet potato makes a delicious change.

Each filling serves 1

55g (2oz) tuna in brine blended with 1 tsp cottage cheese or natural yoghurt

or 115g (4oz) low-fat cottage cheese with chives and spring onions

or 140g (5oz) hummus with a sliced tomato

or 200g (7oz) baked beans

or 1 mug Dhal (Lentil Curry) (see page 345)

or 1 small, roast chicken breast (no skin) tossed in 1 tbsp yoghurt dressing (natural yoghurt blended with paprika, black pepper and fresh chives, basil or parsley)

or 2 tsp Pumpkin Seed Pesto (see page 331) with 55g (2oz) cottage cheese and chopped chives

Fish

Tuna Steak with Black-eyed Bean Salsa

A robust summer dish. Vegetarians could substitute a thick slice of smoked tofu for the fish.

> Serves 2
> 1 tbsp olive oil
> 2 small tuna fillets
> *For the salsa*
> 2 tomatoes, deseeded and chopped
> 400g (14oz) can black-eyed beans, rinsed and drained
> 1 red pepper, finely chopped
> 1 mild, fresh red chilli, deseeded and finely chopped
> 2 garlic cloves, crushed
> juice of 2 limes
> 2 tsp olive oil
> 2 tsp sesame oil
> 2 tbsp fresh coriander or flat-leaf parsley, roughly chopped
> Solo sea salt and ground black pepper

1 Mix together the salsa ingredients. Set to one side while you cook the tuna steaks.
2 Heat a frying pan and spray or lightly drizzle with olive oil. When hot, add the fish and press firmly into the pan to sear on both sides. Reduce the heat and cook for a further 1–3 minutes (until the flesh flakes easily).
3 Serve with the salsa on the side.

Sticky Mustard Salmon Fillets

Salmon not only provides plenty of protein but is also a source of essential fats. Try to go for wild salmon, as it's a healthier option than farmed fish. Vegetarians could marinate tofu slices instead of salmon.

> Serves 2
> juice and grated rind of ½ orange
> 1 tsp clear honey
> 1 tsp wholegrain mustard
> 2 small skinless and boneless salmon fillets
> steam-fried spinach and red or yellow peppers, and boiled baby new
>   potatoes or brown basmati rice, to serve

1 Whisk the orange juice and rind into the honey and mustard.
2 Put the salmon into a shallow dish and pour over the orange mixture. Leave to marinate for 30–60 minutes, in the fridge. Meanwhile, preheat the oven to 180°C/350°F/gas mark 4.
3 Bake for 20–25 minutes and serve with steam-fried spinach and red or yellow peppers, and boiled baby new potatoes (5 ⅁ per small potato serving) or brown basmati rice (5 ⅁ per half-serving).

Trout with Puy Lentils and Roasted Tomatoes on the Vine

A simple but sophisticated dish that is perfectly balanced and smart enough to serve at a supper party.

> Serves 2
> 85g (3oz) dried Puy lentils, washed and drained
> 1 tsp vegetable bouillon powder
> 1 tsp mixed dried herbs (such as Herbes de Provence)
> 2 small trout fillets
> ½ bunch cherry tomatoes on the vine (or 5–6 tomatoes per person)
> 2 slices of lemon
> handful fresh flat-leaf parsley
> ground black pepper

1 Cover the lentils with cold water and bring to the boil, then simmer for about 20 minutes, or until the water is more or less absorbed. Add the bouillon powder and mixed herbs when the lentils are soft to the bite. (Don't worry if the lentils seem a little hard – Puy lentils retain their shape and have a satisfyingly chewy texture when cooked.)
2 Put the fish in a non-stick roasting tin and lay the tomatoes around them, then bake at 190°C/375°F/gas mark 5 for 12–15 minutes or until cooked through.
3 Put a dollop of lentils onto each plate and lay the fish on top. Add a slice of lemon and some chopped parsley to each fillet and put the tomatoes on the side. Sprinkle with black pepper.

Thai Baked Cod

This dish is permeated with classic Thai flavours, which are clean and sharp, yet subtle. You can use any white fish instead of cod if you prefer.

Serves 2
juice and grated rind of 1 lime
½in (1cm) piece fresh root ginger, grated
1 lemon grass stalk, sliced
2 garlic cloves, crushed
1 tsp tamari or soy sauce
1 mild, fresh, red chilli, deseeded and finely chopped
2 small cod fillets

1 Mix the lime juice, rind, ginger, lemon grass, garlic, tamari and chilli.
2 Put the cod fillets in a baking dish.
3 Pour the lime mixture over the fish, turning it so that it is well coated. Leave to marinate in the fridge for up to 2 hours, if time. Meanwhile, preheat the oven to 200°C/400°F/gas mark 6.
4 Cover the dish with a lid or foil and bake for 20 minutes, or until cooked through – this will depend on the thickness of the fish.

Cod Roasted with Lemon and Garlic

A delicious, no-fuss fish dish that is perfect for a light summer supper.

Serves 2
½ tbsp olive oil
½ tbsp chopped fresh parsley
2 garlic cloves, crushed
2 small cod fillets (or haddock or plaice)
1 lemon, sliced thinly
Solo sea salt and ground black pepper

1 Mix the oil, parsley, garlic and seasoning, and rub over the fish. Set aside to marinate for 10 minutes. Preheat the oven to 180°C/350°F/gas mark 4.
2 Put the fish on a baking try and arrange the lemon slices on top. Bake for 8–10 minutes, or until just cooked through and the flesh flakes easily.
3 Serve with the Tomato and Red Onion Salad (see page 320).

Spicy Mackerel with Couscous

The hint of North African cuisine in this spicy sauce is a wonderful complement to the rich taste of mackerel. It's partnered with couscous, an excellent source of carbohydrate, which is very easy to prepare.

Serves 2
425ml (¾ pint) boiling water
115g (4oz) couscous
1 tsp vegetable bouillon powder
1 tbsp olive oil
1 small onion, finely chopped
1 garlic clove, crushed
¼ tsp chilli powder
1 tsp ground cumin
1 red pepper, chopped
1 courgette, sliced
1 tbsp tomato purée
1 tsp lemon juice
2 small smoked mackerel fillets (skinned if you prefer), or ½ medium fillet each

1 Pour the boiling water over the couscous, stir in the bouillon powder, then cover and leave to stand for 15 minutes, to allow it to absorb the water. Fluff up and separate the grains using a fork.
2 Meanwhile, put the oil in a sauté pan over a low–medium heat and add the onion, garlic, chilli powder and ground cumin. Put on the lid and steam-fry for 2 minutes.
3 Add the red pepper and courgette, and sauté for a further 2 minutes.
4 Add the tomato purée and lemon juice and steam-fry with the lid on until the vegetables are tender but still crisp.
5 Arrange each mackerel fillet on a mound of couscous and top with the vegetables.

Grilled Herring

Norwegians are on to something: herrings are one of the best fish for omega-3 essential fats as well as protein and vitamins. The flavour is strong, so it needs little enhancement.

Serves 1
½ lemon
1 small prepared herring
ground black pepper

Squeeze the lemon over the herring, and grind over some black pepper. Cook under a medium grill for 6–7 minutes each side, or until cooked through.

Poached Salmon

Salmon responds well to extremely simple treatments, as in this recipe. Fast food with a difference!

Serves 2
2 small salmon fillets
Solo sea salt and ground black pepper
2 lemon wedges, to garnish

1 Put the salmon fillets in a shallow pan with just enough water to cover, and poach them gently for about 15 minutes, or until cooked through.
2 Season and serve garnished with lemon wedges.

Vegetarian

Borlotti Bean Bolognese

This is a mouthwatering vegetarian alternative to the classic 'spag bol'. It can be prepared in batches and frozen for convenience.

Serves 2
1 tbsp olive oil
1 onion, chopped
2 garlic cloves, crushed
1 tsp mixed dried herbs

115g (4oz) button mushrooms, sliced
1 tsp vegetable bouillon powder
1 tbsp tomato purée
140g (5oz) canned tomatoes
¾ × 400g (14oz) can borlotti beans, drained and rinsed
Solo sea salt and ground black pepper
wholegrain spaghetti or pasta, to serve

1 Put the oil in a pan and sauté the onion, garlic and herbs for 2 minutes, then add the mushrooms and cook until soft.
2 Add the vegetable bouillon powder, tomato purée, canned tomatoes and beans, then season and simmer for 15 minutes.
3 Serve with wholegrain spaghetti or other wholegrain pasta.

Dhal (Lentil Curry)

This dish is a variation on a recipe given to me by a lady from Goa, and is one of my favourites. It always goes down well with meat eaters as well as vegetarians. This is incredibly moreish and leftovers can be kept in the fridge and eaten with a baked potato for lunch the following day, or frozen.

Serves 4
310g (11oz) red lentils, rinsed and drained
1 medium onion, chopped
4 garlic cloves, crushed
4 tsp vegetable bouillon powder
400g (14oz) can tomatoes
1 heaped tsp curry powder

1 Put the lentils in a pan with 600ml (1 pint) of water, the onion, garlic and bouillon powder. Bring to the boil and simmer for 10 minutes.
2 Add the tomatoes and curry powder, and stir well. Cover and simmer for a further 20 minutes, stirring occasionally to make sure the dhal does not stick to the pan. If it starts to get too thick, add a little water or, if it seems too watery, leave uncovered. The lentils should form a porridge-like consistency.

Pasta with Pumpkin Seed Pesto

Serve with a Tomato and Red Onion Salad (see page 320).

Serves 2
175g (6oz) wholewheat or buckwheat pasta
2 servings of Pumpkin Seed Pesto (see page 331)
handful fresh basil leaves
2 tsp pumpkin seeds (toast in a dry pan over a medium heat, shaking from
   time to time until golden)
ground black pepper

1 Cook the pasta according to the pack instructions, then drain well.
2 Stir the pesto through the pasta and divide between serving plates.
3 Top with basil, pumpkin seeds and black pepper.

Chickpea Curry

Nutty-tasting and firm, chickpeas make a delicious curry.

Serves 2
2 tsp olive oil
2 garlic cloves, crushed
1 large white onion, chopped
1 tsp cumin
½ tsp each turmeric and mild or medium curry powder
1 tsp ground ginger
1 celery stick, finely chopped
1 medium carrot, chopped
600ml (1 pint) vegetable stock
400g (14oz) can chickpeas, drained and rinsed
2 tbsp tomato purée
½ tsp Solo sea salt

1 Gently heat the oil in a large frying pan and fry the garlic for 1 minute.
2 Add the onion and dry spices and cook for a further 2 minutes.
3 Toss in the vegetables and add 2 tbsp of the stock. Cover and steam-fry
   for 2 minutes.
4 Add the chickpeas, the tomato purée, the Solo sea salt and the remaining stock and allow the curry to simmer uncovered for 30 minutes, or
   until the vegetables are tender and the sauce has thickened slightly.

Grilled Goat's Cheese on Portabella Mushrooms

Serve this full-flavoured supper with a mixed salad, perhaps with a light dressing of walnut oil and balsamic vinegar or lemon juice.

Serves 2
1 tbsp sun-dried tomato paste
6 Portabella mushrooms, cleaned with a dry brush or kitchen paper
2 tsp olive oil
6 round slices goat's cheese (each about 5mm–1cm/¼–½in thick)
6 large basil leaves, torn
1 tbsp walnuts, roughly chopped
ground black pepper
mixed salad, to serve (dressed if you prefer)

1 Spread the sun-dried tomato paste on the gill sides of the mushrooms. Heat the oil in a frying pan and gently fry the mushrooms on both sides until they start to go brown, taking care when you turn them over not to dislodge too much of the sun-dried tomato paste.
2 Place the mushrooms gill-side up in a grill pan and top each with a slice of goat's cheese. Grill gently until the cheese starts to bubble and turn golden on top. Remove from the heat.
3 Put the mixed salad on a plate and place the mushrooms on top. Scatter the basil and walnuts over and serve immediately.

Chestnut and Mushroom Pilaf

The flavours in this dish go together beautifully.

Serves 2
1 tbsp olive oil
55g (2oz) brown basmati rice
2 garlic cloves, crushed
2.5cm (1in) piece fresh root ginger, finely chopped
1 small onion, chopped
115g (4oz) shiitake or button mushrooms, sliced
150ml (¼ pint) stock made from vegetable bouillon powder
175g (6oz) cooked chestnuts (vacuum-packed or canned)
2 tsp tamari or soy sauce
55g (2oz) frozen peas

1 Gently heat the oil in a heavy frying pan and fry the rice for 3–4 minutes, or until pale brown. Add the garlic and ginger, and stir for 30 seconds, then add the onion, and cook for a further 3 minutes. Add the mushrooms and cook for 3 minutes.
2 Stir in the stock, chestnuts and tamari or soy sauce, then cover and simmer for 35 minutes, or until the liquid is absorbed and the rice just tender.
3 Stir in the frozen peas and allow to cook gently until they turn bright green.

Stuffed Peppers

Pine nuts and mushrooms make an interesting stuffing for peppers, which taste good accompanied by a salad. You don't have to stop at peppers: aubergines and larger courgettes are all excellent stuffed, too.

Serves 2
2 large red peppers
1 tbsp olive oil, plus a little extra for greasing
1 medium onion, finely chopped
2 garlic cloves, crushed
175g (6oz) mushrooms, sliced
1 tsp vegetable bouillon powder, mixed with 2–3 tbsp water
115g (4oz) brown basmati rice, cooked
1 tbsp pine nuts
handful fresh basil, chopped
Solo sea salt and ground black pepper

1 Preheat the oven to 200°C/400°F/gas mark 6 and lightly oil a baking tray. Cut off the tops of the peppers and remove the seeds and pith. Keep the tops to use as lids.
2 Heat the oil in a sauté pan and fry the onion and garlic for 2 minutes. Add the chopped mushrooms and bouillon mixture and fry for a further 2–3 minutes.
3 In a large bowl, combine the cooked mixture with the rice, pine nuts and basil, and season with Solo salt and black pepper.
4 Stuff the peppers with the mixture and put the tops back on.
5 Put on the tray and bake for 35 minutes.

Roasted Vegetables with Mediterranean Quinoa

Quinoa is amazingly versatile and very special, because it is packed full of protein. It's a great foil for these Mediterranean flavours.

Serves 2
1 handful cherry tomatoes
1 medium courgette, cubed
1 red onion, sliced into wedges
1 red pepper, sliced
1 handful button mushrooms
4 tsp olive oil
Solo sea salt

For the quinoa
225g (8oz) quinoa
1 tsp vegetable bouillon powder or ½ stock cube
4 stoned black olives (Kalamata are delicious), roughly chopped
1 tbsp fresh basil leaves, finely chopped
ground black pepper

1 Preheat the oven to 180°C/350°F/gas mark 4. Place all the vegetables on a baking tray, lightly drizzle with the olive oil and sprinkle with Solo salt.
2 Roast for 40–50 minutes until tender, shaking the tray twice during cooking to turn and recoat the vegetables.
3 Meanwhile, rinse the quinoa very well under cold, running water.
4 Put it in a pan with the bouillon powder or crumbled stock cube and 600ml (20fl oz) water. Bring to the boil, cover and simmer for 13 minutes, until the water has boiled away and the grains are light and fluffy.
5 Allow the quinoa to cool, then mix the olives and basil through with a fork.
6 Serve a mound of the quinoa topped with vegetables and freshly ground black pepper.

Grilled Burgers*

Here is a home-made vegetarian alternative to the beefburger.

> Serves 2
> 225g (8oz) tofu, mashed
> 4 tbsp tamari or soy sauce
> 1 medium carrot, peeled and grated
> 1 garlic clove, crushed
> 1 small spring onion, chopped
> 2 slices rye bread, toasted and crumbed
> 1 tbsp tomato purée
> 1 medium free-range egg
> ground black pepper
> 1 tbsp chopped fresh coriander
> 1 tbsp olive oil
> rye bread, sliced tomato and lettuce to serve

1 Mix the tofu and tamari or soy sauce in a bowl, then marinate for 20 minutes. Squeeze out and discard any excess moisture.
2 In a bowl, mix the prepared tofu with the remaining ingredients except the oil and form into four burgers. Chill for 20 minutes.
3 Lightly brush the burgers with oil and cook under a medium grill for 15 minutes, turning frequently.
4 Serve between slices of rye bread with sliced tomato and lettuce.

* Recipe courtesy of Cauldron Foods.

Sweet Potato and Red Onion Tortilla

This variation on a traditional potato tortilla uses sweet potatoes for a lower GL score. Serve with a side salad or steamed broccoli.

> Serves 2
> 1 large sweet potato, peeled and sliced horizontally into thin circles
> 1 tbsp olive oil
> 2 large red onions, chopped
> 2 garlic cloves, crushed
> 4 medium free-range eggs
> Solo sea salt and ground black pepper

1 Steam the sweet potato for 10 minutes, or until tender, then slice thinly.
2 Heat half the oil in a pan and add the onions and garlic. Cover and cook over a very low heat, stirring occasionally, for 12–15 minutes or until soft. Then remove from the heat to cool.
3 Beat the eggs and stir in the sweet potato and half the cooked onion. Season generously with Solo salt and black pepper.
4 Heat the remaining oil in a shallow, non-stick frying pan until hot, then add the reserved onion. Pour in the egg mixture and cook over a very low heat for 6 minutes or until the underneath is golden and the mixture looks set.
5 If the top is set, take a spatula and loosen the edges of the tortilla so that you can slide it onto a plate and serve. However, if the top is still runny when the base has set, slide the tortilla onto a plate, and then tip it back into the pan, topside down, to set the top quickly before serving.

Japanese Noodles

Soba (buckwheat) noodles complement this Japanese sauce and steam-fry perfectly.

Serves 2

For the sauce
4 tbsp dashi (Japanese stock made from bonito flakes, available from Oriental supermarkets)
1 tbsp tamari or soy sauce
1 tsp mirin (Japanese rice wine, available from supermarkets)
1 tsp grated root ginger
4 finely sliced shiitake mushrooms
1 tsp cornflour (optional)
310g (11oz) smoked tofu, cut into bite-sized pieces
finely sliced vegetables, choosing from carrots, sugar snap peas, mangetouts, broccoli or green pepper, or beansprouts
115g (4oz) soba noodles

1 Combine the sauce ingredients and simmer in a pan until thickening but still runny. If necessary, add 1 tsp cornflour.
2 Lightly grill the tofu until it begins to brown, turning to colour both sides.
3 Add the grilled tofu, with the vegetables, to the sauce and simmer for a few minutes, or until the vegetables have softened slightly.
4 Cook the soba noodles according to the pack instructions (they take almost no time), and toss the steam-fry through the noodles.

Sesame Steamed Vegetables with Quinoa

Steaming vegetables brings out their individual delicate flavours, but the dressing in this recipe adds real pizzazz, turning them into a light, delicious feast.

Serves 2
225g (8oz) quinoa
1 tsp vegetable bouillon powder or ½ stock cube

For the dressing
2 tsp sesame oil
2 tsp tamari or soy sauce
1 tbsp sesame seeds (toast in a dry pan over a medium heat, shaking from time to time until golden)
a squeeze of lemon juice

For the vegetables
4 broccoli florets, chopped
2 handfuls mangetouts
handful baby corn
2 spring onions, chopped

1 Rinse the quinoa very well under cold, running water. Put it in a pan with 600ml (1 pint) of water and the bouillon powder or crumbled stock cube. Bring to the boil, cover and simmer for 13 minutes, or until the water has been absorbed. Fluff up the grains using a fork.
2 Mix the dressing ingredients in a cup.
3 Put the broccoli in a vegetable steamer and steam for 4½ minutes, then add the mangetouts and baby corn and cook for a further 2 minutes, or until the vegetables are lightly cooked.
4 Serve the vegetables on a mound of quinoa and pour the dressing over the top, then sprinkle with chopped spring onions.

Chilli

This wonderful dish – just the thing for a crisp autumn evening – has fooled many a hardy meat eater. You can prepare this in double quantities and freeze it. It works well with brown basmati rice, or on a small baked potato, or in a toasted tortilla wrap.

Serves 2
1 tbsp olive oil
1 small onion, sliced
2 garlic cloves, crushed
½ green pepper, sliced
½ tsp chilli powder
1 tsp paprika
1 tsp ground cumin
1 tsp ground coriander
55g (2oz) dried soya mince, soaked, or 175g (6oz) Quorn mince
200g (7oz) canned tomatoes, chopped
1 tbsp tomato purée
115g (4oz) canned red kidney beans, drained and rinsed

1 Put the oil in a large pan and add the onion, garlic and pepper with the chilli powder, paprika, cumin and coriander. Cover and steam-fry over low-medium heat for 5 minutes.
2 Add the soya or Quorn mince and stir for 2 minutes.
3 Add the tomatoes, tomato purée and red kidney beans. Mix well and leave to simmer for 30 minutes, stirring occasionally to prevent it from sticking or burning. If the mixture becomes too thick, add a little water.

Poultry and meat
Indian Spiced Chicken

This simple dish is irresistible.

Serves 2
juice of 1 lemon
1 garlic clove, crushed
½ tsp each ground turmeric and ground cumin
1 tsp ground coriander
pinch of cayenne pepper
2 small skinless chicken breasts

1 Blend the lemon juice with the garlic and spices.
2 Place the chicken in a dish and toss it in the spice blend so that it is well coated. Leave to marinate for at least 30 minutes, or ideally several hours.
3 Cook under a medium grill, turning halfway through, for 15 minutes or until cooked through with no pink juices.

Chicken Tandoori

It's the end of the week and you fancy some spicy food. What better than this fabulous Chicken Tandoori recipe? Even better, the herbs and spices in this dish lend it anti-inflammatory properties. Serve with brown basmati rice and steamed vegetables. (For vegetarians, tofu would work just as well.)

Serves 2
2 small skinless chicken breasts, chopped into bite-sized chunks
85g (3oz) natural yoghurt
handful flaked almonds
½ tbsp lemon juice
2 garlic cloves, crushed
½ tsp grated fresh root ginger
½ tsp ground cumin
½ tsp ground coriander
¼ tsp ground turmeric
pinch of cayenne pepper
Solo sea salt and black pepper

1 Put the chicken pieces in a shallow casserole.
2 Mix together the remaining ingredients and spread over the chicken, then cover the dish and place it in the fridge to marinate for 1–1½ hours. Preheat the oven to 200°C/400°F/gas mark 6.
3 Bake the chicken in the marinade for 35–40 minutes, or until cooked thoroughly.

Chicken Chermoula

Chermoula is a North African spice and herb mix that makes a wonderful marinade for chicken or tofu.

Serves 2
½ tbsp olive oil
1½ tbsp lemon juice
2 garlic cloves, crushed
1 tbsp chopped fresh parsley
½ tbsp chopped fresh coriander
½ tsp ground coriander
½ tsp cayenne pepper

½ tsp ground cumin
½ tsp paprika
2 small skinless chicken breasts
Solo sea salt and ground black pepper
couscous or Quinoa Tabouleh (page 323), or Coleslaw (page 320) and Sweet
Potato Mash (page 334), to serve

1 Mix all the ingredients except the chicken together in a bowl to make a marinade.
2 Cut several slashes in each chicken breast and rub the marinade into the meat. Cover the chicken and place in the fridge for 2 hours.
3 Take out and cook under a medium grill for 10–15 minutes, or until the meat is cooked and the juices run clear, turning the chicken over halfway through.
4 Slice the breasts and arrange on top of couscous or Quinoa Tabouleh, or serve with Coleslaw (3 ⑭) and Sweet Potato Mash (7 ⑭).

Garlic and Lemon Roast Chicken

Organic, free-range chicken is the best available. Once you've roasted the chicken, remove the skin before eating. Leftover meat can be used to make sandwiches or salads the next day.

Serves 2 (with leftovers)
½ lemon
1 tsp olive oil
4 garlic cloves: 2 crushed, 2 whole and unpeeled
1 medium-sized chicken
ground black pepper
coarse sea salt

1 Preheat the oven to 180°C/350°F/gas mark 4. Squeeze the juice from the lemon. Reserve the lemon peel. Mix together the lemon juice, oil and crushed garlic, and rub all over the chicken, then sprinkle with freshly ground black pepper and coarse sea salt. Put the squeezed lemon and whole garlic cloves inside the cavity.
2 Put the chicken on a rack in a roasting dish (to allow the fat to drain) and roast, calculating 20 minutes per 450g (1lb) plus an extra 20 minutes. Baste 2 to 3 times during cooking. Test the chicken is cooked through by piercing the thickest part with the point of a knife; the juices should run clear and the flesh should be white, not pink.

Chicken with Roasted Courgettes and Red Onion

Roasting vegetables with chicken is a great idea, as the veg absorb the flavour of the chicken. This version uses a Mediterranean-inspired mix of aubergine, courgette, new potatoes and red onion.

Serves 2
2 courgettes, cut into chunks
2 red onions, cut into wedges
6 baby new potatoes
1½ tbsp olive oil
1–2 tbsp balsamic vinegar, to taste
4 thyme sprigs
2 garlic cloves, unpeeled
2 small skinless chicken breasts
Solo sea salt and ground black pepper

1 Preheat the oven to 180°C/350°F/gas mark 4. Put the vegetables into a small roasting tin, pour over 1 tbsp of oil and half the vinegar and add a pinch of Solo sea salt and the thyme. Toss together and put the chicken breasts on top, pressing them into the mixture.
2 Drizzle the remaining vinegar and oil over the chicken and season.
3 Roast for 40–45 minutes, shaking the vegetables to turn them and turning the chicken halfway through. Make sure the chicken doesn't dry out on top.

Spiced Turkey Meatballs

A leaner alternative to beef meatballs with a spicy kick, these patties go down well with teenagers.

Serves 4
1 tbsp olive oil
2 large garlic cloves, crushed
1 large green chilli, deseeded and finely chopped
a large pinch of ground cumin
400g (14oz) lean minced turkey
Solo sea salt and ground black pepper
baked beans, grilled mushrooms and tomatoes, or grilled courgettes and
    wholegrain spaghetti, to serve

1 Heat the oil in a pan and gently fry the garlic, chilli and cumin for 2 minutes, then leave to cool.
2 Add to the turkey, season with a little Solo salt and pepper, and mix thoroughly. Shape the mixture into four patties.
3 Cook under a medium grill for 10 minutes, or until cooked thoroughly, turning halfway through.
4 Serve with baked beans and grilled mushrooms and tomatoes, or wholegrain spaghetti and grilled courgette pieces. (To cook the courgettes, slice the courgettes lengthways and drizzle with a little oil and Solo salt, then lightly grill, turning halfway through.)

Ratatouille Sausage Bake

A no-fuss, warming dish, superb as a midweek supper. This seems like a lot of vegetables but they cook down and any leftovers are delicious on a baked potato. Vegetarians could simply omit the sausages and add half a can of kidney beans with a pinch of chilli powder per person to the ratatouille, and serve with baby new potatoes.

Serves 2
4 red, green, yellow and/or orange peppers, chopped
2 red onions, sliced
2 courgettes, sliced
400g (14oz) can chopped tomatoes
2 tbsp tomato purée
2 garlic cloves, crushed
2 tsp dried mixed Italian herbs
4 lean, good-quality sausages (venison are the leanest, otherwise opt for lean pork or beef)
Solo sea salt and ground black pepper

1 Preheat the oven to 180°C/350°F/gas mark 4. Place the peppers, onions and courgettes in a shallow casserole or roasting tin and mix in the tomatoes, tomato purée, garlic, herbs and Solo salt, combining well so that the tomato mixture coats everything.
2 Put the sausages on top of the vegetable base. Bake for 1 hour, add pepper and serve.

Nick's Beefburgers

Created by a cavalry officer friend, this burger is seriously delicious served with the Mexican Bean Dip (4 **⑥**) and lettuce in a toasted pitta bread (5 **⑥** per half-slice).

> Serves 2
> 1 tbsp tamari or soy sauce
> 1 tsp Worcester sauce
> 1 tbsp finely chopped fresh coriander
> ¼ red onion, finely chopped
> ½ free-range egg, beaten
> ½ tsp Solo sea salt
> ½ tsp ground black pepper
> 225g (8oz) extra-lean minced beef

1 Mix all the flavourings together with the egg, then add to the mince.
2 Knead the mixture thoroughly, then divide into four patties and flatten into burger shapes.
3 Cover, then chill to firm for 10 minutes, or until required.
4 Cook under a medium grill for approximately 7 minutes per side.

Chicken Dumplings with Chilli Dipping Sauce

These dumplings are steamed, making them much lower in fat than traditional fried meatballs. Turkey is equally tasty in this recipe.

> Serves 2
> 2 small skinless chicken breasts, cut into chunks
> 1 tbsp tamari or soy sauce
> 1 red chilli, deseeded and finely chopped
> 2cm (¾in) chunk of fresh root ginger, peeled and finely grated
> 4 spring onions, roughly chopped
> 1 garlic clove, finely grated
> 1 tbsp fresh coriander, roughly chopped
> 2 tbsp sweet chilli dipping sauce
> Crunchy Thai Salad (page 319) and soba (buckwheat) noodles, to serve

1 Put the chicken, tamari or soy sauce, chilli, ginger, spring onions, garlic and coriander in a food processor and pulse until the mixture is coarsely chopped and combined.

2 Using your hands, shape the mixture into 12 balls, then cover and chill for at least 20 minutes or up to 8 hours.
3 Put the dumplings into a steamer over a pan of simmering water and cook for 20 minutes, or until cooked through. The chicken is thoroughly cooked when there is no pink flesh showing inside.
4 Serve with chilli dipping sauce, Crunchy Thai Salad (4 ⑨) and soba (buckwheat) noodles (7 ⑨ per small serving).

Fajitas

Here's a low-fat take on this ever-popular Tex-Mex dish. Substitute a can of black-eyed beans if you do not eat meat.

Serves 2

For the fajitas
olive oil
2 onions, sliced
1 garlic clove, crushed
1 red and 1 yellow pepper, topped, seeded and sliced lengthways
⅔ tbsp Old El Paso Fajita Seasoning
2 small skinless chicken breasts, cut into slices
2 soft flour tortillas

For the tomato salsa
2 plum tomatoes, chopped
2 spring onions, finely chopped
1 garlic clove, crushed
2 tbsp finely chopped fresh coriander
1 tbsp lime juice
1 tbsp olive oil
pinch Solo sea salt and ground black pepper

1 Put the oil in a pan and add the onion, garlic and peppers. Cover and steam-fry over a low-medium heat for 5 minutes.
2 Rub the seasoning into the chicken and cook under a medium grill for 5–10 minutes, or until cooked through. Mix into the vegetables. (If you're making the vegetarian version with black-eyed beans, add the fajita seasoning to the steam-fry and cook for a further few minutes, then stir in a 400g-can of black-eyed beans, drained and rinsed. Heat through.)
3 Stir the salsa ingredients together. Divide the salsa between the tortillas and add the filling. Roll up the tortillas.

Thai Green Curry

The aromatic blend of spices and creamy coconut milk in this dish suits a number of protein-rich foods, so you can adapt this recipe whether you eat meat or not (simply add tofu chunks or prawns as directed). If you can't find the lime leaves, the curry will still be delicious.

Serves 2
1 tbsp olive oil
1 small onion, chopped
2 garlic cloves, crushed
2 heaped tsp Thai green curry paste
100g (3½oz) chicken breast meat, cubed or 310g (11oz) firm tofu, cubed or
    175g (6oz) peeled prawns
2 tsp fish sauce (optional)
425ml (¾ pint) canned coconut milk
2 kaffir lime leaves
1 large courgette, chopped
handful fresh basil leaves

1 Put the oil in a pan and add the onion, garlic and curry paste. Cover and steam-fry over a low-medium heat for 2 minutes.
2 Add the chicken or tofu and fry for a further 5 minutes.
3 Add the fish sauce if using the chicken or prawns, the coconut milk and kaffir lime leaves. Stir well, cover and leave to simmer for 20 minutes.
4 Add the courgette and cook for 5 minutes, then add the prawns, if using, and cook for another 5 minutes or until heated through. Add the basil leaves and serve.

Coronation Chicken Salad

A good meal to make with leftover chicken. It's full of crunch with a slightly sweet, spicy flavour. Perfect for packed lunches or picnics.

Serves 2
1 gem lettuce, torn into bite-sized pieces
1½ tbsp low-fat mayonnaise
1½ tbsp low-fat natural yoghurt
2 tsp mango chutney
1 tsp tomato purée

1 tsp paprika
cold meat from ½ small roast chicken, skin removed
½ eating apple, cubed
1 celery stick, chopped
pinch of Solo sea salt

1 Create a bed of lettuce on a large plate.
2 Mix together the mayonnaise, yoghurt, mango chutney, tomato purée, paprika and Solo salt.
3 Combine the sauce with the chicken, apple and celery.
4 Pile on top of the lettuce and serve either with oatcakes or pitta bread, or with cold boiled potatoes.

Tarragon and Lemon Roast Chicken Breast

Tarragon and lemon lend extra flavour to roast chicken.

Serves 2
1 garlic clove, sliced
2 tarragon sprigs
2 small chicken breasts (with skin)
2 tsp olive oil
½ lemon

1 Preheat the oven to 190°C/375°F/gas mark 5. Put the garlic slices and tarragon under the chicken skin.
2 Place the chicken breasts in a baking dish and drizzle with olive oil and lemon juice.
3 Roast for 15–20 minutes, or until cooked through with no pink juices. Before eating, remove the skin.

Spicy Pork Loin

Here is a delicious way to serve pork, which should be lovely and moist. Serve with steam-fried greens and Sweet Potato Mash (7 ⓖⓛ) (page 334).

Serves 2
1 tbsp olive oil
2 tsp tomato purée
1 garlic clove, peeled
3 tbsp tamari or soy sauce
1 large mild, red chilli, deseeded
2.5cm (1in) piece fresh root ginger, peeled
2 tsp honey or dark muscovado sugar
1 small pork loin (fillet), fat trimmed

1 In a blender, whizz the olive oil, tomato purée, garlic, tamari or soy sauce, chilli, ginger and honey or sugar, until it forms a smooth paste.
2 Lightly boil the mixture in a pan for 2 minutes, then cool.
3 Rub this marinade all over the pork, then cover and place in the fridge for 20–30 minutes or until needed. Preheat the oven to 180°C/350°F/gas mark 4.
4 Place the pork on a rack in a roasting tin, cover with the marinade and bake for 30–35 minutes, bashing the pork with the marinade halfway through. Remove from the oven when cooked through and leave to rest for 5 minutes under foil before serving.

Venison Stroganoff

Leaner than beef, venison is very tasty and is not farmed intensively, making it less likely to be contaminated with chemical residues. If you want a vegetarian version, replace the venison with extra mushrooms (allowing 2 handfuls per person), and serve with quinoa to make sure you get adequate protein.

Serves 2
1 tbsp olive oil
85g (3oz) chestnut mushrooms, halved
1 onion, sliced
1 garlic clove, chopped

Solo sea salt and ground black pepper

200g (7oz) venison rump, trimmed of fat and sliced into 2cm (¾in) strips

55g (2oz) natural yoghurt mixed with 1 rounded tsp cornflour

½ rounded tbsp chopped fresh tarragon

¼ tsp paprika

Sweet Potato Mash (see page 333), or brown basmati rice, and steamed
   green beans, to serve

1 Heat half the oil in a frying pan and gently sauté the mushrooms, onion and garlic for about 10 minutes. Season and put in a bowl.

2 Increase the heat to high, add the remaining oil and put in the meat, quickly sealing it and stirring occasionally until cooked through. Season and add to the reserved mushroom mixture, leaving any juices in the pan.

3 Add 50ml (2fl oz) of water to the pan and heat gently for 5 minutes to reduce, stirring to mix in all the juices. Add the yoghurt mixture and cook for another minute.

4 Add the vegetables and venison together with the tarragon and paprika.

5 Serve with Sweet Potato Mash (7 ⓖⓛ) or 70g (2½oz) brown basmati rice (7 ⓖⓛ), sprinkled with paprika, and with steamed green beans on the side.

Desserts

This section is all about people who think life is sweet – and want to celebrate that, not succumb to seesawing blood sugar. You don't have to give up desserts on the Holford Diet. As you can see, cakes, flapjacks, pies and puddings all have a part to play. Once your fatburning capabilities have reached their stride, have one of these a week if you like – or perhaps two, on the maintenance diet. Once your blood sugar is balanced, you can *really* enjoy desserts, because they're not ruling your life.

GL scores

Recipe	Page number	ⓖⓛ
Individual Berry Cheesecake	364	5
Chocolate Coconut Cookies	365	5
Kiwi and Coconut Pudding	365	6
Cinnamon Steamed Pears with Summer Berry Purée	366	5
Almond Macaroons	366	2

Individual Berry Cheesecake

The base of this cheesecake uses chopped fruit and nuts for a much lower GL score. It's an easy-to-prepare pudding that can be made in advance.

Serves 2
20g (¾oz) chopped walnuts and pecan nuts (or other nuts)
4 ready-to-eat dried apricots
½ tsp walnut oil
2 tbsp lemon juice
3 tsp xylitol
grated rind of ½ lemon
200g (7oz) very low-fat plain cream cheese
4 tbsp berries, such as raspberries, blueberries or blackberries
1 tbsp apple juice or water

1 Place the nuts and apricots with the oil in small blender and process until broken into very small pieces and sticking together. Press into the base of two ramekins and chill.
2 In a bowl add the lemon juice to the xylitol and stir to allow the granules to dissolve.
3 Mix the xylitol mixture and lemon rind into the cream cheese until smooth and thoroughly combined, then spoon into the prepared ramekins, level off the top and return to the fridge.
4 Put the berries in a small pan and gently stew them in apple juice or water until they soften and begin to burst. Remove from the heat and cool before pouring onto the cheesecakes.
5 Chill the cheesecakes until ready to serve.

Chocolate Coconut Cookies

These miniature biscuit bars are absolutely scrummy served after a meal.

Makes 12 (serves 4)
140g (5oz) desiccated coconut
3 egg whites
3 tbsp xylitol
1 tsp lime or lemon juice
1 tbsp cornflour
3 small squares of good-quality dark chocolate, such as Green and Black's

1 Preheat the oven to 180°C/350°F/gas mark 4. Line a baking tray with baking parchment. Put the coconut into a bowl with the egg whites, xylitol, lime or lemon juice and cornflour and combine well into a stiff paste.
2 Divide into 12 walnut-sized balls and shape into rectangles or flattish circles. Place on the prepared baking tray and bake for 10 minutes, then reduce the heat to 150°C/300°F/gas mark 2 for a further 5 minutes. Remove from the oven.
3 Melt the chocolate in a heatproof bowl over a pan of gently simmering water, then dip one half of each coconut bar into the chocolate. Alternatively, drizzle the melted chocolate over the bars. Put on a plate covered with baking parchment. Chill in the fridge to set.

Kiwi and Coconut Pudding

This is the easiest pudding ever, but it's special enough for entertaining. It can be made in advance and kept in the fridge until needed.

Serves 2
2 ripe kiwi fruits, peeled and cut into thin slices
4 tbsp Rachel's Organic Coconut Greek-style Live Yoghurt

1 Divide the kiwi slices between two bowls or ramekins (glass dishes look best, because you can see the different layers of the finished pudding).
2 Spoon the yoghurt over the top.

Cinnamon Steamed Pears with Summer Berry Purée

Steaming is much easier than poaching these pears, which are lovely served with puréed summer berries.

Serves 2
2 ripe pears
½ tsp cinnamon
1 tsp xylitol
2 heaped tbsp summer berries

1 Slice the bottom off each pear, so that they can stand upright, then remove the core using either a melon-ball scoop or a teaspoon.
2 Mix together the cinnamon and the xylitol, then sprinkle into the hollow of each pear, where the core has been removed.
3 Lay them in a steamer over a pan of simmering water and steam for about 8–10 minutes, turning halfway through, until they are soft when pierced with a knife. (Do not stand them up or you will lose all of the sweet juices inside.)
4 While the pears are steaming, purée the summer berries in a blender or cook lightly in 1 tbsp water until they burst and release some of their juice.
5 Serve the pears warm, with a dollop of the fruit purée.

Almond Macaroons

These chewy little biscuits will fill the spot if you have a carb craving, but, being made of egg and nuts, have a low GL.

Makes 12 miniature biscuits (serves 3)
1 egg white
½ tsp ground ginger
55g (2oz) ground almonds
55g (2oz) xylitol
12 flaked almonds

1 Preheat the oven to 180°C/350°F/gas mark 4 and line a baking tray with rice paper.
2 Put the egg white into a clean, grease-free bowl and whisk until it forms stiff peaks.

3 Gently fold the ginger, ground almonds and xylitol into the egg white using a metal spoon, taking care not to stir out all the air.

4 Place 12 teaspoonfuls of the mixture onto the baking tray and top each one with a flaked almond.

5 Bake for 15–20 minutes, or until firm to the touch. Cool on the tray.

6 When cooled, remove from the tray and peel or trim the rice paper from the edges of each macaroon.

Fruit Juice Jelly

An all-natural jelly that can be made from your favourite fruit juice, such as cranberry or freshly squeezed orange. Serve with fresh blueberries.

> Serves 6
> 2 tsp agar-agar powder or flakes (vegetarian alternative to gelatine) or 4 tsp powdered gelatine
> 600ml (1 pint) fruit juice, at room temperature

Soak the agar-agar in 3 tablespoons of water in a pan for 5 minutes if using the powder, or for 10–15 minutes if using flakes. Dissolve over a medium heat, stirring constantly, then increase the heat and boil for 2–3 minutes, again stirring constantly. Stir in the fruit juice, pour into a glass bowl or individual ramekins and chill until set.

If using gelatine, put 3 tablespoons of water into a small pan, sprinkle over the powdered gelatine and leave for 5 minutes, or until it becomes spongy, without stirring. Put the pan over a very low heat and wait for the water to become clear (without stirring or boiling). Warm a quarter of the juice and add to the gelatine, stirring it in well, then add the remaining juice, pour into a bowl or ramkins and chill as above.

Apple Flapjack Crumble

Serve this crumble to family and friends and I promise no one will guess that you are on a diet. Experiment by adding different dried fruit and nuts, or pumpkin and sunflower seeds to the crumble.

Serves 2

For the crumble
2 tbsp xylitol
2 tbsp olive oil
175g (6oz) oat flakes
55g (2oz) chopped walnuts

For the filling
2 Bramley (cooking) apples, cored and diced
1 tsp lemon juice
1 tsp xylitol
¼ tsp ground ginger or ½ tsp cinnamon

1 Gently dissolve the xylitol in the oil in a pan over a medium heat, then add the oat flakes and walnuts and mix well. Cook, stirring, for 3 minutes, or until the oats just start to become crisp and golden. Set aside.
2 Put the apples, lemon juice, xylitol and ginger or cinnamon in a pan and gently stew until the apples soften and start to disintegrate.
3 Divide the apple mixture between two ramekins and cover with the flapjack crumble topping. Serve warm.

Ginger Stewed Apricots

These spicy apricots go beautifully with the Coconut Quinoa Pudding (opposite) or simply with a spoon of reduced-fat crème fraîche.

Serves 2
4 ripe apricots, halved and stoned
1 tbsp xylitol
¼ tsp ground ginger
1 tbsp orange juice or water

Stew the apricot halves with the other ingredients until they are soft but retain their shape.

Raspberry Mousse

This fruit fool is light and fresh. It's also good made with strawberries or blackcurrants.

Serves 2
225g (8oz) raspberries (fresh or frozen and thawed)
115g (4oz) low-fat fromage frais
1–2 tsp honey
handful fresh mint leaves

1 Blend the raspberries, fromage frais and honey.
2 Pour into individual serving dishes and garnish with a sprig of mint.

Coconut Quinoa Pudding

A high-protein, low-GL version of the classic comfort-food rice pudding. This is not a glamorous-looking pudding but it does taste delicious, especially served alongside a spoonful of Ginger Stewed Apricots (see opposite).

Serves 2
115g (4oz) quinoa, rinsed
150ml (¼ pint) semi-skimmed milk or soya milk
1 tbsp desiccated coconut
2 tsp xylitol

Put all the ingredients in a pan and bring to the boil, then reduce the heat, cover and simmer until the quinoa is cooked (the grains will look light and fluffy, and will be soft to the bite).

Baked Apple with Spiced Blackberry Stuffing

A warming, fibre-rich pudding for autumn and winter. It also tastes good with blueberries.

Serves 2
¼ tsp cinnamon or ground ginger
2 tsp xylitol
1 heaped tbsp blackberries
2 Bramley (cooking) apples, cored to create a fairly large hole inside

1 Preheat the oven to 180°C/350°F/gas mark 4. Gently mix the cinnamon or ginger and xylitol with the berries.
2 Place the apples in an ovenproof dish or plate and stuff with the mixture.
3 Bake for 35–40 minutes, or until soft right through (test by inserting a skewer) but not collapsing.

Chocolate Ice Cream

This luscious ice cream shines if made with the highest-quality cocoa powder.

Serves 2
75g (2¾oz) xylitol
225ml (8fl oz) milk
1 egg
40g (1½oz) dark chocolate cocoa powder
450ml (16fl oz) cream
1 tsp vanilla extract

1 Mix the xylitol, milk and egg together in a bowl, then pour into a small pan and cook over a medium-low heat, stirring constantly, for 10 minutes, or until the mixture thickens. Take care not to let it boil.
2 Remove from the heat and add the cocoa powder, stirring until the cocoa dissolves and is mixed in well. Transfer to a bowl.
3 Leave to cool for 15 minutes at room temperature then stir in the cream and vanilla extract. Pour into a freezerproof container and put in the freezer for at least 2½ hours. Remove 5 minutes before serving.

Fruit Kebabs

Just the thing for a late-summer barbecue, and a favourite with all ages.

Serves 2
1 apple
a little lemon juice
1 orange
4 black grapes
200g (7oz) natural yoghurt
1 tsp honey

1 Cube the apple and coat with a little lemon juice to prevent the pieces from going brown.
2 Peel the orange, removing all the pith, and cut into chunks. Halve the grapes and remove the pips.
3 Thread the fruit on to skewers and cook under a high grill or on a barbecue.
4 Blend the yoghurt with the honey and use as a dipping sauce.

Drinks

The following drinks can be drunk without limit throughout the day:

- still mineral water
- herbal teas
- dandelion coffee, Barley Cup, Caro, Teeccino

The following drinks are best limited to a glass a day:

- Aqua Libra
- other sugar-free juice blends (best diluted)

Also, you can have one of these a day (within your 5 ⓒⓛ allowance for drinks, sweets and desserts):

- Fruit juices diluted 50 per cent with water (see page 400 for quantities)

If you're prone to overindulge in alcohol, you'll need to stop drinking it for two weeks to a month at the start of the diet for maximum fatburning. Thereafter, limit your consumption of alcohol to a maximum of three units a week. A unit is:

- a small glass of wine
- a half-pint of beer or lager
- a measure of spirits

Snacks

As we saw in Chapter 21, you need never be bored at snack time. Have your snacks mid-morning and mid-afternoon, away from main meals.

- You can have a piece of fruit, plus five almonds or two teaspoons of pumpkin seeds. Choose from apples, pears, plums, cherries, berries, peaches, grapefruit and oranges. You can eat an entire punnet or even more of strawberries (see the table on page 392), but avoid bananas; although they're fine with Get Up & Go for breakfast, they have too high a GL to have as an additional snack.
- Low-GL bread and oatcakes with protein spreads and dips are a good savoury option. Try one thin slice of rye, pumpernickel, sourdough or other low-GL bread, or two oatcakes, with either half a small tub of cottage cheese, half a small tub of hummus, or 1 tbsp sugar-free peanut butter. You could substitute a raw carrot or a selection of crudités for the bread or oatcakes.
- If you like, you can have a small, plain, low-fat bio yoghurt, 140g (5oz), or half a small tub of cottage cheese, with berries.

These should keep you going strong through the day.

Here's another delicious idea – if you bring them to work, you may have to hide them from your colleagues!

Spiced Chickpea Chews

A low-fat, savoury snack rich in combined protein and carb.

> Serves 3 (keep some in an airtight container for a ready snack)
> 400g (14oz) chickpeas, rinsed and drained
> 1 tsp olive oil
> 1 tbsp lemon juice
> 1 tsp paprika or cayenne pepper
> pinch of Solo sea salt and ground black pepper

1 Preheat the oven to 150°C/300°F/gas mark 2. Toss the chickpeas in the oil and put into a roasting tin. Roast for 1 hour, or until crisp, shaking them around in the tin from time to time.
2 Take out and drizzle with lemon juice. Sprinkle with the paprika or cayenne pepper and add seasoning.
3 Shake the chickpeas in the tin to coat thoroughly and then leave to cool.

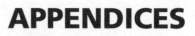

APPENDICES

Appendix 1

Ideal Weight, Body Mass Index and Body Fat Percentage

Weight in relation to height

The following table gives you your ideal weight range depending on your height and sex.

Your ideal weight for height

Men aged 25 and over

Height (ft/m)	Weight (lb/st/kg)
5ft 1in/1.55m	112–129lb/8–9st 3lb/51–59kg
5ft 2in/1.57m	115–133lb/8st 3lb–9st 7lb/52–60kg
5ft 3in/1.6m	118–136lb/8st 6lb–9st 10lb/54–62kg
5ft 4in/1.63m	121–139lb/8st 9lb–9st 13lb/55–63kg
5ft 5in/1.65m	124–143lb/8st 12lb–10st 3lb/56–65kg
5ft 6in/1.68m	128–147lb/9st 2lb–10st 7lb/58–67kg
5ft 7in/1.7m	132–152lb/9st 6lb–10st 12lb/60–69kg
5ft 8in/1.73m	136–156lb/9st 10lb–11st 2lb/62–71kg
5ft 9in/1.75m	140–160lb/10st–11st 6lb/64–73kg
5ft 10in/1.78m	144–165lb/10st 4lb–11st 11lb/65–75kg
5ft 11in/1.8m	148–170lb/10st 8lb–12st 2lb/67–77kg
6ft/1.83m	152–175lb/10st 12lb–12st 7lb/69–79kg
6ft 1in/1.85m	156–180lb/11st 2lb–12st 12lb/71–82kg
6ft 2in/1.88m	160–185lb/11st 6lb–13st 3lb/73–84kg
6ft 3in/1.9m	164–190lb/11st 10lb–13st 8lb/74–86kg

Women aged 25 and over

Height (ft/m)	Weight (lb/st/kg)
4ft 8in/1.42m	92–107lb/6st 8lb–7st 9lb/42–49kg
4ft 9in/1.45m	94–110lb/6st 10lb–7st 12lb/43–50kg
4ft 10in/1.47m	96–113lb/6st 12lb–8st 1lb/44–51kg
4ft 11in/1.5m	99–116lb/7st 1lb–8st 4lb/45–53kg
5ft/1.52m	102–119lb/7st 4lb–8st 7lb/46–54kg
5ft 1in/1.55m	105–122lb/7st 7lb–8st 10lb/48–55kg
5ft 2in/1.57m	108–126lb/7st 10lb–9st/49–57kg
5ft 3in/1.6m	111–130lb/7st 13lb–9st 4lb/50–59kg
5ft 4in/1.63m	114–135lb/8st 2lb–9st 9lb/52–61kg
5ft 5in/1.65m	118–139lb/8st 6lb–9st 13lb/54–63kg
5ft 6in/1.68m	122–143lb/8st 10lb–10st 3lb/55–65kg
5ft 7in/1.7m	126–147lb/9st–10st 7lb/57–67kg
5ft 8in/1.73m	130–151lb/9st 4lb–10st 11lb/59–68kg
5ft 9in/1.75m	134–155lb/9st 8lb–11st 1lb/61–70kg
5ft 10in/1.78m	138–159lb/9st 12lb–11st 5lb/63–72kg

Body mass index

Even better than knowing your ideal weight for your height is to calculate your body mass index, or BMI, a measure of fat based on your height and your weight. Your BMI is a reliable indicator of total body fat. The score is valid for both men and women, but does have some limits:

- It may overestimate body fat in athletes and others who have a muscular build.

- It may underestimate body fat in older people and those who have lost muscle mass.

Your BMI can be used to work out whether you are overweight or obese. Here are the scores:

Underweight = 18.5 or less
Normal weight = 18.5–24.9
Overweight = 25–29.9
Obese = 30 or more

Body Mass Index table – Imperial version

	Normal							Overweight				Obese										Extreme obesity														
BMI	19	20	21	22	23	24	25	26	27	28	29	30	31	32	33	34	35	36	37	38	39	40	41	42	43	44	45	46	47	48	49	50	51	52	53	54
Height (inches)												Body weight (pounds)																								
58	91	96	100	105	110	115	119	124	129	134	138	143	148	153	158	162	167	172	177	181	186	191	196	201	205	210	215	220	224	229	234	239	244	248	253	258
59	94	99	104	109	114	119	124	128	133	138	143	148	153	158	163	168	173	178	183	188	193	198	203	208	212	217	222	227	232	237	242	247	252	257	262	267
60	97	102	107	112	118	123	128	133	138	143	148	153	158	163	168	174	179	184	189	194	199	204	209	215	220	225	230	235	240	245	250	255	261	266	271	276
61	100	106	111	116	122	127	132	137	143	148	153	158	164	169	174	180	185	190	195	201	206	211	217	222	227	232	238	243	248	254	259	264	269	275	280	285
62	104	109	115	120	126	131	136	142	147	153	158	164	169	175	180	186	191	196	202	207	213	218	224	229	235	240	246	251	256	262	267	273	278	284	289	295
63	107	113	118	124	130	135	141	146	152	158	163	169	175	180	186	191	197	203	208	214	220	225	231	237	242	248	254	259	265	270	278	282	287	293	299	304
64	110	116	122	128	134	140	145	151	157	163	169	174	180	186	192	197	204	209	215	221	227	232	238	244	250	256	262	267	273	279	285	291	296	302	308	314
65	114	120	126	132	138	144	150	156	162	168	174	180	186	192	198	204	210	216	222	228	234	240	246	252	258	264	270	276	282	288	294	300	306	312	318	324
66	118	124	130	136	142	148	155	161	167	173	179	186	192	198	204	210	216	223	229	235	241	247	253	260	266	272	278	284	291	297	303	309	315	322	328	334
67	121	127	134	140	146	153	159	166	172	178	185	191	198	204	211	217	223	230	236	242	249	255	261	268	274	280	287	293	299	306	312	319	325	331	338	344
68	125	131	138	144	151	158	164	171	177	184	190	197	203	210	216	223	230	236	243	249	256	262	269	276	282	289	295	302	308	315	322	328	335	341	348	354
69	128	135	142	149	155	162	169	176	182	189	196	203	209	216	223	230	236	243	250	257	263	270	277	284	291	297	304	311	318	324	331	338	345	351	358	365
70	132	139	146	153	160	167	174	181	188	195	202	209	216	222	229	236	243	250	257	264	271	278	285	292	299	306	313	320	327	334	341	348	355	362	369	376
71	136	143	150	157	165	172	179	186	193	200	208	215	222	229	236	243	250	257	265	272	279	286	293	301	308	315	322	329	338	343	351	358	365	372	379	386
72	140	147	154	162	169	177	184	191	199	206	213	221	228	235	242	250	258	265	272	279	287	294	302	309	316	324	331	338	346	353	361	368	375	383	390	397
73	144	151	159	166	174	182	189	197	204	212	219	227	235	242	250	257	265	272	280	288	295	302	310	318	325	333	340	348	355	363	371	378	386	393	401	408
74	148	155	163	171	179	186	194	202	210	218	225	233	241	249	256	264	272	280	287	295	303	311	319	326	334	342	350	358	365	373	381	389	396	404	412	420
75	152	160	168	176	184	192	200	208	216	224	232	240	248	256	264	272	279	287	295	303	311	319	327	335	343	351	359	367	375	383	391	399	407	415	423	431
76	156	164	172	180	189	197	205	213	221	230	238	246	254	263	271	279	287	295	304	312	320	328	336	344	353	361	369	377	385	394	402	410	418	426	435	443

Source: Adapted from Clinical Guidelines on the Identification, Evaluation, and Treatment of Overweight and Obesity in Adults: The Evidence Report.

Body Mass Index table – metric version

Height (cms)	Normal							Overweight				Obese										Extreme obesity														
BMI	19	20	21	22	23	24	25	26	27	28	29	30	31	32	33	34	35	36	37	38	39	40	41	42	43	44	45	46	47	48	49	50	51	52	53	54
												Body weight (kgs)																									
147	41	43	45	48	50	52	54	56	58	61	63	65	67	69	72	74	76	78	80	82	84	87	89	91	93	95	98	100	102	104	106	108	111	112	115	117
150	43	45	47	49	51	54	56	58	60	63	65	67	69	72	74	76	78	81	83	85	88	90	92	94	96	98	101	103	105	108	110	112	114	117	119	121
152	44	46	49	51	53	56	58	60	63	65	67	69	72	74	76	79	81	83	86	88	90	93	95	98	101	103	105	107	109	111	113	116	118	121	123	125
155	45	48	50	53	55	58	60	62	64	67	69	72	74	77	79	82	84	86	89	91	93	96	98	101	103	105	108	110	112	115	117	120	122	125	127	129
158	47	49	52	54	57	59	62	64	66	69	72	74	77	79	82	84	86	89	92	94	97	99	101	104	107	110	112	115	117	119	121	124	126	129	131	134
160	49	51	54	56	59	61	64	66	68	71	74	77	79	82	84	87	89	92	95	97	100	102	105	108	110	112	115	117	120	122	126	128	130	133	136	138
163	50	53	55	58	60	63	65	68	71	73	76	79	82	84	87	90	93	95	98	101	103	106	108	111	114	117	119	122	124	127	129	132	134	137	140	142
165	52	54	57	60	63	65	68	71	73	76	79	82	84	87	90	93	95	98	101	104	106	108	112	114	117	119	122	125	128	131	133	136	139	142	144	147
168	54	56	59	62	64	67	70	73	75	78	81	84	87	90	93	95	98	101	104	107	109	112	115	118	120	123	126	129	132	135	137	140	143	146	149	152
170	55	58	61	64	66	69	72	75	78	81	84	87	90	93	96	98	101	104	107	110	113	116	118	122	124	127	130	133	137	139	142	145	147	150	153	156
173	57	59	63	66	68	72	74	78	80	83	86	89	92	95	98	101	104	107	110	113	116	119	122	125	128	131	134	137	140	143	146	149	152	155	158	161
176	58	61	64	68	70	73	77	80	83	86	89	92	95	98	101	104	107	110	113	117	119	122	126	129	132	135	138	141	144	147	150	153	156	160	162	166
178	60	63	66	68	70	73	77	80	83	86	89	92	95	98	101	104	107	110	113	117	119	122	126	129	132	135	139	141	144	147	150	153	156	160	162	166
180	62	65	68	71	73	76	79	82	85	88	91	95	98	101	104	107	110	113	117	120	123	126	129	132	136	140	143	146	149	153	156	159	162	166	169	172
183	64	67	70	73	77	80	83	87	90	93	96	100	103	107	110	113	117	120	123	127	130	133	137	140	143	147	150	153	157	160	164	167	170	173	177	180
185	65	68	72	75	79	83	86	89	93	96	99	103	107	110	113	117	120	123	127	131	134	137	141	144	147	151	154	158	161	165	168	171	175	178	182	185
188	67	70	74	78	81	84	88	92	95	99	102	106	109	113	116	120	123	127	130	134	137	141	145	148	152	155	159	162	166	169	173	176	179	183	187	190
191	69	73	76	80	83	87	91	94	98	102	105	109	112	116	119	123	126	130	134	137	141	145	148	152	156	160	163	167	170	173	177	181	185	188	192	196
193	71	74	78	82	86	89	93	97	100	104	108	112	115	119	123	127	130	134	138	142	145	149	152	156	160	163	167	171	175	179	182	186	190	193	197	201

Measuring percentage of body fat

A more important statistic than your BMI is your body fat percentage. Opposite is an equation to work out an approximation of this percentage. (Your local gym may offer a service for measuring your body fat percentage more accurately using callipers or testing equipment.) An ideal percentage of fat for a man is less than 15 per cent; for a woman it's less than 22 per cent. You can reduce your body fat percentage by around 10 per cent a month on the Holford Diet.

Step 1
Find your body weight (BW) on the chart opposite and write down the corresponding conversion factor. For every pound over the figures given, add 1.08 to the conversion factor.

So: if you weigh 175lb, your conversion factor is 189.36.

If you weigh 132lb, your conversion factor is 142.83 (140.67 plus 2 × 1.08).

Step 2
Find your waist girth on the chart and write down the corresponding conversion factor.

So: if you have a 35in waist, your conversion factor is 145.26.

Step 3
Subtract the waist conversion factor from the body weight conversion factor.

So: 189.36 − 145.26 = 44.1.

Step 4
To the result, add 98.42 for men or 76.76 for women. This gives you your lean body weight (LBW).

So: 44.10 + 98.42 (for a man) = 142.52.

Step 5
To calculate your fat weight (FW), subtract the LBW from the BW: BW − LBW = FW.

So: 175 − 142.52 = 32.48.

Step 6

To determine the actual percentage of your body fat, divide FW by BW and multiply by 100:

$$FW \div BW \times 100 = \%BF.$$

So: $32.48 \div 175 \times 100 = 19\%$.

Body fat percentage calculation chart

Body weight (pounds)	Conversion factor	Waist girth (in)	Conversion factor
100	108.21	25	103.75
105	113.62	25.5	105.83
110	119.03	26	107.9
115	124.44	26.5	109.98
120	129.85	27	112.05
125	135.26	27.5	114.13
130	140.67	28	116.2
135	146.08	28.5	118.28
140	151.49	29	120.35
145	156.9	29.5	122.43
150	162.31	30	124.51
155	167.72	30.5	126.58
160	173.13	31	128.66
165	178.54	31.5	130.73
170	183.95	32	132.81
175	189.36	32.5	134.88
180	194.77	33	136.96
185	200.18	33.5	139.03
190	205.59	34	141.11
195	211	34.5	143.18
200	216.41	35	145.26
205	221.82	35.5	147.33
210	227.23	36	149.41
215	232.64	36.5	151.48
220	238.05	37	153.56

continued

Body weight (pounds)	Conversion factor	Waist girth (in)	Conversion factor
225	243.46	37.5	155.63
230	248.87	38	157.71
235	254.28	38.5	159.78
240	259.69	39	161.86
245	265.1	39.5	163.93
250	270.51	40	166.01
255	275.92	40.5	167.08
260	281.33	41	170.16
265	286.74	41.5	172.23
270	292.15	42	174.31
275	297.56	42.5	176.38
280	302.97	43	178.46
285	308.38	43.5	180.53
290	313.79	44	182.61

Appendix 2

The Complete Glycemic Load of Foods

Glycemic index

The glycemic index is about the *quality* of the carbohydrate within a food, not the *quantity*. In other words, the glycemic index (GI) of a food remains the same whether you eat 10 grams or 100 grams. It is a comparison of how one type of carbohydrate (for example, that in bread) compares to another type of carbohydrate (for example, sugar). It's worked out by feeding volunteers however much of the food in question they would need to eat to consume 50 grams of 'available' carbohydrate. (Some carbohydrate, such as fibre, is not available to the body for its energy needs.)

If, for example, half a food's carbohydrate is 'available', the volunteers would be fed 100 grams of the food to obtain 50 grams of the available carbohydrate. The extent to which this raises blood sugar levels (see the diagrams on page 146), compared to the extent to which 50 grams of glucose does, determines its GI score. Glucose, by definition, scores 100 on the GI Index. So, if a food creates half the increase in blood sugar compared to glucose, its GI score will be 50. This means that you could eat twice as much carbohydrate in the form found in this food to match the effect of glucose on your blood sugar level.

Glycemic load

The Glycemic Load of a food (GL) is basically the GI of a food multiplied by the serving size. So, the GL actually tells you what that specific serving, biscuit or slice of bread will do to your blood sugar.

The GL of a food is worked out as follows:

GI score divided by 100, multiplied by the available carbohydrate (carbohydrates minus fibre) in grams.

So, in our example above this would be:
50 (GI score) ÷ 100 × 50 (50 grams of carbohydrate in 100 gram serving) = 25
So a 100 gram serving of our example food has a GL of 25

Take watermelon as another example. Its glycemic index (GI) is pretty high, about 72. According to the calculations by the people at the University of Sydney's Human Nutrition Unit, in a serving of 120 grams it has 6 grams of available carbohydrate per serving, so its glycemic load is pretty low, 72 ÷ 100 × 6 = 4.32 (rounded to 4).

So, as long as you know the glycemic index of a food, the size of the serving you wish to use, and the amount of available carbohydrate in the food, you can calculate the GL yourself. However, I have calculated the GL for a comprehensive range of foods, which can be found in the chart on pages 386–399.

Please note that the glycemic index for some foods has not been published. In these instances we have estimated the GL based on the GI for very similar foods. These foods are marked 'E'.

The most accurate way to gauge whether or not you should eat a food is the glycemic load of a food, which is a calculation based on both the quantity of carbohydrate in a food, and the quality of that carbohydrate.

A GL of 10 or less is good, and is **shown in bold**
A GL of 11–14 is OK, shown in normal text
A GL of 15 or more is bad, *shown in italics*

However, even this is only a guide because the amount you eat of a food will obviously alter its effect on your blood sugar, and hence your weight. So, while generally I say liberally eat the **bold** foods with low GLs, limit the normal-text foods and avoid the *italic* foods, what is most important is to limit the total glycemic load of your diet.

If you want to lose weight and feel great, eat no more than 40 ⓖ a day. This means roughly 10 for breakfast, 10 for lunch, 10 for dinner and 5 each for your two snacks, mid-morning and mid-afternoon. You can also drink 5 ⓖ, so your total daily intake from food and drink is 45 ⓖ. If you choose the good, low-GL foods you'll be able to eat more food. If you choose the bad high-GL foods you'll have to eat much less.

In the chart below mainly select from the bold foods, then use the right-hand column to work out how much to eat for 5 ⓖ, which is the serving for a snack, or 10 ⓖ, which is a serving for a main meal. If you are not sure what a 'serving' means look at the amounts of grams for 5 ⓖ and check the grams on the packet of the food in question. Foods containing no carbohydrate, composed entirely of protein or fat (meat, fish, eggs, cheese, mayonnaise) have, in effect, a GL of 0, and are not included in this chart. Remember that foods marked with an 'E' have an estimated value, whereas other foods have measured values. As the GLs of more foods are calculated, this table will be updated on www.theholforddiet.com. You can also input a selection of foods into this database and it will calculate the GL of a particular recipe for you.

THE GLYCEMIC LOAD OF COMMON FOODS

Item	Serving size (in g)	GLs per serving	10 GLs	5 GLs	5 GLs
Bakery products					
Muffin – apple, made without sugar	**60**	**9**	**1 muffin**	**½ muffin**	**33g**
Muffin – apple muffin, made with sugar	60	13	1 small muffin	½ small muffin	23g
Crumpet	50	13	1 crumpet	½ crumpet	19g
Muffin – apple, oat, sultana, made from packet mix	50	14	1 small muffin	½ small muffin	18g
Muffin – bran	57	15	½ muffin	¼ muffin	18g
Muffin – blueberry	57	17	½ muffin	¼ muffin	17g
Muffin – banana, oat and honey	50	17	½ muffin	¼ muffin	15g
Muffin – carrot	57	20	½ muffin	¼ muffin	14g
Banana cake, made without sugar	80	16	1 small slice	⅓ slice	25g
Croissant	57	17	½ croissant	¼ croissant	17g
Doughnut	47	17	½ doughnut	¼ doughnut	14g
Sponge cake, plain	63	17	½ slice	¼ slice	19g

Item	Serving size (in g)	GLs per serving	10 GLs	5 GLs	5 GLs
Breads					
Rye kernel (pumpernickel) bread	30	6	2 slices	1 slice	25g
Sourdough rye	30	6	2 slices	1 slice	25g
Volkenbrot, wholemeal rye bread	30	7	2 slices	1 slice	21g
Rice bread, high-amylose	30	7	2 small slices	1 small slice	21g
Rice bread, low-amylose	30	8	2 thin slices	1 thin slice	19g
Wholemeal rye bread	30	8	2 thin slices	1 thin slice	19g
Wheat tortilla (Mexican)	50	8	1½ tortillas	Less than 1 tortilla	31g
Chapatti, white wheat flour, thin, with green gram	50	8	1½ chapattis	1 chapatti	31g
White, high-fibre	30	9	1 thick slice	1 thin slice	17g
Wholemeal (wholewheat) wheat flour bread	30	9	1 thick slice	1 thin slice	17g
Gluten-free fibre-enriched	30	9	1 thick slice	½ thick slice	17g
Gluten-free multigrain bread	30	10	1 slice	½ slice	15g
Light rye	30	10	1 slice	½ slice	15g
White wheat flour bread	30	10	1 slice	½ slice	15g
Pitta bread, white	30	10	1 pitta	½ slice	15g
Wheat flour flatbread	30	10	1 slice	½ slice	15g
Gluten-free white bread	30	11	1 slice	½ slice	14g

Item	Serving size (in g)	GLs per serving	10 GLs	5 GLs	5 GLs
Corn tortilla	50	12	1 tortilla	½ tortilla	21g
Middle Eastern flatbread	30	15	⅔ slice	⅓ slice	10g
Baguette, white, plain	30	15	1/20 baton	1/40 baton	10g
Bagel, white, frozen	70	25	½ bagel	¼ bagel	14g

Breakfast cereals

Item	Serving size (in g)	GLs per serving	10 GLs	5 GLs	5 GLs
Holford Oat Muesli Mix (see page 313) (E)	30	1	As much as you like	As much as you like	100g
Porridge made from rolled oats	30	2	As much as you like	1 very large bowl	75g
Get Up & Go with strawberries and ½ pint milk (E)	30	5	½ pint drink	½ pint drink	5fl oz/ 150ml
All-Bran™	30	6	2 small servings	1 small serving	25g
Muesli, gluten-free	30	7	2 small servings	1 small serving	21g
Muesli (Alpen)	30	10	1 serving	½ serving	15g
Muesli, Natural	30	10	1 serving	½ serving	15g
Raisin Bran™ (Kellogg's)	30	12	1 small serving	⅓ serving	13g
Weetabix™	30	13	2 biscuits	1 biscuit	12g
Bran Flakes™	30	13	1 small serving	½ serving	12g

Item	Serving size (in g)	GLs per serving	10 GLs	5 GLs	5 GLs
Sultana Bran™ (Kellogg's)	30	14	1 small serving	½ serving	11g
Special K™ (Kellogg's)	30	14	1 small serving	½ serving	11g
Shredded Wheat	30	15	*1 biscuit*	*½ serving*	*10g*
Cheerios™	30	15	*1 very small serving*	*½ serving*	*10g*
Frosties™, sugar-coated cornflakes (Kellogg's)	30	15	*1 very small serving*	*½ serving*	*10g*
Grapenuts™	30	15	*1 very small serving*	*½ serving*	*10g*
Golden Wheats™ (Kellogg's)	30	16	*1 very small serving*	*½ serving*	*9g*
Puffed Wheat	30	16	*1 very small serving*	*½ serving*	*9g*
Honey Smacks™ (Kellogg's)	30	16	*1 very small serving*	*½ serving*	*9g*
Cornflakes, Crunchy Nut™ (Kellogg's)	30	17	*1 very small serving*	*½ serving*	*9g*
Coco Pops™ (cocoa-flavoured puffed rice)	30	20	*½ serving*	*¼ serving*	*8g*
Rice Krispies™ (Kellogg's)	30	21	*½ serving*	*¼ serving*	*7g*
Cornflakes™ (Kellogg's)	30	21	*½ serving*	*¼ serving*	*7g*

Cereal grains

Item	Serving size (in g)	GLs per serving	10 GLs	5 GLs	5 GLs
Semolina	150	6	1 very large serving	small serving	125g
Taco shells, cornmeal-based, baked (Old El Paso)	20	8	2 shells	1 shell	13g
Quinoa	150	8	1½ cup	⅔ cup	94g
Cornmeal	150	9	1 very large serving	1 small serving	83g

Item	Serving size (in g)	GLs per serving	10 GLs	5 GLs	5 GLs
			1 very large serving	1 small serving	
Kamut (E)	**150**	**9**	1 very large serving	1 small serving	**83g**
Pearl Barley	150	11	1 serving	½ serving	68g
Cracked wheat (bulgur/bourghul)	150	12	1 serving	½ serving	63g
Brown basmati rice	150	13	1 small serving	½ serving	58g
Buckwheat	*150*	*16*	*1 small serving*	*⅓ serving*	*47g*
Rice, brown	*150*	*18*	*1 small serving*	*⅓ serving*	*42g*
Rice, long grain, white, precooked microwaved 2 min.					
(Express Rice, Uncle Ben's)	*150*	*19*	*½ serving*	*¼ serving*	*39g*
Basmati, white, boiled	*150*	*22*	*½ serving*	*¼ serving*	*34g*
Couscous	*150*	*23*	*½ serving*	*¼ serving*	*33g*
Rice, white	*150*	*23*	*½ serving*	*¼ serving*	*33g*
Long grain, boiled	*150*	*23*	*½ serving*	*¼ serving*	*33g*
Millet, porridge	*150*	*25*	*½ serving*	*¼ serving*	*30g*

Crispbreads and crackers

Item	Serving size (in g)	GLs per serving	10 GLs	5 GLs	5 GLs
Oatcakes	**25**	**8**	**4 oatcakes**	**2 oatcakes**	**16g**
Digestives	**25**	**10**	**1 biscuit**	**½ biscuit**	**13g**
Cream cracker	25	11	2 biscuits	1 biscuit	11g
Rye crispbread	25	11	2 biscuits	1 biscuit	11g

Item	Serving size (in g)	GLs per serving	10 GLs	5 GLs	5 GLs
Water cracker	25	17	2 biscuits	1 biscuit	7g
Puffed rice cakes	*25*	*17*	*2 biscuits*	*1 biscuit*	*7g*

Dairy products and alternatives

Item	Serving size (in g)	GLs per serving	10 GLs	5 GLs	5 GLs
Plain yoghurt (no sugar)	200	3	3 small pots	1½ small pots	333g
Non-fat yoghurt (plain, no sugar)	200	3	3 small pots	1½ small pots	333g
Milk, full-fat	250ml	3	833ml	416ml	416ml
Milk, skim (Canada)	250ml	4	625ml	312ml	312ml
Soya yoghurt (Provamel)	200	7	2 small pots	1 small pot	150g
Soya milk (no sugar)	250ml	7	2 small cups	1 small cup	178ml
Custard, homemade from milk	100ml	7	1 small cup	½ cup	71ml
Ice cream, regular	50ml	8	2 scoops	1 scoop	31ml
Soya milk (sweetened with apple juice concentrate)	250ml	8	2 small cups	1 small cup	156ml
Soya milk, reduced-fat (1.5%), 120mg calcium	250ml	8	2 small cups	1 small cup	156ml
Soya milk (sweetened with sugar)	250ml	9	1½ small cups	⅔ small cup	138ml
Low-fat yoghurt, fruit, sugar, (Ski™)	200	10	1½ small pots	⅔ of small pot	100g
Rice milk, E	250ml	14	1 small cup	½ cup	90ml
Milk, condensed, sweetened (Nestlé)	*50ml*	*17*	*1 tsp*	*½ tsp*	*14ml*

Fruit and fruit products

Item	Serving size (in g)	GLs per serving	10 GLs	5 GLs	5 GLs
Blackberries E	120	1	2 large punnets	1 large punnet	600g
Blueberries E	120	1	2 large punnets	1 large punnet	600g
Raspberries E	120	1	2 large punnets	1 large punnet	600g
Strawberries, fresh, raw	120	1	2 large punnets	1 large punnet	600g
Cherries, raw	120	3	2 punnets	1 punnet	200g
Grapefruit, raw	120	3	1 large	1 small	200g
Pear, raw	120	4	2 large pears	1 large pear	150g
Melon/cantaloupe, raw	120	4	1 small melon	½ small melon	150g
Watermelon, raw	120	4	2 big slices	1 big slice	150g
Peaches raw (or canned in natural juice)	120	5	2 peaches	1 peach	120g
Apricots, raw	120	5	8 apricots	4 apricots	120g
Oranges, raw	120	5	2 large	1 large	120g
Plum, raw	120	5	8 plums	4 plums	120g
Apples, raw	120	6	2 small	1 small	100g
Kiwi fruit, raw	120	6	2 kiwis	1 kiwi	100g
Pineapple raw	120	7	2 thin slices	1 thin slice	85g
Grapes, raw	120	8	20 grapes	10 grapes	75g

Item	Serving size (in g)	GLs per serving	10 GLs	5 GLs	5 GLs
Mango, raw	120	8	½ mango	1 slice	75g
Apricots, dried	60	9	6 apricots	3 apricots	33g
Fruit Cocktail, canned (Delmonte)	120	9	Small can	Half a small can	66g
Pawpaw/papaya, raw	120	10	Half a small papaya	1 slice	60g
Prunes, pitted	60	10	6 prunes	3 prunes	30g
Apple, dried	60	10	6 rings	3 rings	30g
Banana, raw	120	12	1 banana	½ banana	50g
Apricots, canned in light syrup	120	12	Less than 1 small can	⅓ small can	50g
Lychees, canned in syrup and drained	120	16	½ 200g can	¼ 200g can	37g
Figs, dried, tenderised, Dessert Maid brand	60	16	2 figs	1 fig	19g
Sultanas	60	25	20	10	12g
Raisins	60	28	20	10	11g
Dates, dried	60	42	2 dates	1 date	7g

Jams and spreads

Item	Serving size (in g)	GLs per serving	10 GLs	5 GLs	5 GLs
Pumpkin seed butter E	16	1	3 large pots	1½ large pots	765g
Peanut butter (no sugar) E	16	1	3 large pots	1½ large pots	765g
Blueberry spread (no sugar) E	30	4	4 tbsp	2 tbsp	21g
Apricot fruit spread, reduced sugar	30	7	8 tsp	4 tsp	21g

Item	Serving size (in g)	GLs per serving	10 GLs	5 GLs	5 GLs
Orange marmalade	30	9	8 tsp	4 tsp	17g
Strawberry jam	30	10	2 tbsp	2 heaped tsp	15g

Legumes and nuts

Item	Serving size (in g)	GLs per serving	10 GLs	5 GLs	5 GLs
Hummus (chickpea dip)	30	1	4 large tubs	4 small tubs	765g
Soya beans	150	1	6 cups	3 cups	750g
Peas, dried, boiled	150	2	3 cups	1½ cups	375g
Pinto beans, boiled in salted water	150	4	2 cups	1 cup	187g
Borlotti beans, boiled, canned	150	4	1½ cans	⅔ can	187g
Lentils	150	5	2 cups	1 cup	150g
Butter beans	150	6	1½ cup	⅔ cup	125g
Split peas, yellow, boiled 20 min.	150	6	1½ cup	⅔ cup	125g
Baked beans, canned	150	7	½ can	¼ can	107g
Kidney beans, canned	150	7	¾ can	⅓ can	107g
Chickpeas (Bengal gram), boiled	150	8	1½ cups	⅔ cup	94g
Chickpeas, canned in brine	150	9	¾ can	⅓ can	83g
Chestnuts, cooked E	150	8	1½ cups	⅔ cup	94g
Flageolet beans, canned in brine E	150	8	¾ can	⅓ can	83g
Haricot/navy beans, canned	150	12	½ can	¼ can	62g
Black-eyed beans, boiled	150	13	1 cup	½ cup	58g

Pasta and noodles*

Item	Serving size (in g)	GLs per serving	10 GLs	5 GLs	5 GLs
Ravioli, durum wheat flour, meat filled, boiled	90	7.5	½ packet	1 small serving	60g
Vermicelli, white, boiled	90	8	1 large serving	½ large serving	56g
Spaghetti, wholemeal, boiled	90	8	1 large serving	½ large serving	56g
Pasta, wholemeal, boiled	90	8	1 large serving	½ a serving	56g
Fettuccine, egg, boiled	90	9	1 serving	½ a serving	50g
Spirali, durum wheat, white, boiled to *al dente* texture	90	9	1 serving	½ serving	47g
Spaghetti, white, boiled	90	9	1 serving	½ serving	47g
Instant noodles	90	9	1 serving	½ serving	47g
Spaghetti durum wheat, boiled 10-15 min,	90	10	1 serving	½ serving	43g
Gluten-free pasta, maize starch, boiled 8 min.	90	11	1 small serving	½ small serving	41g
Macaroni, plain	90	11	1 very small serving	½ very small serving	39g
Rice noodles, dried, boiled	90	11	1 very small serving	½ very small serving	39g
Udon noodles, plain (buckwheat/wheat)	90	15	⅔ serving	⅓ serving	30g
Corn pasta, gluten-free	90	16	1 small serving	½ small serving	28g
Gnocchi	90	16	1 very small serving	½ small serving	27g
Rice pasta, brown, boiled 16 min.	90	17	1 very small serving	½ small serving	26g

Item	Serving size (in g)	GLs per serving	10 GLs	5 GLs	5 GLs
Snack foods (savoury)					
Olives, in brine E	**50**	**1**	4 cups	2 cups	270g
Peanuts	**50**	**1**	1 large pack	1 medium or 2 small packs	250g
Cashew nuts, salted	**50**	**3**	1½ small packs	Less than 1 small pack	83g
Popcorn, salted, no sugar	**20**	**8**	1 small pack	½ small pack	12g
Potato crisps, plain, salted	50	11	1½ small packs	⅔ small pack	23g
Pretzels, oven-baked, traditional wheat flavour	30	16	8 pretzels	4 pretzels	9g
Corn chips, plain, salted	50	17	13 chips	7 chips	15g
Snack foods (sweet)					
Fruitus apple cereal bar E	35	5	2	1	35g
Rebar fruit and veg bar E	50	8	1	½	25g
Muesli bar containing dried fruit	30	13	Less than 1 bar	Less than ½ bar	12g
Chocolate, milk, plain (Mars/Cadburys/Nestlé)	50	14	Less than ½ bar	Less than ¼ bar	18g
Apricot fruit bar (dried apricot filling in wholemeal pastry)	*50*	*17*	*1 bar*	*½ bar*	*15g*

Item	Serving size (in g)	GLs per serving	10 GLs	5 GLs	5 GLs
Twix ® Cookie Bar, caramel (M&M/Mars, USA)	*60*	*17*	*1 stick*	*½ stick*	*18g*
Snickers Bar ®	*60*	*19*	*⅔ bar*	*⅓ bar*	*16g*
Polos – peppermint sweets	*30*	*21*	*8 polos*	*4 polos*	*7g*
Jellybeans, assorted colours	*30*	*22*	*4 jellybeans*	*2 jellybeans*	*7g*
Pop Tarts™, double choc	*50*	*24*	*21g*	*10g*	*10g*
Mars Bar ®	*60*	*26*	*½ bar*	*¼ bar*	*13g*

SOUPS

Item	Serving size (in g)	GLs per serving	10 GLs	5 GLs	5 GLs
Tomato soup	**250**	**6**	**1 can**	**½ can**	**208g**
Minestrone	**250**	**7**	**1 can**	**½ can**	**179g**
Lentil, canned	**250**	**9**	**⅔ can**	**⅓ can**	**139g**
Split pea, canned	*250*	*16*	*½ can*	*¼ can*	*78g*
Black bean, canned	*250*	*17*	*½ can*	*¼ can*	*74g*
Green pea, canned	*250*	*17*	*½ can*	*¼ can*	*74g*

Sugars

Item	Serving size (in g)	GLs per serving	10 GLs	5 GLs	5 GLs
Xylitol	**20**	**2**	**6 tbsp**	**3 tbsp**	**50g**
Blue agave cactus nectar (liquid sweetener in drinks)	**20**	**2**	**100ml**	**50ml**	**50g**

Item	Serving size (in g)	GLs per serving	10 GLs	5 GLs	5 GLs
Fructose	20	4	3 tbsp	5 tsp	25g
Sucrose	*20*	*14*	*3 tsp*	*1½ tsp*	*7g*
Honey	*20*	*16*	*2 tsp*	*1 tsp*	*6g*
Glucose	*20*	*20*	*2 tsp*	*1 tsp*	*5g*
Maltose (malt)	*20*	*22*	*2 tsp*	*1 tsp*	*5g*

Vegetables

Item	Serving size (in g)	GLs per serving	10 GLs	5 GLs	5 GLs
Tomato E	70	2	5 medium	2½ medium	175g
Broccoli E	100	2	5 handfuls	2½ handfuls	250g
Kale E	75	1	10 handfuls	5 handfuls	375g
Avocado E	190	1	10	5	950g
Onion E	180	2	5 medium	2½ medium	450g
Asparagus E	125	2	5 handfuls	2½ handfuls	315g
Green beans E	75	1	10 handfuls	5 handfuls	375g
Carrots	80	3	2 carrots	1 carrot	133g
Green peas	80	3	5 tbsp	2–3 tbsp	133g
Pumpkin	80	3	3 servings	1½ serving	133g
Beetroot	80	5	4 beets	2 beets	80g
Swede	150	7	½ swede	1 serving	107g

Item	Serving size (in g)	GLs per serving	10 GLs	5 GLs	5 GLs
Banana/plantain, green	120	8	1 small	½ small	75g
Broad beans	80	9	89g	1 tbsp	44g
Sweetcorn	80	9	1 serving	½ serving	44g
Parsnips	80	12	1 small	½ small	33g
Yam	150	13	1 small serving	½ small serving	58g
Boiled potato	150	14	107g	1 small	53g
Microwaved potato	150	14	107g	1 small	53g
Mashed potato	150	15	2 tbsp	1 tbsp	50g
New potato, unpeeled and boiled 20 min.	150	16	4 very small	2 very small	47g
Instant mashed potato	150	17	88g	2 tsp	44g
Sweet potato	150	17	1 small	½ small	44g
Baked potato, white, baked in skin	150	18	83g	⅔ medium	42g
French fries	150	22	68g	4–5	34g
Baked potato, baked without fat	150	26	½ a medium	¼ a medium	29g

TABLE OF GLYCEMIC LOAD (GL) OF COMMON DRINKS

DRINKS

Item	Serving size in ml	GL per serving	10 GLs	5 GLs	5 GLs
Tomato juice, canned, no added sugar	250	4	625ml	½ pint	315ml
Yakult ®, fermented milk drink with Lactobacillus casei	65	6	108ml	⅔ × 65ml bottle	30ml
Smoothie drink, soy, banana	250	7	357ml	⅔ × 250ml carton	175ml
Smoothie drink, soy, chocolate hazelnut	250	8	313ml	⅗ × 250ml carton	150ml
Carrot juice, freshly made	250	10	250ml	⅕ pint or ⅓ cup	125ml
Grapefruit juice, unsweetened	250	11	227ml	⅕ pint or ⅓ cup	115ml
Apple juice, pure, unsweetened	250	12	208ml	⅙ pint or ⅓ cup	105ml
Orange juice	250	13	192ml	⅙ pint or ⅓ cup	95ml
Cordial, orange, reconstituted	250	13	192ml	⅙ pint or ⅓ cup	95ml
Smoothie, raspberry	250	14	179ml	⅖ 250ml carton or ⅓ cup	90ml
Pineapple juice, unsweetened	250	16	156ml	¼ pint or ½ cup	80ml
Cranberry juice drink, Ocean Spray®	250	16	156ml	¼ pint or ½ cup	80ml
Coca Cola ®, soft drink/soda	250	16	156ml	⅕ × 330ml can	80ml
Fanta ®, orange soft drink	250	23	109ml	⅙ pint or ⅓ cup	50ml
Lucozade ®, original	250	40	63	⅛ pint or ¼ cup	30

Most of the GL values of foods listed here are derived from research published in 2002 by K. Foster-Powell, S. H. Holt and J. C. Brand-Miller in 'International table of glycemic index and glycemic load values: 2002', *American Journal of Clinical Nutrition* Vol 76(1) (2002), pp. 5–56 or from the University of Sydney online database at http://www.glycemicindex.com/ (database pages created by A/Prof. Gareth Denyer and Scott Dickinson using data collected by Professor Jennie Brand-Miller & SUGIRS). Last modified: 13 December 2005.

Notes

Serving sizes:

* All pasta serving sizes are for cooked food. For the equivalent of dry weight, halve the amount – so, if you're cooking spaghetti and the serving size is 120g, that means you put 60g in the pan.

Appendix 3

The Dangers of High-Protein Diets

There are big problems with high-protein diets, especially in the long term, that I'd like you to know about. Although I agree that high-protein diets do help balance your blood sugar, and hence cause weight loss, the reason I'm not a fan of this approach is that I believe the risks and the restrictions outweigh the benefits. The most famous high-protein diet is the Atkins Diet. Headlines the world over have issued warnings of heart and cancer risk, kidney damage and bone mass loss – and quite rightly so. Let's examine these causes of concern.

Kidney problems

Protein produces breakdown products that are hard work for the kidneys. If your kidneys are healthy and your protein excess isn't too high, there's no problem. But how far can you push it? Researchers found that about 30 per cent of women between the ages of 42 and 68 had a mild kidney problem. They also found that in women who had normal kidney function there was no link between high protein intakes and a decline in renal function.

However, those who already had a mild kidney problem and ate a high-protein diet – particularly one high in meat protein – showed some deterioration. Interestingly, dairy and vegetable proteins were not associated with worsening kidney function. And the parameters here for 'high protein' were much less than you'd normally eat on the Atkins Diet. Ironically, one of the first signs of poor kidney function is water retention (see Chapter 15), which leads to weight gain. However, the consequences are much more serious as kidney function starts to decline, leading to the need for dialysis.

Bone problems

Protein is acidic, and excess amounts need to be neutralised. The Nurse's Health Study, conducted in the US and analysed by the Harvard School of Public Health, recently found that women who consumed 95g (3¼oz) of protein a day, as compared with those who consumed less than 68g (2½oz) a day, had a 22 per cent greater risk of forearm fractures.[1] In another study, eating more than 80g (2¾oz) of protein a day, which is equivalent to bacon and eggs for breakfast and a steak for dinner, was found to increase your risk of osteoporosis.[2]

This happens because protein is made of amino acids. Too much acid is neutralised by the body's release of calcium, an alkaline mineral, from the bones – a finding that has been confirmed by 'metabolic ward' studies in which people are kept in a controlled environment, fed precise diets and measured for their calcium loss. Such studies have found that a negative calcium balance is created when 95g (3¼oz) of protein is consumed while a person eats 500mg of calcium. The calcium intake must be raised to 800mg before calcium balance is achieved – that is to say, when the calcium entering the body is the same as the amount leaving.

Dr Shalini Reddy from the University of Chicago conducted a six-week study on 10 healthy adults eating a low-carb diet. Volunteers lost an average of 4kg (9lb) over the course of the study – that's 680g (1½lb) a week.

That's the good news. The bad news was that the acid excretion in the urine, which is an indication of acid levels in the blood, rose by 90 per cent in some volunteers. There was also a sharp rise in the amount of calcium excreted in the urine during the low-carbohydrate, high-protein diets, and even the 'maintenance' diets for these regimes, despite only a slight decrease in calcium intake. This means the people were losing calcium from the body. Also, urinary citrate – a compound that inhibits kidney stone formation – decreased, implying an increased risk of kidney stone formation.[3]

According to Dr Reddy, 'Consumption of a low-carbohydrate, high-protein diet for six weeks delivers a marked acid load to the kidney, increases the risk for stone formation, decreases estimated calcium balance, and may increase the risk for bone loss.' These studies all suggest that such high-protein diets may increase the risk of bone loss over the long term. Of course, we are going to have to wait a while to find out, but I'd rather you weren't the guinea pig.

Breast and prostate cancer risk

After reviewing thousands of studies on diet and cancer, the World Cancer Research Fund states that there is an unequivocal link between high meat consumption and cancer incidence, especially for breast, colon and prostate cancer.[4] For breast and prostate cancer the link is strongest in relation to high dairy and dairy meat (beef) consumption. People in countries where beef and dairy products are not eaten have a fraction of the risk. In China, for example, the chances of a woman dying from breast cancer are one in 10,000, whereas her chance in the UK is one in 10. For prostate cancer the difference is even greater. In rural China the incidence is 0.5 in 100,000, yet it is estimated that, by 2015, one in four men in the UK will have a diagnosis of prostate cancer at some point in his life! Why?

The main likely cause of prostate and breast cancer is that these hormone-sensitive cells go into overgrowth due to exposure to abnormal levels of hormones or hormone-like substances, which include many of the man-made pollutants, from pesticides to PCBs, and dioxins to DDT. These tell a cell to continue growing. The hormone oestrogen does this too, which is why oestrogen HRT increases the risk of developing breast cancer.

Milk is high in oestrogen, but it's also high in other growth-stimulating chemicals, which, as we've seen, is hardly surprising, since milk is designed to make baby calves grow massively. It's called insulin-like growth factor. There are different types – IGF-1, IGF-2 and so on, although much of the focus is on IGF-1, which is abundant in milk and beef. The amount in modern milk is double this, partly because cows have been selectively reared to produce milk during pregnancy. On top of that, in the US cows are treated with BST (bovine somatotrophin), a growth hormone capable of further increasing milk yield by about 12 per cent.

All this means a cow's daily milk production has gone from 3 litres (5¼ pints) to 30 litres (52¾ pints). Not surprisingly, this milk has two to five times the amount of IGF-1, whereas the beef from a BST-treated animal has about double the IGF. Casein, the protein in milk, then helps to carry the IGF into us.

But what does IGF-1 do and why is it a strong candidate for increasing the risk of cancer? We make IGF, but very little in adulthood. It's produced mainly in childhood to stimulate growth. Normally, it is produced by the liver, especially during puberty. In girls it stimulates the growth of breast tissue, encouraging cells to divide and grow. In boys it stimulates growth of the prostate. There's nothing wrong with IGF-1, just as there's nothing wrong with oestrogen. It's a perfectly normal hormone. It's just that we aren't designed to be eating sources of it in adulthood. And that makes me very worried when a nation of dieters starts living off meat and cheese.

When levels of IGF in the blood increase by 8 per cent, the risk of prostate cancer increases seven times. Levels of IGF are, on average, 9 per cent higher in meat-eating omnivores and dairy-eating vegetarians compared with vegans. Recent research from Shangai, China, has found that the higher a woman's IGF-1 levels, the higher her risk of breast cancer. This study found that women in the top 25 per cent of IGF-1 scores had two to three times the risk of women in the bottom 25 per cent of IGF-1 levels.[5]

A study from York University in the UK on the link between IGF and prostate cancer risk in men found a similar result. Men in the top 25 per cent of IGF levels had three times the risk of prostate cancer.[6] These are just two of a dozen trials finding a strong link between circulating levels of IGF-1 and prostate cancer. There are many more linking IGF with breast cancer, with the combination of being insulin-resistant and having high IGF and excessive levels of oestrogen increasing the risk most greatly.[7] The way to reverse this risk is to correct insulin resistance by eating low-GL carbohydrates, reducing milk and beef consumption, eating organic where possible and staying away from HRT.

Underactive thyroid

What's more, high-protein diets can lead to an underactive thyroid. Just two weeks without carbohydrates suppresses the body's production of thyroxine, which controls your metabolic rate. It also promotes the stress hormone cortisol, which makes you even more insulin resistant (see page 169). This, in turn, even further reduces thyroxine production, the major symptom of which is weight gain. Thyroxine is now the second most commonly prescribed drug in the US. So don't be surprised if your metabolism slows down, and you experience rebound weight gain after being on a high-protein, very low-carb diet.

Other problems

Cancer is not the only disease associated with this type of high-protein, high-meat and high-dairy diet. Other research strongly suggests that high consumption of meats and dairy products can lead, or at least contribute to, heart disease, type-2 diabetes, gallbladder disease, osteoporosis, kidney failure, kidney stones, multiple sclerosis, rheumatoid arthritis, constipation, diverticulosis, haemorrhoids and hiatal hernia.[8] Recent research in mice has also shown substantial reduction in the ability to conceive in females placed on high-protein diets.[9]

Dr Atkins argued, justifiably, that if you can correct blood sugar problems, you can reduce your risk for many of these diseases. And, while you *can* correct blood sugar problems with a high-fat, high-protein diet, unless caution is exercised you may put yourself at risk of all of the negative effects associated with such a diet. The fact is, you can control your blood sugar just as well, if not better, by eating the right kinds of carbohydrate, the right kinds of fat, plus sufficient, not excessive, protein and less saturated fat. That's what I'm recommending to you in the Holford Diet because I believe it's safer, tastier, easier and more effective.

Ironically, if you follow the development of the Atkins Diet, you'll see that it is edging in this direction. The earliest version was really low on carbs, whereas the latest version ends up with 30 per cent carbohydrates, 30 per cent protein and 40 per cent fat. In my opinion, this still falls short of the ideal diet for painless weight loss, weight maintenance and overall lifelong health.

The other argument sometimes given in favour of high-protein, high-fat diets is that they mimic the diets of our hunter-gather ancestors. I would dispute this. Even in the most carnivorous phases of our evolution, our ancestors would never have eaten the amount of fat advised on a conventional high-protein, high-fat diet. Why? Because it wasn't in the meat. Today's animals are fattened up. Almost all meat you buy is marbled with fat, even if you buy the lean stuff. Real meat, as our ancestors ate, was real *lean* meat. However, our ancestors really thrived when they switched from the higher-protein 'hunter-gatherer' diets to the lower-protein, higher-carbohydrate 'peasant farmer' diet. That's when humanity multiplied and become dominant. Of course, these diets were also low-GL.

Appendix 4

Keeping Track

Follow the instructions in Chapter 29 to monitor your progress week by week using the Holford Diet Progress Report on the following pages. There's a Progress Report for each of the first four weeks, and a spare Progress Report that you can photocopy and use for subsequent weeks.

Holford Diet Feedback and Research

You can help with ongoing Holford Diet research. If you've completed the diet for four or more weeks, let me know your results by going online at www.holforddiet.com, selecting 'share your experience'. I value your feedback as it helps refine and improve the Holford Diet.

The Holford Diet progress reports

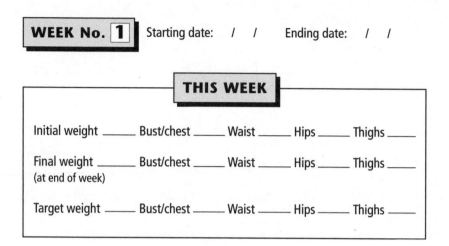

WEEK No. 1   Starting date: /   /   Ending date: /   /

THIS WEEK

Initial weight _____ Bust/chest _____ Waist _____ Hips _____ Thighs _____

Final weight _____ Bust/chest _____ Waist _____ Hips _____ Thighs _____
(at end of week)

Target weight _____ Bust/chest _____ Waist _____ Hips _____ Thighs _____

PROGRESS THIS WEEK

Weight lost _____ Total inch loss _____

How many aerobic sessions? _____ How many toning sessions? _____

How well did you follow the diet? _____ % the exercises? _____ %

PROGRESS TO DATE

Initial weight _____ Initial total inches _____
(at start of diet)   (bust+waist+hips+thighs)

Weight lost to date _____ Inches lost to date _____

WEEK No. 2   Starting date: /   /   Ending date: /   /

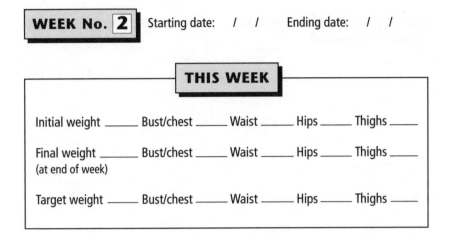

THIS WEEK

Initial weight _____ Bust/chest _____ Waist _____ Hips _____ Thighs _____

Final weight _____ Bust/chest _____ Waist _____ Hips _____ Thighs _____
(at end of week)

Target weight _____ Bust/chest _____ Waist _____ Hips _____ Thighs _____

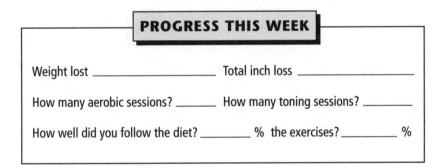

PROGRESS THIS WEEK

Weight lost _____ Total inch loss _____

How many aerobic sessions? _____ How many toning sessions? _____

How well did you follow the diet? _____ % the exercises? _____ %

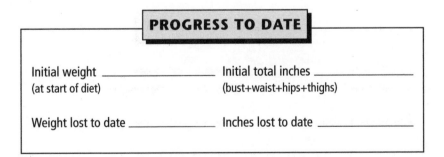

PROGRESS TO DATE

Initial weight _____ Initial total inches _____
(at start of diet)   (bust+waist+hips+thighs)

Weight lost to date _____ Inches lost to date _____

WEEK No. 3   Starting date: /   /   Ending date: /   /

THIS WEEK

Initial weight _____ Bust/chest _____ Waist _____ Hips _____ Thighs _____

Final weight _____ Bust/chest _____ Waist _____ Hips _____ Thighs _____
(at end of week)

Target weight _____ Bust/chest _____ Waist _____ Hips _____ Thighs _____

PROGRESS THIS WEEK

Weight lost _____ Total inch loss _____

How many aerobic sessions? _____ How many toning sessions? _____

How well did you follow the diet? _____ % the exercises? _____ %

PROGRESS TO DATE

Initial weight _____ Initial total inches _____
(at start of diet)   (bust+waist+hips+thighs)

Weight lost to date _____ Inches lost to date _____

WEEK No. 4   Starting date: /   /   Ending date: /   /

THIS WEEK

Initial weight _____ Bust/chest _____ Waist _____ Hips _____ Thighs _____

Final weight _____ Bust/chest _____ Waist _____ Hips _____ Thighs _____
(at end of week)

Target weight _____ Bust/chest _____ Waist _____ Hips _____ Thighs _____

PROGRESS THIS WEEK

Weight lost _____ Total inch loss _____

How many aerobic sessions? _____ How many toning sessions? _____

How well did you follow the diet? _____ % the exercises? _____ %

PROGRESS TO DATE

Initial weight _____ Initial total inches _____
(at start of diet)   (bust+waist+hips+thighs)

Weight lost to date _____ Inches lost to date _____

WEEK No. [ ]   Starting date: /   /   Ending date: /   /

THIS WEEK

Initial weight _____ Bust/chest _____ Waist _____ Hips _____ Thighs _____

Final weight _____ Bust/chest _____ Waist _____ Hips _____ Thighs _____
(at end of week)

Target weight _____ Bust/chest _____ Waist _____ Hips _____ Thighs _____

PROGRESS THIS WEEK

Weight lost _____ Total inch loss _____

How many aerobic sessions? _____ How many toning sessions? _____

How well did you follow the diet? _____ % the exercises? _____ %

PROGRESS TO DATE

Initial weight _____ Initial total inches _____
(at start of diet)   (bust+waist+hips+thighs)

Weight lost to date _____ Inches lost to date _____

Appendix 5

Working Out Your Training Heart-rate Zone

The best way to know that you are exercising at an intensity that will burn fat and boost your metabolism is to measure your pulse while exercising. If it is within your training heart-rate zone for 15 minutes or more then your exercising is having a fatburning effect.

To find your training heart-rate zone, you need to subtract your age from 220, then calculate 65 per cent of this amount for the lower end of your training zone and 80 per cent for the upper limit:

220 − [age] × .65 = lower limit
220 − [age] × .80 = upper limit

For example, for a 30-year-old:

220 − 30 = 190 × .65 = lower limit = 124 beats per minute
220 − 30 = 190 × .80 = upper limit = 152 beats per minute

To find your pulse rate, you will need a watch with a second hand. There are several points at which the pulse can be felt easily: the neck (the carotid pulse) on either side of the Adam's apple; or the wrist (the radial pulse). To find your pulse, apply light pressure with your fingers. Normally, for medical examinations your pulse is taken for 60 seconds. But to find your pulse while exercising, stopping for this long would lower your pulse and give you a false reading. So taking your pulse for only 10 seconds and multiplying the result by 6 will give you the number of beats in one minute without giving your heart rate a chance to slow down. This will be your exercising pulse rate.

When you first embark on your aerobic exercise sessions, you will need to stop briefly every 10–15 minutes to monitor your pulse. After a while you will become familiar with how the correct pulse feels for you. See the chart below to find your exercise heart rate for your age.

Training heart-rate zone chart (while exercising)

Age	65–80% of maximum heart rate (beats in 1 minute)	(beats in 10 sec.)
20	130–160	22–27
22	129–158	22–26
24	127–157	21–26
26	126–155	21–26
28	125–154	21–26
30	124–152	21–25
32	122–150	20–25
34	121–149	20–25
36	120–147	20–25
38	118–146	20–24
40	117–144	20–24
45	114–140	19–23
50	111–136	19–23
55	107–132	18–22
60	104–128	17–21
65	101–124	17–21
70	98–120	16–20

The centre column shows how many beats you should have in one minute; beginners should aim for the lower figure on the left-hand side (that is, 65 per cent of their maximum heart rate for their age), then slowly increase to 80 per cent. Do not exceed this higher level. The column on the far right gives you how many beats you should have in a 10-second pulse count. Again, beginners should stay at the lower end of their exercise range.

References

Introduction

1 Q. Chen, et al., Abstract, 'Pharmacologic doses of ascorbate act as a prooxidant and decrease growth of aggressive tumor xenografts in mice', Proc Natl Acad Sci. Vol 105(32) (12 August 2008), pp.11105–9; see also Q, Chen, et al., 'Pharmacologic ascorbic acid concentrations selectively kill cancer cells: Action as a pro-drug to deliver hydrogen peroxide to tissues', Proc Natl Acad Sci, Vol 102(38) (20 September 2005), pp. 13604–9; see also Sebastian J. Padayatty, Hugh D. Riordan, Stephen M. Hewitt, Arie Katz, L. John Hoffer and Mark Levine, 'Intravenously administered vitamin C as cancer therapy: Three cases', *Canadian Medical Association Journal*, Vol 174 (7) (28 March 2006)

Part One

1 ONUK survey, 'A Comparison of the health and nutrition of over 37,000 people in Britain and the effects of improving nutrition in a Cohort over 3 months', Institute for Optimum Nutrition, London (2004)

2 P. Holford et al., 'The effects of a low glycemic load diet on weight loss and key health risk indicators', *Journal of Orthomolecular Medicine*, Vol 21(2) (2006), pp. 71–8

3 M. Pereira et al., 'Effects of a low-glycemic load diet on resting energy expenditure and heart disease risk factors during weight loss', *Journal of the American Medical Association*, Vol 292(20) (2004), pp. 2482–90

4 D. Pawlak et al., 'Effects of dietary glycaemic index on adiposity, glucose homoeostasis, and plasma lipids in animals', *Lancet*, Vol 364 (9436) (2004), pp. 778–85

5 Anne-Helen Harding et al., 'Plasma vitamin C level, fruit and vegetable consumption, and the risk of new-onset type 2 diabetes mellitus: The European prospective investigation of cancer – Norfolk prospective study', *Archives of Internal Medicine*, Vol 168(14) (2008), pp. 1493–9

6 L. Henderson et al., 'MAFF national food survey', HMSO, 1996; 'The national diet and nutrition survey', Trading Standards Office, 2003; 'Health survey for England', Department of Health (data relating to 1995–2002)

7 J. Brand-Miller et al., 'Glycemic index and obesity', *American Journal of Clinical Nutrition*, Vol 76(1) (2002), pp. 281S–285S

8 D. Pawlak et al., 'Effects of dietary glycaemic index on adiposity, glucose homoeostasis, and plasma lipids in animals', *Lancet*, Vol 364 (9436) (2004), pp. 778–85

9 M. Slabber et al., 'Effects of a low-insulin-response, energy-restricted diet on weight loss and plasma insulin concentrations in hyperinsulinemic obese females', *American Journal of Clinical Nutrition*, Vol 60(1) (1994), pp. 48–53

10 I. Shai et al., 'Weight loss with a low-carbohydrate, Mediterranean, or low-fat diet', *New England Journal of Medicine*, Vol 359 (3) (2008), pp. 229–41

11 D. S. Ludwig, 'The Glycemic Index', *Journal of the American Medical Association*, Vol 287(18) (2002), pp. 2414–23

12 M. Pereira et al., 'Effects of a low-glycemic load diet on resting energy expenditure and heart disease risk factors during weight loss', *Journal of the American Medical Association*, Vol 292(20) (2004), pp. 2482–90

13 M. Pereira et al., 'Effects of a low-glycemic load diet on resting energy expenditure and heart disease risk factors during weight loss', *Journal of the American Medical Association*, Vol 292(20) (2004), pp. 2482–90

14 F. Samaha et al., 'A low-carbohydrate as compared with a low-fat diet in severe obesity', *New England Journal of Medicine*, Vol 348(21) (2003), pp. 2074–81

15 G. D. Foster et al., 'A randomized trial of a low-carbohydrate diet for obesity', *New England Journal of Medicine*, Vol 348(21) (2003), pp. 2082–90

16 H. Truby et al., 'Randomised controlled trial of four commercial weight loss programmes in the UK: Initial findings from the BBC diet trials', *British Medical Journal*, Vol 332 (3 June 2006), pp. 1309–14

17 D. M. Bravata et al., 'Efficacy and Safety of Low-Carbohydrate Diets: A Systematic Review', *Journal of the American Medical Association*, Vol 289(14) (2003), pp. 1837–50

18 C. S. Johnston et al., 'Ketogenic low-carbohydrate diets have no metabolic advantage over nonketogenic low-carbohydrate diets', *American Journal of Clinical Nutrition*, Vol 83(5) (2006), pp. 1055–61

19 Y. W. Aude et al., 'The national cholesterol education program diet vs a diet lower in carbohydrates and higher in protein and monounsaturated fat: A randomized trial', *Archives of Internal Medicine*, Vol 164(19) (2004), pp. 2141–6

20 M. Noakes et al., 'Effect of an energy-restricted, high-protein, low-fat diet relative to a conventional high-carbohydrate, low-fat diet on weight loss, body composition, nutritional status, and markers of cardiovascular health in obese women', *American Journal of Clinical Nutrition*, Vol 81(6) (2005), pp. 1298–306

21 H. Hull, 'The effect of food combining on weight loss', ION Research Project, 1997

22 N. Moussavi et al., 'Could the quality of dietary fat, and not just its quantity, be related to risk of obesity?', *Obesity*, Vol 16(1) (2008), pp. 7–15. See also C. Beermann et al., 'Short term effects of dietary medium-chain fatty acids and n-3 long-chain polyunsaturated fatty acids on the fat metabolism of healthy volunteers', *Lipids in Health and Disease*, Vol 2(10) (2003); and M. Kunesová et al., 'The influence of n-3 polyunsaturated fatty acids and very low calorie diet

during a short-term weight reducing regimen on weight loss and serum fatty acid composition in severely obese women', *Physiological Research*, Vol 55(1) (2006), pp. 63–72

23 Ann Louise Gittleman, *Beyond Pritikin*, Bantam (1996)

24 M. Appelbaum, 'Influences of level of energy intake on energy expenditure in man', reported in *Dieting Makes You Fat*, G. Cannon and H. Einzig, Simon and Schuster (1985)

25 R. Leibel et al., 'Changes in energy expenditure resulting from altered body weight', *New England Journal of Medicine*, Vol 332 (1995), pp. 621–8

26 M. and A. Wynn, 'How dieting can damage your health', *Which? Way to Health* (February 1995), pp. 22–4

27 M. H. Pitler et al., 'Randomized, double-blind trial of chitosan for body weight reduction', *European Journal of Clinical Nutrition*, Vol 53 (1999), pp. 379–81

28 E. Wuolijoki et al., 'Decrease in serum LDL cholesterol with microcrystalline chitosan', *Methods and Findings in Experimental and Clinical Pharmacology*, Vol 21(5) (1999), pp. 357–61

29 S. C. Ho et al., 'In the absence of dietary surveillance, chitosan does not reduce plasma lipids or obesity in hypercholesterolaemic obese Asian subjects', *Singapore Medical Journal*, Vol 42 (2001), pp. 6–10

30 W. McArdle, *Medical Aspects of Clinical Nutrition*, Keats Publishing (1983)

31 Department of Environment, Food and Rural Affairs (DEFRA) data on http://www.defra.gov.uk/farm/arable/sugar/sugar05.htm#consumption

32 P. Clayton and J. Rowbotham, 'An unsuitable and degraded diet? Part one: Public health lessons from the mid-Victorian working class diet', *Journal of the Royal Society of Medicine*, Vol 101(6) (2008), pp. 282–9

33 Health Survey for England, National Centre for Social Research (1998)

34 Z. B. Andrews et al., 'UCP2 mediates ghrelin's action on NPY/AgRP neurons by lowering free radicals', *Nature*, Vol 454(7206) (2008), pp. 846–51

35 ONUK survey, 'A Comparison of the health and nutrition of over 37,000 people in Britain and the effects of improving nutrition in a Cohort over 3 months', Institute for Optimum Nutrition, London (2004)

36 The Action to Control Cardiovascular Risk in Diabetes Study Group, 'Effects of intensive glucose lowering in type 2 diabetes', *New England Journal of Medicine*, Vol 358 (24), pp. 2545–59

37 G. Reaven, 'Role of insulin resistance in human disease', *Diabetes*, Vol 37 (1988), pp. 1595–1607

38 B. Thomas and J. Bishop (eds), British Diabetic Association, *Manual of Dietetic Practice*, 2003 edition, Blackwell Publishing.

39 Department of Health, 'Extra £372 million increases opportunity for all to make healthier choices' (January 2008)

40 T. Jones et al., 'Enhanced adrenomedullary response and increased susceptibility to neuroglycopenia: Mechanisms underlying the adverse effects of sugar ingestion in healthy children', *Journal of Pediatrics*, Vol 126(2) (1995), pp. 171–7

41 T. MacKenzie et al., 'Metabolic and hormonal effects of caffeine: Randomized, double-blind, placebo-controlled crossover trial', *Metabolism: Clinical and Experimental*, Vol 56(12) (2007), pp. 1694–8

42 L. L. Moisey et al., 'Caffeinated coffee consumption impairs blood glucose homeostasis in response to high and low glycemic index meals in healthy men', *American Journal of Clinical Nutrition*, Vol 87(5) (2008), pp. 1254–61; see also D. S. Battram et al., 'Caffeine's Impairment of insulin-mediated glucose disposal cannot be solely attributed to adrenaline in humans', *Journal of Physiology*, Vol 583(3) (2007), pp. 1069–77

43 D. E. Thomas, E. J. Elliott and L. Baur, 'Low glycemic index or low glycemic load diets for overweight and obesity', *Cochrane Database of Systematic Reviews*, Issue 3 (2007), Art. No.: CD005105. DOI: 10.1002/14651858.CD005105.pub2

44 M. Slabber et al., 'Effects of a low-insulin-response, energy-restricted diet on weight loss and plasma insulin concentrations in hyperinsulinemic obese females', *American Journal of Clinical Nutrition*, Vol 60(1) (1994), pp. 48–53

45 C. Bouché et al., 'Five-week, low-glycemic index diet decreases total fat mass and improves plasma lipid profile in moderately overweight nondiabetic men', *Diabetes Care*, Vol 25(5) (May 2002), pp. 822–8

46 C. Ebbeling et al., 'A reduced glycemic load diet in the treatment of adolescent obesity', *Archives of Pediatrics and Adolescent Medicine*, Vol 157 (2003), pp. 773–9

47 S. A. La Haye et al., 'Comparison between a low glycemic load diet and a Canada Food Guide diet in cardiac rehabilitation patients in Ontario', *Canadian Journal of Cardiology*, Vol 21(6) (2005), pp. 489–94

48 Y. W. Aude et al., 'The national cholesterol education program diet vs a diet lower in carbohydrates and higher in protein and monounsaturated fat: a randomized trial', *Archives of Internal Medicine*, Vol 164(19) (2004), pp. 2141–6

49 B. Brehm et al., 'A randomized trial comparing a very low carbohydrate diet and a calorie-restricted low-fat diet on body weight and cardiovascular risk factors in healthy women', *Journal of Clinical Endocrinology and Metabolism*, Vol 88(4) (2003), pp. 1617–23

50 I. Shai et al., 'Weight loss with a low-carbohydrate, Mediterranean, or low-fat diet', *New England Journal of Medicine*, Vol 359(3) (2008), pp. 229–41

51 A. E. Field et al., 'Relation between dieting and weight change among preadolescents and adolescents', *Pediatrics*, Vol 112(4) (2003), pp. 900–6

52 M. and A. Wynn, 'How dieting can damage your health', *Which? Way to Health* (February 1995), pp. 22–4

53 P. Holford et al., 'The effects of a low glycemic load diet on weight loss and key health risk indicators', *Journal of Orthomolecular Medicine*, Vol 21(2) (2006), pp. 71–8

54 P. Maconaghie, 'A comparison of the metabolic diet with the Unislim diet for inducing weight loss', ION, 1988

Part Two

1 A.W. Barclay et al., 'Glycemic index, glycemic load, and chronic disease risk – a meta-analysis of observational studies', *American Journal of Clinical Nutrition*, Vol 87(3) (2008), pp. 627–37

2 Nutrient Data Laboratory, Beltsville Human Nutrition Research Center (BHNRC), Agricultural Research Service (ARS), US Department of Agriculture (USDA) in collaboration with Arkansas Children's Nutrition Center, ARS, USDA, Little Rock, AR *Oxygen Radical Absorbance Capacity (ORAC) of Selected Foods* (2007)

3 S. E. Vollset et al., 'Plasma total homocysteine and cardiovascular and noncardiovascular mortality: The Hordaland Homocysteine Study', *American Journal of Clinical Nutrition*, Vol 74(1) (2001), pp. 130–6

4 D. Xu, R. Neville and T. Finkel, 'Homocysteine accelerates endothelial cell senescence', *Federation of European Biochemical Societies Letters*, Vol 470 (2000), pp. 20–4

5 D. Fergusson et al., 'Association between suicide attempts and selective serotonin reuptake inhibitors: Systematic review of randomised controlled trials', *British Medical Journal*, Vol 330 (2005), pp. 396–9

6 R. Wurtman and J. Wurtman, 'Carbohydrates and depression', *Scientific American*, Vol 260(1) (1989), pp. 68–75

7 Dr Malcolm McLeod, *Lifting depression: The chromium connection*, Basic Health Publications (2005)

8 J. R. Davidson et al., 'Effectiveness of chromium in atypical depression: A placebo-controlled trial', *Biology, Psychiatry*, Vol 53(3) (2003), pp. 261–4

9 J. Docherty et al., 'A double-blind, placebo-controlled, exploratory trial of chromium picolinate in atypical depression', *Journal of Psychiatric Practice*, Vol 11(5) (2005), pp. 302–14

10 D. Benton et al., 'Mild hypoglycaemia and questionnaire measures of aggression', *Biological Psychology*, Vol 14(1–2) (1982), pp. 129–35; A. Roy et al., 'Monoamines, glucose metabolism, aggression toward self and others', *International Journal of Neuroscience*, Vol 41(3–4) (1988), pp. 261–4; A. G. Schauss, *Diet, Crime and Delinquency*, Parker House (1980); M. Virkkunen, 'Reactive hypoglycaemic tendency among arsonists', *Acta Psychiatrica Scandinavica*, Vol 69(5) (1984), pp. 445–52; M. Virkkunen and S. Narvanen, 'Tryptophan and serotonin levels during the glucose tolerance test among habitually violent and impulsive offenders', *Neuropsychobiology*, Vol 17(1–2) (1987), pp. 19–23; J. Yaryura-Tobias and F. Neziroglu, 'Violent behaviour, brain dysrythmia and glucose dysfunction: A new syndrome', *Journal of Orthomolecular Psychiatry*, Vol 4 (1975), pp. 182–5

11 M. Bruce and M. Lader, 'Caffeine abstention and the management of anxiety disorders', *Psychological Medicine*, Vol 19 (1989), pp. 211–14; W. Wendel and W. Beebe, 'Glycolytic activity in schizophrenia', in D. Hawkins and L. Pauling (eds), *Journal of Orthomolecular Psychiatry* (1973)

12 R. Prinz and D. Riddle, 'Associations between nutrition and behaviour in 5 year old children', *Nutrition Reviews*, Vol 43 (1986), suppl.

13 L. Christensen, 'Psychological distress and diet – effects of sucrose and caffeine', *Journal of Applied Nutrition*, Vol 40(1) (1988), pp. 44–50

14 Fullerton et al., 'Sugar, opionoids and binge eating', *Brain Research Bulletin*, Vol 14(6) (1985), pp. 273–80

15 L. Christensen, 'Psychological distress and diet – effects of sucrose and caffeine', *Journal of Applied Nutrition*, Vol 40(1) (1988), pp. 44–50

16 M. Colgan and L. Colgan, 'Do nutrient supplements and dietary changes affect learning and emotional reactions of children with learning difficulties? A controlled series of 16 cases', *Nutrition and Health*, Vol 3 (1984), pp. 69–77; J. Goldman et al., 'Behavioural effects of sucrose on preschool children', *Journal of Abnormal Child Psychology*, Vol 14(4) (1986), pp. 565–77; M. Lester et al., 'Refined carbohydrate intake, hair cadmium levels and cognitive functioning in children', *Nutrition and Behaviour*, Vol 1 (1982), pp. 3–13; S. Schoenthaler et al., 'The impact of low food additive and sucrose diet on academic performance in 803 New York City public schools', *International Journal of Biosocial Research*, Vol 8(2) (1986), pp. 185–95

17 M. Morris et al., 'Vitamin E and vitamin C supplement use and risk incident Alzheimer disease', *Alzheimer's Disease and Associated Disorders*, Vol 12 (1998), pp. 121–6; M. Morris et al., 'Dietary intake of antioxidant nutrients and the risk of incident AD', *Journal of the American Medical Association*, Vol 287(24) (2002), pp. 3230–7; see also pp. 3223–61; M. Sano et al., 'A controlled trial of selegiline, alpha tocopherol or both as treatment of AD', *New England Journal of Medicine*, Vol 336 (1997), pp. 1216–22

18 N. Scarmeas, 'Mediterranean diet and risk for Alzheimer's disease', *Annals of Neurology*, Vol 59(6) (2006), pp. 912–21; also see N. Scarmeas et al., 'Mediterranean diet and Alzheimer disease mortality', *Neurology*, Vol 69(11) (2007), pp. 1084–93

19 S. Seshadri et al., 'Plasma homocysteine as a risk factor for dementia and AD', *New England Journal of Medicine*, Vol 346(7) (2002), pp. 476–83

20 R. M. Sapolsky, 'Why stress is bad for your brain', *Science*, Vol 273(5276) (1996), pp. 749–50

21 P. Holford et al., 'The effects of a low glycemic load diet on weight loss and key health risk indicators', *Journal of Orthomolecular Medicine*, Vol 21(2) (2006), pp. 71–8

22 D. S. Ludwig, 'The Glycemic Index', *Journal of the American Medical Association*, Vol 287(18) (2002), pp. 2414–23

23 A. L. Albright (President for HealthCare and Education) and E. Gregg (Chief of Diabetes Epidemiology, CDC), 'Economic Cost of Diabetes in the U.S. in 2007', American Diabetes Association (2008)

24 D. S. Ludwig et al., 'Hepatic steatosis and increased adiposity in mice consuming rapidly vs. slowly absorbed carbohydrate', *Obesity*, Vol 15(9) (2007), pp. 2190–9

25 C. L. Rohlfing et al., 'Use of GHb (HbA1c) in screening for undiagnosed diabetes in the U.S. Population', *Diabetes Care*, Vol 23(2) (2000), pp. 187–191; see also D. Edelman et al., 'Utility of hemoglobin A1c in predicting diabetes risk', *Journal of General Internal Medicine*, Vol 19(12) (2004), pp. 1175–80

26 Tao Xia, 'Hypoglycaemic role of *Cucurbita ficifolia* (Cucurbitaceae) fruit extract in streptozotocin-induced diabetic rats', *Journal of the Science of Food and Agriculture*, Vol 87(9) (2007), pp. 1753–7

27 K. W. Liu et al., 'Metformin-related vitamin B12 deficiency', *Age and Ageing*, Vol 35 (2006), pp. 200–1

28 S. Hexeberg and F. Lindberg, 'Insulin using woman with type 2 diabetes and weight problems', *Tidsskrift for den Norske laegeforening*, Vol 128(4) (2008), pp. 443–5

29 C. Ebbeling, 'Effect of a low-glycemic load vs low-fat diet in obese young adults: A randomized trial', *Journal of the American Medical Association*, Vol 297(19) (2007), pp. 2092–102

30 S. W. Rizkalla et al., 'Improved plasma glucose control, whole-body glucose utilization, and lipid profile on a low-glycemic index diet in type 2 diabetic men: A randomized controlled trial', *Diabetes Care*, Vol 27(8) (2004), pp. 1866–72

31 D. Bell et al., 'Do sulfonylurea drugs increase the risk of cardiac events?', *The Canadian Medical Association Journal*, Vol 174(2) (2006), pp. 185–6

32 J. D. Williamson et al., 'The action to control cardiovascular risk in diabetes memory in diabetes study (Accord-Mind): Rationale, design, and methods', *The American Journal of Cardiology*, Vol 99(12A) (2007), pp. 112i–122i

33 No authors listed, 'The University Group Diabetes Program: A study of the effects of hypoglycemic agents on vascular complications in patients with adult-onset diabetes. V. Evaluation of pheniformin therapy', *Diabetes*, Vol 24(suppl. 1) (1975), pp. 65–184

34 T. Orchard et al., 'The effect of Metformin and intensive lifestyle intervention on the metabolic syndrome: The diabetes prevention program randomized trial', *Annual of International Medicine*, Vol 142(8) (2005), pp. 611–19

35 C. K. Roberts et al., 'Effect of a diet and exercise intervention on oxidative stress, inflammation, MMP-9, and monocyte chemotactic activity in men with metabolic syndrome factors', *Journal of Applied Physiology* (2005/2006)

36 J. Wylie-Rosett et al., 'Lifestyle intervention to prevent diabetes: Intensive and cost effective, *Current Opinion in Lipidology*, Vol 17(1) (2006), pp. 37–44

37 D. E. Thomas et al., 'Exercise for type 2 diabetes mellitus', *Cochrane Database of Systematic Reviews (online)*, Vol (3) (July 2006), CD002968

38 J. R. Palmer et al., 'Sugar-sweetened beverages and incidence of type 2 diabetes mellitus in African American women', *Archives of Internal Medicine*, Vol 168(14) (2008), pp. 1487–92; L. F. Tinkler et al., 'Low-fat dietary pattern and risk of treated diabetes mellitus in postmenopausal women: The Women's Health Initiative randomized controlled dietary modification trial', *Archives of Internal Medicine*, Vol 168(14) (2008), pp. 1500–11

39 R. Villegas et al., 'Prospective study of dietary carbohydrates, glycemic index, glycemic load, and incidence of type 2 diabetes mellitus in middle-aged Chinese women', *Archives of Internal Medicine*, Vol 167(21) (2007), pp. 2310–16

40 K. Murakami et al., 'Dietary glycemic index and load in relation to metabolic risk factors in Japanese female farmers with traditional dietary habits', *American Journal of Clinical Nutrition*, Vol 83(5) (2006), pp. 1161–9

41 A. W. Barclay et al., 'Glycemic index, dietary fiber, and risk of type 2 diabetes in a cohort of older Australians', *Diabetes Care*, Vol 30(11) (2007), pp. 2811–13

42 T. Halton et al., 'Low-carbohydrate-diet score and risk of type 2 diabetes in women', *American Journal of Clinical Nutrition*, Vol 87(2) (2008), pp. 339–46

43 I. Shai et al., 'Weight loss with a low-carbohydrate, Mediterranean, or low-fat diet', *New England Journal of Medicine*, Vol 359(3) (July 2008), pp. 229–41

44 H. M. Dashti et al., 'Beneficial effects of ketogenic diet in obese diabetic subjects', *Molecular and Cellular Biochemistry*, Vol 302(1–2) (2007), pp. 249–56; Y. Miyashita et al., 'Beneficial effect of low carbohydrate in low calorie diets on visceral fat reduction in type 2 diabetic patients with obesity', *Diabetes Research and Clinical Practice*, Vol 65(3) (2004), pp. 235–41; see also, J. V. Nielsen and E. Joensson, 'Low-carbohydrate diet in type 2 diabetes. Stable improvement

of bodyweight and glycaemic control during 22 months follow-up', *Nutrition & Metabolism*, Vol 3(22) (2006)

45 Prof. M. A. Mart'nez-González et al., 'Adherence to Mediterranean diet and risk of developing diabetes: Prospective cohort study', *British Medical Journal*, Vol 336 (2008), pp. 1348–51

46 V. M. Montori, 'Waking up from the DREAM of preventing diabetes with drugs', *British Medical Journal*, Vol 334 (2007), pp. 882–4

47 R. A. Anderson et al., 'Elevated intakes of supplemental chromium improve glucose and insulin variables in individuals with type 2 diabetes, *Diabetes*, Vol 46(11) (1997), pp. 1786–91

48 H. Rabinovitz et al., 'Effect of chromium supplementation on blood glucose and lipid levels in type 2 diabetes mellitus elderly patients', *International Journal of Vitamin and Nutrition Research*, Vol 74(3) (2004), pp. 178–182

49 N. Cheng et al., 'Follow-up survey of people in China with type 2 diabetes mellitus consuming supplemental chromium', *Journal of Trace Elements in Experimental Medicine*, Vol 12(2) (1999), pp. 55–60

50 E. Balk et al., 'Effect of chromium supplementation on glucose metabolism and lipids: A systematic review of randomized controlled trials', *Diabetes Care*, Vol 30(8) (2007), pp. 2154–63

51 Food Standards Agency, 'Agency revises chromium picolinate advice' (2004), (see www.food.gov.uk)

52 H. Rabinovitz et al., 'Effect of chromium supplementation on blood glucose and lipid levels in type 2 diabetes mellitus elderly patients', *International Journal of Vitamin and Nutrition Research*, Vol 74(3) (2004), pp. 178–82

53 R. A. Anderson, 'Elevated intakes of supplemental chromium improve glucose and insulin variables in individuals with type 2 diabetes', *Diabetes*, Vol 46 (1997), pp. 1786–91; see also A. Ravina et al., 'Clinical use of the trace element chromium (III) in the treatment of diabetes mellitus', *Journal of Trace Elements in Medicine and Biology*, Vol 8 (1995), pp. 183–190

54 A. H. Harding et al., 'Plasma vitamin C level, fruit and vegetable consumption, and the risk of new-onset type 2 diabetes mellitus: The European prospective investigation of cancer – Norfolk Prospective Study', *Archives of Internal Medicine*, Vol 168(14) (2008), pp. 1493–9

55 M. Afkhami-Ardekani and A. Shojaoddiny-Ardekani, 'Effect of vitamin C on blood glucose, serum lipids and serum insulin in type 2 diabetes patients', *Indian Journal of Medical Research*, Vol 126(5) (2007), pp. 471–4

56 E. J. Verspohl et al., 'Antidiabetic effect of *Cinnamoncassia* and *Cinnamomum zeylanicum* in vivo and in vitro', *Phytotherapy Research*, Vol 19 (2005), pp. 203–6

57 S. H. Kim et al., 'Anti-diabetic effect of cinnamon extract on blood glucose in db/db mice', *Journal of Ethnopharmacology*, Vol 104(1–2) (2006), pp. 119–23

58 T. N. Ziegenfuss et al., 'Effects of a water-soluble cinnamon extract on body composition and features of the metabolic syndrome in pre-diabetic men and women', *Journal of the International Society of Sports Nutrition*, Vol 3(2) (2006), pp. 45–53

59 A. Khan et al., 'Cinnamon improves glucose and lipids of people with type 2 diabetes', *Diabetes Care*, Vol 26(12) (2003), pp. 3215–18

60 R. J. Sigal et al., 'Physical activity/exercise and type 2 diabetes', *Diabetes Care*, Vol 27 (2004), pp. 2518–39

61 L. Djoussé and J. M. Gaziano, 'Egg consumption in relation to cardiovascular disease and mortality: The Physicians' Health Study 1–3, *American Journal of Clinical Nutrition*, Vol 87 (2008), pp. 964–9

62 S. B. Kritchevsky, 'A review of scientific research and recommendations regarding gs', *Journal of American College of Nutrition*, Vol 23(6) (2004), pp. 596S–600S; also see A. L. Qureshi et al., 'Regular egg consumption does not increase the risk of stroke and cardiovascular diseases', *Medical Science Monitor*, Vol 13(1) (2007), pp. CR1–8; see also Y. Nakamura et al., 'Egg consumption, serum total cholesterol concentrations and coronary heart disease incidence: Japan Public Health Center-based prospective study', *British Journal of Nutrition*, Vol 96(5) (2006), pp. 921–8

63 J. V. Wal et al., 'Egg breakfast enhances weight loss', *International Journal of Obesity*, (August 2008); see also J. S. Vander et al., 'Short term effect of eggs on satiety in overweight and obese subjects', *Journal of the American College of Nutrition*, Vol 24(6) (2005), pp. 510–15; see also N. V. Dhurandhar, 'Egg breakfast enhances weight loss', *International Journal of Obesity*, (August 2008)

64 H. R. Hellstrom, 'The altered homeostatic theory: A hypothesis proposed to be useful in understanding and preventing ischemic heart disease, hypertension, and diabetes – including reducing the risk of age and atherosclerosis', *Medical Hypotheses*, Vol 68(2) (2007), pp. 415–33

65 S. Boseley, 'Heart disease: US doctors back statins for 8 year olds', *Guardian* (9 July 2008)

66 T. L. Halton et al., 'Low-carbohydrate-diet score and the risk of coronary heart disease in women', *New England Journal of Medicine*, Vol 355 (2006), pp. 1991–2002

67 S. Liu et al., 'A prospective study of dietary glycemic load, carbohydrate intake and risk of coronary heart disease in US women', *American Journal of Clinical Nutrition*, Vol 6 (2000), pp. 1455–61

68 D. Ludwig, 'The glycemic index', *Journal of the American Medical Association*, Vol 287(18) (2002), pp. 2414–23

69 D. E. Thomas, E. J. Elliott, L. Baur, 'Low glycaemic index or low glycaemic load diets for overweight and obesity', *Cochrane Database of Systematic Reviews*, issue 3. Art. No.: CD005105. DOI: 10.1002/14651858.CD005105.pub2. (2007)

70 C. B. Ebbeling et al., 'Effects of an *ad libitum* low-glycemic load diet on cardiovascular disease risk factors in obese young adults', *American Journal of Clinical Nutrition*, Vol 81(5) (2005), pp. 976–82; also see B. Sloth et al., 'No difference in body weight decrease between a low-glycemic-index and a high-glycemic-index diet but reduced LDL cholesterol after 10-wk *ad libitum* intake of the low-glycemic-index diet', *American Journal of Clinical Nutrition*, Vol 80(2) (2004), pp. 337–47

71 J. McMillan-Price et al., 'Comparison of 4 Diets of varying glycemic load on weight loss and cardiovascular risk reduction in overweight and obese young adults', *Archives of Internal Medicine*, Vol 166, pp. 1466–75

72 David Jenkins et al., 'Effect on blood lipids of very high intakes of fiber in diets low in saturated fat and cholesterol', *New England Journal of Medicine*, Vol 329 (1999), pp. 21–6

73 D. J. Jenkins, 'A dietary portfolio approach to cholesterol reduction: Combined effects of plant sterols, vegetable proteins, and viscous fibers in hypercholesterolemia', *Metabolism*, Vol 51(12) (2002), pp. 1596–1604

74 D. J. Jenkins et al., 'Direct comparison of a dietary portfolio of cholesterol-lowering foods with a statin in hypercholesterolemic participants', *American Journal of Clinical Nutrition*, Vol 81(2) (2005), pp. 380–7; see also: D. J. Jenkins et al., 'Assessment of the longer-term effects of a dietary portfolio of cholesterol-lowering foods in hypercholesterolemia', *American Journal of Clinical Nutrition*, Vol 83(3) (2006), pp. 582–91

75 M. W. Brands et al., 'Obesity and hypertension: Roles of hyperinsulinemia, sympathetic nervous system and intrarenal mechanisms', *Journal of Nutrition*, Vol 125(6) (1995), pp. 1725–31

76 P. Holford et al., 'The effects of a low glycemic load diet on weight loss and key health risk indicators', *Journal of Orthomolecular Medicine*, Vol 21(2) (2006), pp. 71–8

77 G. Yang et al., 'Longitudinal study of soy food intake and blood pressure among middle-aged and elderly Chinese women', *American Journal of Clinical Nutrition*, Vol 81(5) (2005), pp. 1012–17

78 Department of Health, 'Nutritional aspects of cardiovascular disease' (1994)

79 World Cancer Research Fund, 'Food, nutrition and the prevention of cancer: A global perspective' (1997)

80 P. Lichtenstein et al., 'Environmental and heritable factors in the causation of cancer—analyses of cohorts of twins from Sweden, Denmark, and Finland', *New England Journal of Medicine*, Vol 343(2) (2000), pp. 78–85

81 A. Eliassen et al., 'Adult weight change and risk of postmenopausal breast cancer', *Journal of the American Medical Association*, Vol 296(2) (2006), pp. 193–201

82 A. Tavani et al., 'Consumption of sweet foods and breast cancer risk in Italy', *Annals of Oncology*, Vol 17(2) (2006), pp. 341–5; see also S. Sieri et al., 'Dietary glycemic index, glycemic load, and the risk of breast cancer in an Italian prospective cohort study', *American Journal of Clinical Nutrition*, Vol 86(4) (2007), pp. 1160–6

83 S. E. McCann et al., 'Dietary patterns related to glycemic index and load and risk of premenopausal and postmenopausal breast cancer in the Western New York Exposure and Breast Cancer Study', *American Journal of Clinical Nutrition*, Vol 86(2) (2007), pp. 465–71; see also M. Lajous, 'Carbohydrate intake, glycemic index, glycemic load, and risk of postmenopausal breast cancer in a prospective study of French women', *American Journal of Clinical Nutrition*, Vol 87(5) (2008), pp. 1384–91

84 S. A. Silvera et al., 'Glycaemic index, glycaemic load and ovarian cancer risk: A prospective cohort study', *Public Health Nutrition*, Vol 10(10) (2007), pp. 1076–81

85 S. A. Silvera et al., 'Glycaemic index, glycaemic load and risk of endometrial cancer: A prospective cohort study', *Public Health Nutrition*, Vol 8 (7) (2005), pp. 912–19; see also S. C. Larsson et al., 'Carbohydrate intake, glycemic index and glycemic load in relation to risk of endometrial cancer: A prospective study of Swedish women', *International Journal of Cancer*, Vol 120(5) (2007), pp. 1103–7

86 G. Randi et al., 'Glycemic index, glycemic load and thyroid cancer risk', *Annals of Oncology*, Vol 19(2) (2008), pp. 380–3

87 J. A. Darbinian, 'Glycemic status and risk of prostate cancer', *Cancer Epidemiology, Biomarkers and Prevention*, Vol 17(3) (2008), pp. 628–35

88 P. Gnagnarella et al., 'Glycemic index, glycemic load, and cancer risk: A meta-analysis', *American Journal of Clinical Nutrition*, Vol 87(6) (2008), pp. 1793–801

89 G. C. Kabat et al., 'Dietary carbohydrate, glycemic index, and glycemic load in relation to colorectal cancer risk in the Women's Health Initiative', *Cancer Causes and Control* (July 2008) [Epub ahead of print]

Part Three

1 Y. Granfeldt et al., 'On the importance of processing conditions, product thickness and egg addition for the glycaemic and hormonal responses to pasta: A comparison of bread made with "pasta ingredients"', *European Journal of Clinical Nutrition*, Vol 45 (1991), pp. 489–99

2 M. Sadiq Butt et al., 'Oat: unique among the cereals', *European Journal of Nutrition*, Vol 47(2) (2008), pp. 68–79

3 H. Delargy et al., 'Effects of amount and type of dietary fibre (soluble and insoluble) on short-term control of appetite', *International Journal of Food Sciences and Nutrition*, Vol 48 (1997), pp. 67–77

4 H. Kissilef, *American Journal of Physiology*, 238 (1980), pp. 14–22; S. Konnyyaku, *Agricultural Biological Chemistry*, Vol 34(4) (1970), pp. 641–3; M. Matsuura, *Japanese Diabetic Association*, Vol 23(3) (1980), pp. 209–17

5 A. Mito, data held in ION library, source unknown

6 D. Walsh, unpublished study at GNC Research Center, Fargo, North Dakota (1982)

7 P. Holford, 'The Effects of Glucomannan on Weight Loss', ION (1983)

8 D. Jenkins et al., 'Glycemic index of foods: A physiological basis for carbohydrate exchange', *American Journal of Clinical Nutrition*, Vol 34 (1980), pp. 362–6

9 C. B. Pert, *The Molecules of Emotion*, Pocket Books (1999)

10 J. Cleary et al., 'Naloxone effects of sugar-motivated behaviour', *Psychpharmacology*, Vol 176 (1996), pp. 110–14; S. A. Czirr and L. D. Reid, 'Demonstrating morphine's potentiating effects on sucrose-intake', *Brain Research Bulletin*, Vol 17 (1986), pp. 639–42; E. Blass et al., 'Interactions between sucrose, pain, isolation distress', *Pharmacology, Biochemistry of Behaviour*, Vol 26 (1986), pp. 483–9; L. Leventhal et al., 'Selective actions of central mu and kappa opioid antagonists upon sucrose intake in sham-fed rats', *Brain Research*, Vol 685 (1995), pp. 205–10; A. Moles and S. Cooper, 'Opioid modulation of sucrose intake in CD-1 mice', *Physiology and Behaviour*, Vol 58 (1995), pp. 791–96; E. Cheraskin and W. M. Ringsdorf, 'A biochemical denominator in the primary prevention of alcoholism', *Journal of Orthomolecular Psychiatry*, Vol 9(3) (1980), pp. 158–63

11 G. B. Keijzers et al., 'Caffeine can decrease insulin sensitivity in humans', *Diabetes Care*, Vol 25(2) (2002), pp. 364–9

12 N. J. Richardson et al., 'Mood and performance effects of caffeine in relation to acute and chronic caffeine deprivation', *Pharmacology, Biochemistry and Behavior*, Vol 52(2) (1995), pp. 313–20

13 L. L. Moisey et al., 'Caffeinated coffee consumption impairs blood glucose homeostasis in response to high and low glycemic index meals in healthy men', *American Journal of Clinical Nutrition*, Vol 87(5) (2008), pp. 1254–61

14 A. Hartz et al., 'Randomized controlled trial of Siberian ginseng for chronic fatigue', *Psychological Medicine*, Vol 34 (2004), pp. 51–61

15 ONUK survey, 'A Comparison of the health and nutrition of over 37,000 people in Britain and the effects of improving nutrition in a Cohort over 3 months', Institute for Optimum Nutrition, London (2004)

16 C. Ebbeling et al., 'A reduced-glycemic load diet in the treatment of obesity', *Archives of Pediatrics and Adolescent Medicine*, Vol 157(8) (2003), pp. 773–9

17 P. Y. Lin and K. P. Su, 'A meta-analytic review of double-blind, placebo-controlled trials of antidepressant efficacy of omega-3 fatty acids', *Journal of Clinical Psychiatry*, Vol 68(7) (2007), pp. 1056–61

18 J. N. Din et al., 'Omega-3 fatty acids and cardiovascular disease: Fishing for a natural treatment', *British Medical Journal*, Vol 328 (2004), pp. 30–5

19 R. J. Goldberg and J. Katz, 'A meta-analysis of the analgesic effects of omega-3 polyunsaturated fatty acid supplementation for inflammatory joint pain', *Pain*, Vol 129(1–2) (2007), pp. 210–23

20 A. Garg, 'High mono-unsaturated fat diets for patients with diabetes mellitus: A meta-analysis', *American Journal of Clinical Nutrition*, Vol 67 (suppl) (1998) pp. 577S–582S; T. Hung et al., 'Fat versus carbohydrate in insulin resistance, obesity, diabetes and cardiovascular disease', *Current Opinion in Clinical Nutrition and Metabolic Care*, Vol 6(2) (2003), pp. 165–76

21 C. Bolton-Smith et al., 'Dietary composition and fat to sugar ratios in relation to obesity', *International Journal of Obesity*, Vol 18 (1994), pp. 820–8

22 David Frahm, 'How to help your thyroid with virgin coconut oil' *Health Quarters Monthly*, Vol 58, August 2003

23 C. M. Albert et al., 'Blood levels of long-chain n-3 fatty acids and the risk of sudden death', *New England Journal of Medicine*, Vol 346(15) (2002), pp. 1113–18

24 M. Morris et al., 'Consumption of fish and n-3 fatty acids and risk of incident Alzheimer disease', *Archives of Neurology*, Vol 60(7) (2003), pp. 940–6

25 J. Geleijnse et al., 'Reduction on blood pressure with a low sodium, high potassium, high magnesium salt in older subjects with mild to moderate hypertension', *British Medical Journal*, Vol 309 (1994), pp. 436–40

26 Wilders-Truschnig et al., 'IgG antibodies against food antigens are correlated with inflammation and intima media thickness in obese juveniles', *Experimental and Clinical Endocrinology and Diabetes*, Vol 116(4) (2008), pp. 241–5

27 T. Gerarduzzi et al., 'Celiac disese in USA among risk groups and general population in USA', *Journal of Pediatric Gastroenterology and Nutrition*, Vol 31 (2000), pp. 104

28 R. Sur et al., 'Avenanthramides, polyphenols from oats, exhibit anti-inflammatory and anti-itch activity', *Archives of Dermatalogical Research* (2008) [Epub ahead of print]

29 R. Williams, *The Wonderful World Within You*, BioCommunications Press (1998)

30 'The Vitamin Controversy', ION (1988)

31 R. Wunderlich, *Sugar and Your Health*, Good Health Publications (1982)

32 S. Davies, 'Zinc, nutrition and health', *1984/5 Yearbook of Nutritional Medicine* (1985)

33 S. Davies et al., 'Age-related decreases in chromium levels in 51,665 hair, sweat and serum samples from 40,872 patients – implications for the prevention of cardiovascular disease and type II diabetes mellitus', *Metabolism*, Vol 46(5) (1997), pp. 1–4

34 G. Evans, 'The effect of chromium picolinate on insulin controlled parameters in humans', *International Journal of Biosocial & Medical Research*, Vol 11(2), 1989, pp. 163–80

35 E. Balk et al., 'Effect of chromium supplementation on glucose metabolism and lipids: A systematic review of randomized controlled trials', *Diabetes Care*, Vol 30(8) (2007), pp. 2154–63; see also R. Riales et al., 'Effects of chromium chloride supplementation on glucose tolerance and serum lipids including high density lipoprotein of adult men', *American Journal of Clinical Nutrition*, Vol 34 (1981), pp. 2670–8; A. Abraham et al., 'The effects of chromium supplementation on serum glucose and lipids in patients with and without non-insulin-dependent diabetes', *Metabolism*, Vol 41 (1992), p. 768; W. Glinsmann et al., 'Effects of trivalent chromium on glucose tolerance', *Metabolism*, Vol 15 (1966), pp. 510–15; R. Levine et al., 'Effects of oral chromium supplementation on the glucose tolerance of elderly human subjects', *Metabolism*, Vol 17 (1968), pp. 114–24; K. Hambidge, 'Chromium: A review', in *Disorders of Mineral Metabolism Vol 1: Trace Minerals*, Academic Press (1981), pp. 272–94

36 M. H. Pittler, C. Stevinson and E. Ernst, 'Chromium picolinate for reducing body weight: Meta-analysis of randomized trials', *International Journal of Obesity Related Metabolic Disorders*, Vol 27(4) (2003), pp. 522–9

37 S. D. Anton et al., 'Effects of chromium picolinate on food intake and satiety', *Diabetes Technololgy and Therapeutics*, Vol 10(5) (2008), pp. 405–12

38 J. R. Davidson et al., 'Effectiveness of chromium in atypical depression: A placebo-controlled trial', *Biological Psychiatry*, Vol 53(3) (2003), pp. 261–4

39 T. Larsen et al., 'Efficacy and safety of dietary supplements containing CLA for the treatment of obesity: Evidence from animal and human studies', *Journal of Lipid Research*, Vol 44(12) (2003), pp. 2234–41

40 D. Clouatre and M. Rosenbaum, *The Diet and Health Benefits of HCA*, Keats Publishing (1994)

41 M. S. Westerterp-Plantenga and E. M. Kovacs, 'The effect of hydroxycitrate on energy intake and satiety in overweight humans', *International Journal of Obesity Related Metabolic Disorders*, Vol 26(6) (2002), pp. 870–2

42 H. G. Preuss et al., 'An overview of the safety and efficacy of a novel, natural(-)-hydroxycitric acid extract (HCA-SX) for weight management', *Journal of Medicine*, Vol 35(1–6) (2004), pp. 33–48

43 A. Amer et al., '5-Hydroxy-L-tryptophan suppresses food intake in food-deprived and stressed rats', *Pharmacology, Biochemistry and Behavior*, Vol 77(1) (2004), pp. 137–43

44 C. Cangiano et al., 'Eating behavior and adherence to dietary prescriptions in obese adult subjects treated with 5-hydroxytryptophan', *American Journal of Clinical Nutrition*, Vol 56(5) (1992), pp. 863–7

45 C. Cangiano et al., 'Effects of oral 5-hydroxy-tryptophan on energy intake and macronutrient selection in non-insulin dependent diabetic patients', *International Journal of Obesity Related Metabolic Disorders*, Vol 22(7) (1998), pp. 648–54

46 P. Holford et al., 'The effects of a low glycemic load diet on weight loss and key health risk indicators', *Journal of Orthomolecular Medicine*, Vol 21(2) (2006), pp 71–8

47 A. Prentice and S. Jebb, 'Obesity in Britain: Gluttony or sloth?', *British Medical Journal*, Vol 311 (1995), pp. 437–9

48 W. McArdle, chapter in *Medical Aspects of Clinical Nutrition*, Keats Publishing (1983)

49 D. E. Thomas et al., 'Exercise for type 2 diabetes mellitus', *Cochrane Database of Systematic Reviews*, Issue 3. Art. No.: CD002968. DOI: 10.1002/14651858.CD002968.pub2 (2006)

50 D. Broughton et al., 'Review: Deterioration of glucose tolerance with age: The role of insulin resistance', *Age and Ageing*, Vol 20 (1991), pp. 221–5

51 J. E. Manson et al., 'Physical activity and incidence of non-insulin-dependent diabetes mellitus in women', *Lancet*, Vol 338(8770) (1991), pp. 774–8

52 C. Hollenbeck et al., 'Effect of habitual exercise on regulation of insulin stimulated glucose disposal in older males', *Journal of American Geriatrics Society*, Vol 33 (1986), pp. 273–7

53 P. Ebelin et al., 'Mechanism of enhanced insulin sensitivity in athletes', *American Society for Clinical Investigations*, Vol 92 (1993), pp. 1623–31

Part Four

1 J. Warren et al., 'Low glycemic index breakfasts and reduced food intake in preadolescent children', *Pediatrics*, Vol 112(5), (2003) p. 414

2 D. Ludwig, 'Dietary glycemic index and regulation of body weight', *Lipids*, Vol 38(2) (2003), pp. 117–21

3 K. Heaton et al., 'Particle size of wheat, maize and oat test meals: Effects on plasma glucose and insulin responses and on the rate of starch digestion in vitro', *American Journal of Clinical Nutrition*, Vol 47 (1988), pp. 675–82

4 E. Cheraskin, 'The breakfast/lunch/dinner ritual', *Journal of Orthomolecular Medicine*, Vol 8(1) (1993), pp. 6–10

5 J. T. Braaten et al., 'High beta-glucan oat bran and oat gum reduce postprandial blood glucose and insulin in subjects with and without type 2 diabetes', *Diabetic Medicine*, Vol 11(3) (1994), pp. 312–18

Appendices

1 E. Knight et al., 'The effect of dietary protein intake on kidney function in women with normal or mildly abnormal kidneys', *Annals of Internal Medicine*, Vol 138(6) (2003), pp. 460–7

2 D. Feskanich et al., 'Protein consumption and bone fractures in women', *American Journal of Epidemiology*, Vol 143(5) (1996), pp. 472–9

3 L. Allen et al., 'Protein-induced hypercalcuria: A longer-term study', *American Journal of Clinical Nutrition*, Vol 32 (1979), pp. 741–9; C. Anand et al., 'Effect of protein intake on calcium balance of young men given 500mg calcium daily', *Journal of Nutrition*, Vol 104 (1974), pp. 695–700; S. Reddy et al., 'Effect of low-carbohydrate high-protein diets on acid-base balance, stone-forming propensity, and calcium metabolism', *American Journal of Kidney Diseases*, Vol 40 (2002), pp. 265–74

4 *Food, Nutrition and the Prevention of Cancer*, World Cancer Research Fund, American Institute for Cancer Research (1997)

5 A. Malin et al., 'Evaluation of the synergistic effect of insulin resistance and IGF on the risk of breast carcinoma', *Cancer*, Vol 100(4) (2004), pp. 694–700

6 S. E. Oliver et al., 'Screen-detected prostate cancer and IGF', *International Journal of Cancer*, Vol 108(6) (2004), pp. 887–92

7 H. Seeger, D. Wallwiener and A. O. Mueck, 'Influence of stroma-derived growth factors on the estradiol-stimulated proliferation of human breast cancer cells', *European Journal of Gynaecological Oncology*, Vol 25(2) (2004), pp. 175–7; D. W. Voskuil et al., 'Insulin-like growth factor (IGF)-system mRNA quantities in normal and tumor breast tissue of women with sporadic and familial breast cancer risk', *Breast Cancer Research and Treatment*, Vol 84(3) (2004), pp. 225–33; A. Malin et al., 'Evaluation of the synergistic effect of insulin resistance and insulin-like growth factors on the risk of breast carcinoma', *Cancer*, Vol 100(4) (2004), pp. 694–700

8 S. B. Sondike et al., 'Effects of a low-carbohydrate diet on weight loss and cardiovascular risk factor in overweight adolescents', *Journal of Pediatrics*, Vol 142(3) (2003), pp. 253–8

9 D. Gardner, presentation at European Society of Human Reproduction and Embryology, awaiting publication

Recommended Reading

CHAPTER 2
Geoffrey Cannon, *Dieting Makes You Fat*, Virgin Books (2008)
Jane Plant, *The Plant Diet*, Virgin (2003)

CHAPTER 5
Antony Haynes, *The Insulin Factor*, Thorsons (2004)

CHAPTER 7
Patrick Holford, *Beat Stress and Fatigue*, Piatkus (1999)

CHAPTER 9
Patrick Holford, *Optimum Nutrition Bible*, Piatkus (2004)
Patrick Holford, *New Optimum Nutrition For the Mind*, Piatkus (2007)

CHAPTER 10
Charles Clarke and Maureen Clarke, *Diabetes Revolution*, Vermilion (2008)
Dr Fedon Lindberg, *Greek Doctor's Diet*, Rodale International Ltd (2005)

CHAPTER 11
Patrick Holford and Dr James Braly, *The H Factor*, Piatkus (1999)
Patrick Holford and Jerome Burne, *Food is Better Medicine than Drugs*, Piatkus (2008)

CHAPTER 12
Patrick Holford, *Say No to Arthritis*, Piatkus (1999)

CHAPTER 13
Anthony Leeds et al., *The GI Factor*, Hodder & Stoughton (1996)

CHAPTER 14
Udo Erasmus, *Fats that Heal, Fats that Kill*, Alive Books (1987, rev. 1994)

CHAPTER 15
Patrick Holford and Dr James Braly, *Hidden Food Allergies*, Piatkus (2005)
Dr James Braly and Ron Hoggan, *Dangerous Grains*, Avery Publishing Group (2002)

CHAPTER 16
Patrick Holford, *The Optimum Nutrition Bible*, Piatkus (1997, rev. 2004)

CHAPTER 28
Oscar Ichazo, *Master Level Exercise: Psychocalisthenics*, Sequoia Press (1993)
Brian Sharkey, *Fitness and Health*, Human Kinetics Europe Ltd (2003)

CHAPTER 30
Barry Durrant-Peatfield, *The Great Thyroid Scandal and How to Survive It*, Barons Down Publishing (2003)
Kate Neil and Patrick Holford, *Balancing Hormones Naturally*, Piatkus (1998)

CHAPTERS 32–34
Patrick Holford and Judy Ridgway, *The Optimum Nutrition Cookbook*, Piatkus (2001)
Patrick Holford and Fiona McDonald Joyce, *The Low-GL Diet Cookbook*, Piatkus (2005)
Patrick Holford and Fiona McDonald Joyce, *Food GLorious Food*, Piatkus (2008)
Patrick Holford and Fiona McDonald Joyce, *The Holford Low-GL Diet Made Easy*, Piatkus (2006)

Resources

Eating disorders

If you have a concern about eating disorders I recommend you contact BEAT, 103 Prince of Wales Road, Norwich NR1 1DW. Adult helpline: 0845 634 1414; Youthline: 0845 634 7650 or go to www.beat.co.uk.

Institute for Optimum Nutrition (ION)

The Institute for Optimum Nutrition (ION) offers a three-year foundation degree course in nutritional therapy that includes training in the optimum nutrition approach to mental health. There is a clinic, a list of nutrition practitioners across the UK, an information service and a quarterly journal: *Optimum Nutrition*.

Contact ION at Avalon House, 72 Lower Mortlake Road, Richmond TW9 2JY, or call 020 8614 7800, or visit www.ion.ac.uk.

To find a nutritional therapist near you who we recommend, visit www.patrickholford.com and click on 'consultations'.

Nutrition Consultations

For a personal referral by Patrick Holford to a nutritional therapist in your area, visit www.patrickholford.com and select 'consultations' for an immediate online referral. This service gives details on whom to see in the UK as well as internationally. If there is no one available near by you can always do an online assessment – see below.

Nutrition Assessment Online

You can have your own personal health and nutrition assessment online using my 100% Health Check. This gives you a personalised assessment of your current health, and what you most need to change in order to lose weight and feel great. Visit www.patrickholford.com and go to 'free on-line assessment'.

Psychocalisthenics

The excellent exercise system Psychocalisthenics takes less than 20 minutes a day, develops strength, suppleness and stamina, and generates vital energy. The best way to learn it is to do the Psychocalisthenics Training. See www.patrickholford.com (seminars and workshops) for details on these, or call +44 (0)1252 782661. Also available is the book *Master Level Exercise: Psychocalisthenics*, and the *Psychocalisthenics* CD and DVD. For further information please see www.metafitness.com.

Salt alternatives – Solo Sodium Sea Salt

The average person gets far too much sodium because we eat too much salt (sodium chloride) and salted foods, and not enough potassium and magnesium, found in fruits and vegetables. Not all salt, however, is bad for you. Solo Low Sodium Sea Salt contains 60 per cent less sodium and is high in the essential minerals of magnesium and potassium. Solo Low Sodium Sea Salt is sold in UK, Ireland, Spain, the Netherlands, Singapore, Hong Kong, Japan, Bahrain, Saudi Arabia, United Arab Emirates, Jordan, the Baltic States and the United States of America. Visit their website, www.soloseasalt.com, for more information or call their international helpline on: +44 (0)845 130 4568.

Sugar alternatives – Xylitol

Although it is best to avoid sugar and sugar alternatives as much as possible, there are two natural sugars that have the lowest GL score. These are blue agave syrup, which is used to sweeten healthier drinks, and xylitol. Xylitol has a GL score of one-seventh of that of regular sugar and tastes the same. Therefore, if you need to sweeten a food or drink use xylitol. Xylitol is available from health-food shops, some good supermarkets and also from Totally Nourish on +44 (0)20 8874 8038, or go to www.totallynourish.com.

Skincare products

Environ products were developed by the cosmetic surgeon Dr Des Fernandes to prevent skin cancer and address the damaging effects of the environment on our skin. Formulated with scientifically proven active ingredients, including vitamin A and antioxidant vitamins C, E and betacarotene, which are used in progressively higher concentrations, Environ will maintain a normal healthy skin or effectively treat and prevent the signs of ageing, pigmentation, problem skin and scarring.

Environ products can be purchased by contacting Totally Nourish on: +44 (0)20 8874 8038, or go to www.totallynourish.com. For international enquiries call +27 21 683 1034; email environc@ iafrica.com.

Water filters

There are many water filters on the market. One of the best is offered by the **Fresh Water Filter Company**, who produce mains-attached water-filtering units. For details visit www.totallynourish.com or call 020 8871 2949.

Zest4Life

Zest4life is a 12-week weight loss and nutrition programme for people who are serious about losing weight and improving their health and who need the right support and motivation to do it. Trained practitioners and weight loss coaches provide weekly motivational group sessions, teaching clients how to follow Patrick's highly successful low-GL diet and to overcome barriers to success. To find out more about Zest4life and to find your nearest practitioner, call 0845 603 9333 or visit our website: www.zest4life.eu.

Tests

Food Intolerance, Allergies, Homocysteine and glycosylated haemoglobin

YorkTest Laboratories sells FoodScan, a convenient finger-prick mail-order service with the added benefit of clinical laboratory analysis, and is the only food-intolerance test endorsed by Allergy UK.

Designed as a simple two-step process, FoodScan helps identify the foods that may be contributing to your symptoms by testing for food-specific reactions in your body (called IgG antibody reactions).

The First Step FoodScan is an indicator test that will generate a positive or negative result as to whether or not there is a food specific reaction. If positive, your sample is then upgraded to the Second Step FoodScan 113 test.

The Second Step FoodScan 113 is a comprehensive service that tests for 113 foods. The FoodScan 113 identifies the actual foods causing the intolerance and the level of intolerance (from 1–4). In addition, the service includes nutritionist consultations and comprehensive support and advice on managing your elimination diet.

YorkTest Laboratories also sell home testing kits for homocysteine, food and inhalant allergies (AllergyCheck) and glycosylated haemoglobin (GLCheck).

To order, call YorkTest Laboratories on 0800 074 6185 or visit www.yorktest.com.

Supplement, remedy and supplier directory

Finding your own perfect supplement programme can be confusing, but my website, www.patrickholford.com, offers useful guidance.

The backbone of a good supplement programme is:

- A high-strength multivitamin.

- Additional vitamin C.

- An all-round antioxidant complex.

- An essential-fat supplement containing omega-3 and omega-6 oils.

Supplement resources

The following companies produce good-quality supplements that are widely available in the UK.

Totally Nourish offers a wide range of excellent health products, including the BioCare supplements listed below, and many other health products, from Udo's Choice Oil and low-GL foods to water filters, by mail and online. Order by phone on +44 (0) 20 8874 8038, or visit www.totallynourish.com.

BioCare is available from all good health-food shops. They make my low-GL Get Up & Go shake and also GL Support, which contains chromium, 5-HTP and *Garcinia cambogia*. BioCare's Optimum Nutrition Pack with GL Support provides a daily blister strip, each containing a high potency multivitamin, vitamin C, essential fats plus GL Support. Taking two a day provides all the nutrients to support you during your low-GL diet. Available in most health-food shops. Tel: +44 (0)121 433 3727. Website: www.BioCare.co.uk.

Health Plus sell konjac fibre, a source of glucomannan. Health Plus Ltd, Dolphin House, 27 Cradle Hill Industrial Estate, Seaford, BN25 3JE. Phone +44 (0)1323 872277.

Higher Nature sell Omega 3:6:9 Balance Oil. Visit www. highernature.co.uk.

And in other regions ...

Australia. Solgar supplements are available in Australia. Contact Solgar on 1800 029 871 (free call) for your nearest supplier, or visit www.solgar.com.au. Another good brand is Blackmores.

New Zealand. BioCare products are available in New Zealand. Contact Aurora Natural Therapies, 4 La Trobe Track, KareKare, Waitakere City, Auckland 1232, or visit www.Aurora.org.nz.

Singapore. BioCare and Solgar products are available in Singapore. Contact Essential Living on 6276 1380 for your nearest supplier or visit www.essliv.com.

South Africa. Bioharmony produce a wide range of products in South Africa and other African countries. For details of your nearest supplier contact 0860 888 339 or visit www.bioharmony.co.za.

Index

Please note that references to diagrams are in *italic* print

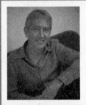

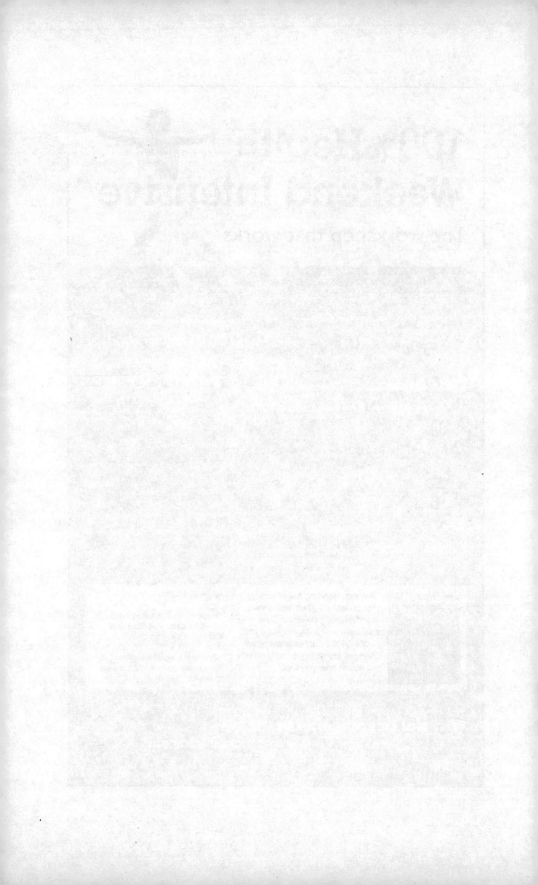